MORE FIRE

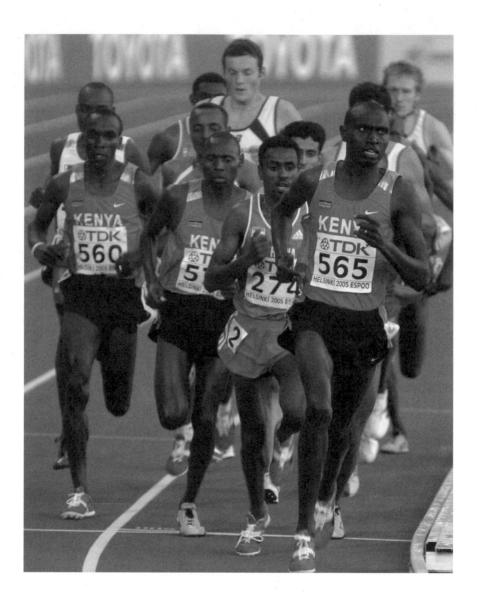

MORE FIRE

How to Run the Kenyan Way

Toby Tanser

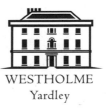

WESTHOLME
Yardley

Frontispiece: Benjamin Limo leads in helsinki. Isaac Songok and Eliud Kipchoge (#560) in pursuit. (*Flanagan/PrettySporty*)

Westholme Publishing, LLC
Eight Harvey Avenue
Yardley, Pennsylvania 19067
Visit our Web site at www.westholmepublishing.com

First Printing: October 2008
10 9 8 7 6 5 4 3

ISBN: 978-1-59416-074-5

Printed in United States of America

To the Runner: Begin with having a compelling dream, burn with desire to succeed. Your watchword is discipline and your password is perseverance. More painful than stumbling, as we all must, is to have never strode out. At the end of the run, at the close of the day, you will remember not the results of a position or stopwatch, but how intensely you tried, and at what velocity you lived in your life. Run, and live, with More Fire.

This book is dedicated to four amazing friends: Pieter "Starbucks" Langerhorst, Lornah "Simba" Kiplagat, Anthony (Tony) Edwards, and dear Sally (Barsosio).

All of the author royalties from this book go directly to building a children's hospital in Kenya.

"Toby Tanser knows and understands Kenya, its land, its people, and most of all, its magnificent runners. As an elite runner and coach, he shows us what we can learn from the Kenyan training camps to improve, enrich, and inspire our own running."—George A. Hirsch, Chairman of the Board, New York City Marathon

"The best thing I've read, because it is so direct and factual.
—Bruce Tulloh, coach, author of the *Complete Distance Runner*

"Quite simply the best book on running I have ever seen. Read *More Fire*."—Moses Tanui

"If you want to know how we do it, then read Toby's book. Here are all the recipes for our success."—Ezekiel Kemboi

"Toby opened his heart to Kenya, and as you will read, this is beyond a mere running book. This is Kenya."—Moses Kiptanui,

"This is *the* book on Kenyan running. He lived with us, ate with us, and trained with us. This is our story."—Sally Barsosio

"The whole Kenyan way of training in one book."—Jackson Kabiga

Contents

Introduction

To learn the principles of physics one looks to the unchanging laws of Newton; to study how to optimize your running, it would be foolish to dismiss the methodology of the world's finest runners. This book may not be riddled with fandangled formulas of lactic acid and percentages of your pulse rate, however it is a book that teaches, tells stories, makes documentation of a history far passing athletics, is visual and beyond about a running nation and its memorable people.

The advice, theories, and ideas of the runners in this book are pure genius. I may be biased but I think we can learn more from the running in Kenya than the laboratories in the West.

The title of this book comes from a misty morning in Eldoret, Kenya, at a time before the Sun had risen. A group of men stood at a lofty thin altitude of 2000 meters ready for an 18-kilometer foot race. Perhaps the best conditioned aerobic athletes the world could offer on this given day. Athletes who can elevate that central muscle we call a heart, tell it to beat to its utter maximum, then run like the very Gods for a full 26.2 miles.

They had known about this race for two weeks, and everyone was prepared to their best. There were no members of the press present, no prizes on offer, and no spectators to applaud their efforts, or offer words of encouragement.

The start was a mere quick shout command and the men accelerated, kicking dust on the dirt road that would provide less than perfect footing for speed as they flew along the undulating path, in rhythm with life. Robert Cheruiyot, the tall 4-time Boston Marathon winner was easy to pick out with that powerful stride as he immediately took the lead, punishment promised with each of his flicking footsteps, flames blazing in those spiritual eyes. Martin Lel ran over the ground as if he was a ballet dancer, nimble and defined — running like Lel the Gazelle three-time London Marathon, two-time ING New York winner should do. Patrick Ivuti was up there, the reigning Chicago Marathon winner whose life had begun when running to collect firewood as a determined youngster, Boston runner-up James Kwambai who had paced and pushed Gebrselassie to his marathon world record... the names combined would have bankrupted any major marathon's budget for appearance fees alone.

As the dawn broke the runners were now silently sweeping passed many unassuming folk walking to work. Nobody cheered these Kings of Kenya, no one even glanced at the steeds of fire who raced onward at tempo. With their chests roaring for oxygen they hold pose seemingly without fatigue, as they continued to push, hurling their bodies forward at an alarming swiftness, defying all barriers of threshold and despair.

At 17-km the group was still packed together, the Honolulu champion Jimmy Muindi is the only one with apparent labored legs. This race is a fast moving journey to wrench the body past its mortal restrictions, it starts with the recognition that pain is the validation of accomplishment. Each one of this dozen or so runners renews their faith daily when they afflict the doubts and torment their limbs in a quest to be the very best they can, best beyond the mind's own pitiful limitations.

When the sun rises over the equator it does so with a quick and sharp brilliance. As flashes of golden sunlight lit Martin Lel it sparked certain acute acceleration to his lithe legs; he distanced himself from the pack by a clear 100m before the competition had a chance to adjust their stride, running himself blind and covering the final kilometer in a staggering 2-minutes 30-seconds pace. Impossible speed exists in Kenya.

Talent does not ensure success; each triumph has to be earned. What was truly grueling to tolerate is now reward for Lel. His first words, with a smile, he tells all, "That's More Fire!"

The Kenyan Way

In the senior ranks, there were well over 500 sub 2:20 performances in 2006 by Kenyan marathon runners, far greater than any other nation. Britain, with roughly double the population of Kenya, had eleven sub 2:20 men in 2006. 20 of the top 30 fastest times in 2008 so far are by Kenyan men. The current marathon world champion Luke Kibet and William Kipsang, who tried to qualify by running the eighth fastest time ever at the marathon four months prior, were not able to make their national 2008 Olympic team, but in the final week before competition, Kibet was added as a reserve. In the 1988-2007 World Cross-Country Championships there have been 291 individual medals on offer; Kenyans have taken 134 medals. If you look at the medals on offer for males, the number is 147, and Kenyan runners took 86 of those medals, 58.9%. Kenyan women are following. Never in one single sport has one country dominated the way Kenya has, and does, in distance running.

This is one small country against the rest of the world. One nation that, in recent years, has also lost a good number of its best athletes to other countries. Where life expectancy hovers between 45 and 48 years depending on whose reports you follow, and where the population is only around 34 million. Where poverty, disease, and desperation are the median and more people than not live on less than $2 per day. Where mere literacy and education are a luxury never taken for granted. That was turned upside down in 2008 by extreme riots and destruction. And, against all the odds, this indigent country, in the sport of the Gods, still reigns supreme.

The statistics, per capita, illuminate Kenyan supremacy at all distances from 800m to the marathon. Many people put the success down to plain hard work, but can it really be that simple, as hard work in athletic training is a universally accepted trait of the sport, and why then is there also a hoard of hardworking Kenyan runners who do not prevail? Many questions are asked in this book, and various answers, if not watertight conclusions, are given.

I hope the information presented here gives you some insight into their lifestyle and training. Their philosophies and running routines were startling to me, very different from the conventional approaches I had read and witnessed elsewhere in the world. Having trained with many Olympic champions, national team members, and squads from literally all over the world on training camps, in my opinion, the Kenyan method of running is by far the best. I try, in this book, to convey Kenyan running to you. The way they run is ultimately with *More Fire*.

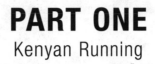

PART ONE
Kenyan Running

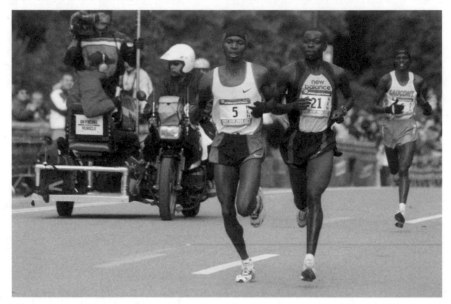

Kenyans Rodgers Rop, Laban Kipkemboi, and Christopher Cheboiboch, go 1, 3, and 2, in the ING New York City Marathon, 2002. (*New York Road Runners*)

Why Do Kenyans Run with More Fire?

The Kenyan marvel of, to put it nicely, "The talent of the moving feet" first came to light in the 1960s. Although there was a slight melancholic era following the two boycotted Olympics of 1976 and 1980, the upsurge that had flowed from the sixties had been gaining thrust to a crescendo when at the 1988 Seoul Olympics, Kenya took the men's gold in the 800m, 1500m, 5000m, and steeplechase; the bronze in the 10,000m; and the silver in the steeplechase and the marathon. "Based on population statistics applied to the Seoul results, the chances of Kenyan men winning the 800, 1500, 3000, and 5000 were one in 1,600,000,000," wrote Amby Burfoot, the senior editor of *Runner's World*.

Unlike the long-distance Finns of the 1920s, the Swedish milers of the 1940s, or the middle-distance Brits of the 1980s, Kenyans have sustained their claim of being *the* dominant force for all those distances combined, for longer than a decade.

It is important to remember that in the amateur days, athletes worldwide trained exclusively for the Olympic Games; lucrative meets like the IAAF Grand Prix were only a twinkle of hope in an athlete's mind. To illustrate this point, the real flood of Kenyan athletes to hit the world's stage, outside the Olympics, came after a two-fold change. First, track and field opened up to include not only amateurism and the Olympics but also professional meetings with appearance and prize monies. Second, when Dr. Mike Boit was elected sports commissioner of Kenya in 1990, he created opportunity by opening up the free market for athletes to travel without the shackles of needing the federation's permission, and commission. If earlier Kenyans had had the opportunities that the Westerners were privy to, chances are good that the boom would have occurred a lot earlier than it did (Trying to get a visa in modern-day Kenya can still be a nightmare; the well-traveled and financially secure internationalists Susan Chepkemei and John Korir tried to travel to the 2005 Peachtree Road Race—visas denied. Back in the 1950s, forget it!)

So, why is Kenya so densely populated with distance running talent? Scientists have suggested that the Kenyans' thin legs, narrow hips, and amazingly strong ankles constitute the perfect biomechanical machine for distance running, but is that enough? Not enough for the nearly identical-bodied Tanzanian tribe of the Jaluo that borders Kenya. After extensive recent studies of elite Kenyans, including Felix Limo, Dr. Yannis Pitsiladis, PhD, says, "I am not convinced by the East African thin-calf theory, although it may be part of the answer. A small part, and not a prerequisite to success."

Some say that because Kenyans were on-foot cattle farmers in pastoral highlands, they developed into super runners because they had to round up stray cattle on foot. As any dairy farmer will tell, if you put a 1,000-pound cow in a grassy field to eat its twenty-five pounds worth of grass, it will not run ten miles to the north. Cattle rustling, another given reason, was not an everyday occurrence, and the old rustlers probably covered the mileage Paul Tergat covers in one day over a whole month.

Another theory is superior running "engines," yet field tests dismiss this theory. "There is no major difference in peak maximum VO_2 uptake between Kenyans and Caucasians," says physiologist Bengt Saltin, whose studies found that the physical makeup of the "driving system" (cardiovascular) of a Kenyan runner is very similar to that of a European Caucasian elite athlete.

The genetic standpoint, given by many as a carte blanche explanation of Kenyan running magic, also does not explain why Sweden, which led the world in distance running in the 1940s, now led the world, per capita, at the Athens 2004 events for the technical heptathlon, high jump, and triple-jump disciplines. Furthermore, in 2006 a Swedish high jumper, Kajsa Bergqvist, led the world's rankings; and Swedish men, Stefan Holm and Linus Thörnblad, had the second- and fourth-highest leaps of the year. No Swedish milers appeared in the IAAF rankings. Will scientists, who may have theorized in the 1940s about "Swede miler" genes, now be arguing that Swedes have jumping genes? These athletes may have been inspired and motivated to train when watching their countryman, Patrick Sjöberg, who not only set a world record when they were youngsters at school but also won three Olympic medals and was the world champion in 1987.

The Kenyan Marathon Phenomena

In 2007, 67 percent of the top 100 men's times at the marathon distance were run by Kenyan athletes.

Number of sub-2:20 marathon performances among Kenyan, British, and American runners, 1975–2005.

Year	1975	1985	1995	2000	2005
Kenya	0	17	86	296	490
Britain	23	74	34	13	12
USA	34	103	59	27	22

The huge explosion of Kenyan marathon running success occurred in the mid-1990s, somewhat later than the track success. This was due to a number of factors: a strong belief that marathon training led to infertility, no real tradition of marathon events in Kenya, and no training plans for marathoners in Kenya. In the pre-1990 era, most Kenyans competing on the world stage were athletes attending American colleges, and as Runner's World writer Peter Gambaccini reasoned, "You have to remember that a lot of the Kenyans that were running here in the eighties were running the collegiate disciplines, and also that the big marathons were essentially invitational, where people like Fred Lebow would invite people with public relations values. Somebody like Ibrahim Hussein [winner of the New York Marathon in 1987] probably got in the field under the radar."

In addition, the vast amounts of marathon money was not advertised as it is today. Gambaccini says, "The money was still good, say $25,000, but at that time a lot of the marathon money was still under-the-table payments." It was other disciplines where the big money lay, like lucrative "golden miles" or a 10K in Indonesia that was offering $500,000 for a world record. (John Ngugi, at 27:29, and the late Paul Kipkoech, at 27:31, came exceedingly close—seven and nine seconds, respectively—from collecting that pot on April 2, 1988.)

Advocates of the gene-pool theory note that the majority of the success comes from one small area in Kenya: One tribe, the Kalenjin, who number about 3 million, make up about 75 percent of all Kenyan national track and field teams. At the 2007 World Cross Country Championships, Kenya won eight of 12 individual medals, and the Kalenjin tribe took seven of those. Since running is global, unlike speed skating or ice hockey, rugby, or baseball (all of which are regionally based), this is the greatest phenomenon in sports today.

Another statistic that really highlights the Kalenjin supremacy is that since 1968, Kenya has dominated the Olympic steeplechase event (barring the Kenyan-boycotted years of 1976 and 1980), and only once during this era has a non-Kalenjin runner taken the gold. When the sole non-Kalenjin winner, Julius Kariuki of Nyahururu, was asked about this phenomenon, he said, "It is likely that my relatives came from the Kalenjins." Enough said.

However, before theories are made based on the Kalenjins, the world record-holder at the half-marathon, the first Kenyan to break 27 minutes for the 10,000m, and the only three Kenyan men to win Olympic marathon medals are all non-Kalenjin. And so are John Ngugi and Catherine Ndereba, the reigning world marathon champion.

"Kenyans have the perfect location and altitude" is often heard to explain the phenomenon; however, the high-altitude towns of Lokitaung and Lodiwar in the Rift Valley have yet to produce any championship-caliber athletes. One could easily ask, with tongue in cheek, "was there a Rift Valley in the north of England, where Olympic distance-running medalists Sebastian Coe, Peter Elliot, Brendan Foster, Mike McLeod, Derek Ibbotson, and Steve Cram (to name but a handful) came from, which has now disappeared, since England can no longer produce such great runners?" Tibetan marathon runners, born and bred at high altitude, are yet to be seen breaking the tape at any marathons worldwide. The Bolivian national marathon record is nearly thirteen minutes slower than the Kenyan record, despite a perfect runner's climate in Bolivia, and the high altitude of the Andes.

The weather in the runner-rich areas of Kenya is conducive to running. The lowlands, such as the coastal region, have produced no high-caliber distance runners. The climate of such places is highly unfavorable to long-distance running. The climate of the highlands is conducive to training almost year-round. Although the sun is hot, a low humidity makes running pleasantly comfortable. During the rainy period, June to August, the mud roads can be challenging to run on as they become like sticky dough—though the Kenyans believe that this helps to build leg strength. By mid-morning, the powerful sun has usually dried the roads again for the runner wishing to avoid such surfaces.

At high altitudes, the nights and early mornings can be chilly. Some coaches use the shivery 6:00 a.m. sessions to acclimatize runners to the weather that they'll find in European cross-country races. The Kenyans do not like to run in the rain. There is a belief that the water will get into the chest and cause a cold. "It is better to miss one training session than a whole week through catching flu," explained Nicholas Twolongut, a

Kenyan Air Force marathoner. "We sleep in if we hear the rain," relates Kirwa Tanui, explaining why the camp was without movement one rainy morning. The previous day, more than 80 runners had sat in their tents, waiting to see if the weather would clear up sufficiently for their mid-morning training run. Usually it does, since the rain in Kenya falls most often in the afternoon. Kenyan athletes who spend the summer in London, for example, have to adapt to training in the rain. On returning to Kenya, they soon revert to Kenyan ways.

Furthermore, over the past few years, the latest take on high altitude and its effect on athletic performance is that living at high altitude but training at low altitude is the most effective method for enhancing performance. Thus, it can be argued that any of the many Western athletes who now use altitude chambers/tents have an advantage over the Kenyans, who are literally "stuck" at high altitude.

Putting the altitude issue aside, it could be said that Kenya is not the ideal locale for training; considering many of its inhabitants are stricken by bleak poverty (the young Richard Yatich), haunted by hunger (the young Robert Cheruiyot), infected with malaria (Wilson Kipketer) or typhoid fever (the young Stephen Cherono). The AIDS prevalence in Kenya is nothing to boast about. Playing devil's advocate, one *could* ask, is this the perfect location?

Another theory: Kenyans are good at running because they have no other sport. False! As is true the world over, there is a high participation in the sport of running in Kenya. It is a high-participation event, especially for children. However, one can at once dismiss the argument that Kenyans are good runners because the rest of the world does not pump as much membership into the sport. Dr. Norbert Sander, CEO of the New Balance Armory Track and Field Center in New York City, points out, "If you combine track and field with cross-country running in American schools, then the discipline becomes the nation's most participatory event, above basketball, baseball, and football." Furthermore, many of Kenya's finest runners preferred soccer to running while at school, like Moses Kiptanui and the Kirui family. Today, even with enhanced global communications that let Kenyans watch the national track team compete, though they can not watch the national soccer team (as it never qualifies for World Championships), soccer remains the national sport of Kenya. To be a member of the Harambee Stars is the dream of the majority of schoolchildren throughout the country.

The mind is where Tim Noakes thinks the Kenyans have a distinct advantage: "The Ferrari can't go 300 mph without a driver, right?" He continues, "The outcome of the performance is there, from what you really believe, before the first step is taken. The body will always give up; you have to make the mind run the body. Kenyans are *great* believers." An example: at the junior level, Titus Kemboi Masai, who hangs behind his illustrious training partners in practice, literally knocked on the door of a seasoned veteran. Coming to Iten in 2005, after he started running in Kapsokwyo School, he sought out sub-13-minute 5,000m runner James Kwalia and asked if he could join Kwalia's training group, "I can make it, just watch me. Give me a race to prove it!" One year later, running at altitude and barely seventeen years old, Masai ran a stunning 13:47 for the 5000m in Nairobi. Ask about goals, and he mentions winning the next Senior Championships on the calendar.

Another possible premise for the Kenyans prowess is that they have a high level of pain tolerance. Most Kenyan runners are rural-based Africans who have been circumcised in the traditional fashion. Boys and girls are subjected to this ritual—none gets anesthetics. Showing any form of pain or suffering is not accepted. The thirteen to fifteen year old sits in complete silence while the village elders perform the task. "Whenever I think I am in pain during running, I remember the pain of my circumcision," says Nicholas Twolongut. "The pain when running does not compare. A Kenyan has no pain barrier after circumcision. My father told me to remember the pain and gain knowledge that I could face any pain with my eyes open after that ceremony." One problem with this theory is that the circumcision tradition crosses over into Ugandan/Tanzanian lands, yet the runners of those countries cannot come anywhere near the Kenyan runners.

There is no single fact that can produce a watertight conclusion, yet the steely focus of the Kenyan mindset is hard to dismiss. Stephen Cherono, a millionaire with a luxury house in Eldoret's Elgon View, spends the week in Iten living in the most basic of conditions in one room with a cheap foam mattress and a blanket. A padlock closes his plank door to the outside passageway; next door in a similar room lives his brother, Abraham Cherono. They share a communal room and take turns cooking food. There are no cell phones or Internet in this home. Even in the town of Iten, where the concentration of runners is perhaps at its highest in Kenya, there is not one movie house or theater. When I visited in January 2007, there was no Internet café or other public Web access (there had been for a short while at the local post office). No chance for passing the day cyberloafing.

William Kiplagat, a 2:06:50 marathoner, tells a good tale: "I ran well, had some good results then the times started slipping. I realized I was getting distracted, not enough time training, just running. So I turned off the cell phone and went back to being a Kenyan. The good results then came back—I won my next marathon."

Another argument is that Kenyans see Kenyans winning; of course this is a factor. If a young European Caucasian child sits in front of the television to watch the Kenyans sweeping the Olympic steeplechase final or the Boston Marathon, this can set limitations in the mind. The child flips the channel and sees David Beckham scoring a goal, and immediately a more tangible reality is created. Swedish 1976 Olympic steeplechase champion Anders Gärderud did not grow up watching Kenyans dominate the event. However, a British woman holds the women's marathon record. Why? Clearly, hard work, genetics, diet, and adequate rest can add up to greatness for an athlete from someplace other than Kenya. Lifestyle choices, environment, and talent all play roles.

Kenyans are excellent at keeping training simple. "I have a heart rate monitor," begins Brother Colm O'Connell, an Irish priest who has lived in Kenya for decades and coached generations of Olympians. "It was given to me by some Swedish scientists to use, oh, I'd say about twenty, twenty-five years ago. Still got it; it's still in the box in my room." Reflecting the irrelevance of monitors and other modern-day equipment is the fact not one of some 200 runners was using such equipment in the mid-nineties at the Kenyan Armed Forces Camps. However, running wristwatches that double as virtual portable computers are now becoming commonplace in the Western world, where runners return from a workout to record all kinds of data into a training log and/or send infrared beams from the watch into a computer! Only once at the aforementioned camps did I see a piece of heart rate equipment: the chest strap was stretched between two bushes as a washing line. When the owner was asked, he said that he had been given the apparatus in Norway. It had never been on his chest since he left Scandinavia.

The simplistic approach is even seen with the altitude factor. European athletes often spend a certain specific time at sea level after training at altitude, sports scientists having stating that a seven- or fourteen-day return to sea level is optimal for the body's adaptations. Before the Boston Marathon in 1996, Moses Tanui joked, "We Kenyans use the science of the plane ticket; when the race directors send the ticket for us to come, then we travel."

Born to Run, or Born to Train Hard?

A film crew arrived in Eldoret prior to the 1996 Olympics to film a documentary about Kenyan runners. The director wanted a few changes. "Can you please remove your track suits and run with bare legs?" came the request. "Can we have some cows roaming free on the field where the runners are training?" "Can you sing while you run in the group?" And finally, "Can you remove your shoes and run barefoot?" In my previous month of training with this group of students, there had been no bare legs on training runs, no cows mingling with runners, absolutely no singing (or talking) during running, and not a single barefoot runner! This "documentary" film wouldn't be interesting enough, in the mind of the director, if it didn't conform to his preconceived notions.

For every Kenyan runner who succeeds, there are dozens who fail, as is true everywhere. It's a minority who make the national level. The Rift Valley AAA held a track meet in Eldoret when I was there. The signature Kenyan event, the steeplechase, had more than 25 entrants. Fewer than ten made it to the finish!

Paul Tergat says, "You will see why we win if you train with us." Kenyans work harder and have the inspiration of Kenyan middle- and long-distance records being broken year after year. All but one of the British records were set in the 1980s. The longest-standing Kenyan distance record dates to 1996!

If there is any one factor to emphasize, it is hard training, followed by more hard training. Kenyans set no limits. A single week may involve seven straight days of hard workouts. "Rest when the body is tired and worn down, not when your body is strong and can take more training," reasons Christopher Koskei. Julius Korir adds, "I trained hard, hard, hard before I could run well at all; people think we were born running but it is not true."

There is an internal force in Kenyans, a driving brave intrinsic spirit. In 1909, Theodore Roosevelt, with a cadre of hundreds armed with rifles and shotguns, went on a hunting rampage in Kenya, shooting more than 500 animals. It is reported that he was amazed to see a group of Nandis attack and kill a lion with a mere spear. Roosevelt, on his brave hunt, obviously did not feel inclined to try this method. The Kenyan mentality is to work hard, always accepting the challenge or task. Even a novice Kenyan will not

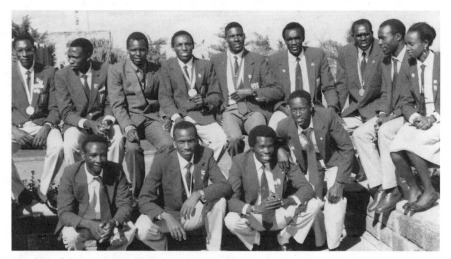

Members of the glorious 1988 Seoul Olympic Team. Back row: Julius Kariuki (gold, steeplechase), John Ngugi (gold, 5000m), Kip Cheruiyot (#7, 1500m), Peter Rono (gold, 1500m), Paul Ereng (gold, 800m), Lucas Sang (400m), Peter Koech (silver, steeplechase), Yobes Ondieki (#12, 5000m), Pascaline Wangui (#49, marathon). Front row: Joseph Kipsang (Marathon), Douglas Wakiihuri (silver, marathon), Robert Wangila (gold, boxing), and Joseph Maritim (#5, 400-m hurdles, semis). (*Author*)

blink an eye when the coach instructs the group about the day's training. As is noted throughout this book, Kenyans relish hard training. They never shirk from the given quota. It is not a matter of simple compliance; the ethic seems to be a commitment to working to achieve the prescribed load.

Poverty is another cited cause for running success, yet Kenya is not among the twenty poorest countries in the world. If this poverty theory explained excellence, then where are all the East Timor runners, or for that matter, Malawi runners?

An active lifestyle does play an obvious part, and a Third-World income makes this more of a necessity: One Kenyan in 260 (according to an article in the *East African Standard*) owns a car, and furthermore, many remote villages are barely reachable with a four-wheel-drive vehicle. Thus the reliance on one's legs is paramount. According to a recent survey by the U.S. Department of Transportation, only 8 percent of U.S. households do not have a car, and the average is 1.9 cars per household. Patrick Sang tells how, while he was out running, a woman with a sack of vegetables started running alongside him at a six-minute-mile pace. The woman did not look like an athlete, nor did she appear to be troubled by the speed.

To walk from Iten to the home of Jebiwott Keitany (a medalist at the World Junior's 10,000m) in Kapkei took over three hours of tramping through the countryside. This was done in the morning hours after an hour-long training run. After lunch with the family, it was time to walk home. Upon reaching Iten, the visitors went straight to the late-afternoon training run at 5 p.m. This occurrence was not unusual for many of the athletes residing in Iten. Jebiwott did not even mention possible fatigue to Brother Colm before

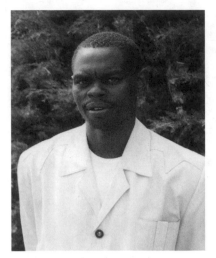

Daniel Komen, the only man in history to run
two consecutive four-minute miles. (*Author*)

the evening's tempo run began. To an outsider, this manner of living might seem like one of hardship. However, it would be wrong to hypothesize that the Kenyans dislike this lifestyle.

The heritage of most tribes in Rift Valley Province is pastoral, with the common activity being working with large herds of livestock. The stock must often be moved to new grazing grounds, since water can be scarce and often great distances must be covered to fine it. From a young age, children are saddled with that responsibility and can find themselves walking vast distances in the process. Nicholas Twolongut remembers his childhood: "I had to take the sheep to the market. The walk would take all morning. I would begin at daylight and reach the market near midday. On the days when there was no market, I was walking with the goats. If I didn't do these jobs, I would be beaten by my father. These tasks began when I was six years old."

The speed of the journey is dictated by the urgency of the destination. "I ran to school to avoid a caning for being late," says Lydia Cheromei. If she was early leaving the house, she would walk to school, but more often than not (for which today she is thankful), she was late and ran most of the way. "I never ran to school; I lived only 400 meters away," says one of Kenya's most successful female runners, Rose Cheruiyot, dispelling the myth that all Kenyan runners travel, if not run, great distances to school. It is the same story with Paul Tergat! Some run to school because they enjoy running but the percentage is low. It's undeniable, however, that early dependence on shank's mare makes a great foundation for an endurance-based sporting future.

This way of life does result in strong legs and a superb aerobic base. Peter Snell, New Zealand's triple Olympic middle-distance gold medalist says, "I believe, that the Western world has it all wrong. There is too much emphasis placed on speed work, and not enough on building a strong aerobic base. If you have two equal athletes, the one with the greater aerobic base will win."

Inactivity and obesity are on the rise in most Western countries, our dependence on pharmaceutical aids grows stronger with each new scientific discovery, and although talent, genetics, and interest exist in the West, the desire people express for hard competitive running, , compared to the what the Kenyans do, is like chalk and cheese. Virtually every starting runner in Kenya wants to set a world record or win a major city marathon and believes this is a viable proposition. Having spent years lecturing beginner runners in New York for the New York Road Runners, I have found that by far, the most common goal is merely to complete a race.

Read the stories in this book—for example, pick out the amiable Robert Cheruiyot—and decide for yourself who will win a big race. Kenyans don't sit at home and think, "The runners are so good in my country, I will never make it myself; there are far too many great athletes, how can I ever be as good as them?" *Au contraire!*

The Kenyan way of training, compared to the Western way, is to say, "Why not?" If Kelly Holmes and Sebastian Coe did it, if Svetlana Masterkova and Steve Cram did it, and if Ronaldo DaCosta and Paula Radcliffe did it, then . . . why not me?"

The Kenyan mentality is not to dwell on the negatives in life. For example, they would not ponder the fact that in the United States or Europe, you will not find as many potential runners as you would in the Rift Valley. Instead, they would reflect that it *is* possible to make yourself a champion wherever you are, or live, in the world. Train hard is the answer: As Brother Colm O'Connell, the famous coach, noted following a particularly grueling hill workout, "This is the bit they [the media] like to ignore when looking for a Kenyan secret!"

Myths of Greatness on the Rim of the Rift Valley

A gene is a biological particle of DNA that controls our hereditary characteristics; according to the national health resource center, the human body is known to have well over 30,000 genes. It has been proposed that Kenyans have a special "fast running gene" that gives them a special advantage. Some believe this; many others do not.

Bengt Saltin, thought by many to be one of the world's leading sports physiologists with an authority on African running, is lucid and articulate upon the matter of genes and running. While in Kenya in 2007, he explained that Kenyans do have significant genetic advantages. He points to a perfect muscular configuration in regard to the running limbs, coupled with a more economical system to convert oxygen to bodily fuel.

Research that is more recent tends to veer away from the running-limbs theories. Although noting that there is "no major difference in peak maximum VO_2 uptake between Kenyans and Caucasians," Saltin says he has seen that Kenyans can and do perform at a higher percentage of their maximum. This, it was thus concluded, was due to their bodies' makeup. In tests he conducted twenty years ago, he saw a comparatively smaller leg volume and higher hemoglobin levels in the East Africans. Saltin has also noted that unlike Europeans tested, the Kenyans do not accumulate ammonia in their bodies. Ammonia has been found to be instrumental in causing fatigue. He told of how Julius Kariuki, tested after a race in Kobenhavn, had the lowest levels he'd ever seen; at that time, Kariuki was the reigning Olympic steeplechase champion. Saltin also added that all his comparisons were between world-class Kenyan and Swedish athletes: "All the Swedes had been in an Olympic or World Championship final, so I had very good study groups." And his concluding comment? "We have no clue if there is one single gene, but we know there is a genetic advantage and that training of the body is a key factor. It is the activation of the genes that is the factor; they play a role but have nothing to do with ethnic groups."

It would seem clear that Kenyans' ability to exploit oxygen to its fullest extent comes from many generations of adapting to the thin air of the high Rift Valley. Thus it can be strongly argued that inherent genetics give a distinct advantage to those living in the Rift Valley. Magic Johnson would never have placed in the Rift Valley cross-country championships, and William Mutwol would never be recruited for college basketball. Half a century after the first Kenyan track and field athlete achieved an Olympic qualifying time, Jason Dunford, at the 2007 world swimming championships in Melbourne, Australia, became the first Kenyan swimmer to do so.

However, the Rift Valley, being 3,000 miles long, and running through Malawi to central Mozambique, includes areas of widely varying running performances: The national marathon records of Malawi are 2:18:05 and 3:16:24. The Turkana tribe resides in the highlands of the Rift Valley and has had scant athletic success, despite being Kenyans who live at high altitude.

As earlier noted, it is also a consideration that Kenya's great athletes are not confined to areas of the Great Rift. Two of Kenya's most distinguished 10,000m runners (the sole Olympic gold medalist to date, and the first man under 27 minutes for the distance) Temu and Ondieki, are both from the Kisii district, and the 2008 Olympic marathon champion, and world half-marathon record holder, Samuel Wanjiru, comes from the central provinces. The first man to break thirteen minutes for the 5000m did not come from the Rift Valley, either; Said Aouita is from Morocco, in north west Africa.

However, to throw genes out of the equation is to totally dismiss the miraculous phenomenon that an amazing number of Rift Valley residents are great distance runners, whereas an equally great number of West Africans have excelled in sprinting.

Among the men's top 50 times ever recorded for the 10,000m, as of January 2007 (discounting one athlete caught for doping), 49 have been run by East African–born athletes, and one by a Moroccan. Among the men's top 50 times for the 100m, not one has been run by an East African. It can be argued that this is not a geographical matter but a tracing of ethnicity. Of course, ignoring the genetic factor would be foolish.

Tim Noakes, the author of *The Lore of Running* says, "I think Kenyan running is something more than genes or exercise physiology."

The same people who tell us it is a gene-pool phenomenon also say Kenyans cannot sprint. A closer look at this theory reveals an interesting fact: it's not true. It could well be that the argument, endorsing a lack of formative technical training, as Evans mentioned, is the main reason that we do not see more Kenyans in the shorter distances.

The proof in the pudding? In the fourteen editions of the men's 4 x 400-meter relay at the African Championships, Kenyan men have taken gold five times. In ten of the Commonwealth Games, the Kenyans have won gold four times. These are unmatched records. Is someone saying that the African and Commonwealth competitions have weak sprint-country representation?

I Want to Do It, and I Can Do It

Kenya is a country far removed from the West, not only in miles. A noticeable attribute of its sportspeople is the "no tomorrows" philosophy. Running in Kenya is like riding the rapids: things move so quickly that if you don't jump in the waters, you'll miss the boat. Typically, Western athletes (excuse the sweeping generalization) work from a long-term plan, a structured program with set goals, and a step-by-step approach to reaching the highest level that can take years. This is not typically the case in Kenya.

Jomo Kenyatta, Kenya's past president, talked a lot of *Harambee*. The word is the maxim of Kenya, and it is inscribed upon the Kenyan coat of arms. It is translated as "pulling together" as a community. The country was founded on that ethic. People work together to achieve success, in life and in sport. On the Kenyan Olympic T-shirts of 1996 was written *Pamoja Tu Tashinda*—Together We Win. This concept is quite removed from the general individualized Western train of thought. The underpinnings of Harambee may well be the lack of a social security system in the country, a land where one never sees advertisements for life insurance or pension plans. People grow up relying on the extended family of a community for survival. To fall from grace in Kenya is to land with a resounding thump. If you stay in bed, there will be no unemployment check in the mail. In the sporting world, the principle of Harambee carries over to the community group training system. The groups of athletes pulling together have a tremendous synergistic power that cannot be overstated. Seeing others' success from the exact training plan one is running creates an attitude of "You can, therefore I can." As the Western world becomes more insular, with the Internet and cell phones becoming primary tools of information and communication, Kenyans' community bonding becomes even stronger.

Winning is Expected

National coach John Ngure explains, "It's a nice idea to take a large team, but there aren't the finances to support such a venture." Kenyans are not sent to international competitions merely to compete; they are sent to win the race. When John Maundu of Kenya started running, at over the age of forty, he did not look for the master's competitions but went straight for the open races; he ran a 2:13:22 marathon. Five years later, he was still in the open division, placing an unbelievable seventh at the Kenyan Armed Forces road championships.

Taking That Opportunity

Another reason for the influx of Rift Valley folk pursuing careers in athletics is the angle of opportunity and prospects. Whereas in the Western world there is an abundance of opportunities, Kenya is the land of narrow openings. The West is spoiled by choice; you want to be a filmmaker, take a class. Got no money, apply for a grant, be discovered. In Kenya, there are no reality TV shows or line-up auditions. Rural East Africans have to think on their feet about continual survival, the fight to have a place in their society. "Chungni Kimiyi" is a popular phrase heard on Kenya that underlines this sentiment: "Standing still does not pay." The surest way to succeed in life is to put foot one foot in front of the other, and Kenyans are excellent at this! Outside the usual day-to-day business of a small town, Rift Valley residents have very few life choices. To be an athlete is possibly one of the easier options to try in Kenya. Not to mention the great earning potential and superstar status it affords.

Demonstrating this "running for dollars" theory is the fact that very, very few Kenyans continue to run, in any capacity, after competitive retirement. One year after she stopped competing, something she had done since childhood, the forty-year-old Esther Kiplagat gained a lot of weight. "I know, I am fat now. [She laughs] I do not run at all. Now I am spending time instead with the family." No easy evening jogs along the back roads of Eldoret, no fitness classes to keep in shape—absolutely nothing. Moses Kiptanui may be the only elite athlete to continue training in Kenya in his post-retirement days. Certainly, Christopher Kosgei, William and Moses Tanui, Ngugi, Sigei, Ondieki, et al. do not run for fun these days.

Running in Numbers

It has been mentioned that the motivation for Kenyans to start running is enhanced because of their immense wealth of role models. the argument is that if, say, Britain had as many stars, more British kids would choose running as a sport. Yet, reading Paul Ereng and Billy Konchellah's stories, one can see that not all Kenyans pick their fellow citizens as role models. Like any 800m man of the 1960s, Mike Boit recalls, "I admired [New Zealander] Peter Snell; I would measure my performance against him. I really wished just to see him, to see he was human, and no more than me."

Moses Kiptanui started running knowing only one other runner, a cousin. Many Kenyan stars grew up far removed from the media, hearing only some runners' names as British kids must hear stories of Ovett, Coe, and Cram. Hilda Kibet notes that there were no newspapers or televisions available where she grew up.

Kenya as a Nation

There is something very likeable and down-to-earth about the Kenyan persona. Kenyans are extremely dependable; they turn up and race when they say they will. Typically, they give a superb effort no matter how small the event is, and they are very team oriented. When they become wealthy, they remain humble and modest. Joyce Chepchumba, who is incredibly wealthy (she once won the biggest prize purse in marathon running when she set the women's world record in London), cannot be distinguished from the next person on the street in Eldoret. She has no airs or attitude, despite her superstar status.

A major advantage for the active, computerless adolescents of Kenya is the development of fitness. Physical exertion in these years can lead to a robust constitution that is perfect for a life in sports. Years of walking and helping on the farms build immense stamina and core strength that are crucial for running. When the Chinese women broke the 1,500-meter, 3,000-meter, and 10,000-meter records in 1993 and swept the World Championship titles, reporters asked their coach, Ma Junren, where he had recruited such a wonder team. Junren replied that he looked for peasant children, who had to face adversity constantly, not established junior athletes. A Kenyan social experiment could be to study the children of the successful post-1990 athletes in Kenya. Currently there are many sons and daughters of accomplished athletes competing, yet these parents competed during the amateur era of running. In the 1970s, at international events, medals and trophies were the only reward. Rose Chepyator Thomson notes that the domestic prizes were "Sufurias [cooking pans] and useful things. It was very good and useful, but certainly not something you would base your career around." This was far from the thousands of dollars that are on offer today at major competitions. The sports stars of today pamper their children by driving them to school. Fifty years after an imaginary oil discovery off Kenyan shores, they might be overfed, underactive, and asking the question, "What is this gene that Europeans runners have that allows them to beat us?"

Running is an immensely desirable career choice in Kenya, arguably a reason why Kenyans work harder to succeed and look for results in a shorter period than their Western counterparts do. The lure of prize money is powerful: a teacher in rural Kenya can make a salary of 4,000 shillings per year (approximately $580). The second female finisher at a recent marathon in Huntsville, Alabama, won $750 in a time slower than the women's marathon group in Iten clocks in their training runs. A successful runner in Eldoret is in the highest income bracket, above financial managers. In New York, the average Goldman Sachs Group, Inc., employee earns $622,000 per year, according to a Wall Street report.

The span of time for earning potential is short for most runners—another reason for making running success happen quickly. Kenya, like most countries, lacks a support system for retired athletes, making for an immediate and aggressive business strategy. In post-athletics, there are few opportunities in Kenya and many candidates to fill those few positions. This was brought to the media's attention in 2003 when the country's first Olympic gold medalist, Naftali Temu, died of prostate cancer in Kenyatta National Hospital at only fifty-seven years of age. Although a diagnosis was made months earlier, he did not have the necessary $600 for medical treatment. Athletes realize that they have to make their own future. Anthony Kiprono, once one of Kenya's brightest talents in road racing, exemplifies the adversity his countrymen can suffer with his story: "After '98, my form fell. I tried to make a comeback in 2000 but then had no money. Chris Cheboiboch gave me a pair of old shoes to train in, but when those wore out, I had nothing to run in." Six years later, Kiprono had not been able to procure training facilities. "In Kenya everyone is needy; I am just waiting in line for my turn."

Tribal Affiliations

Kenya is made up of many different ethnic groups, ranging from huge tribes with millions of members, like the Kikuyu, to small ones with perhaps a thousand members. Most of Kenya's runners come from the tribes listed below.

KALENJIN: Homeland in Western Rift Valley Province. Population about three million, 10–11 percent of the national total, fourth or fifth largest tribe. Examples of runners are listed according to their subtribe.

Nandi: Kip Keino, Henry Rono, Wilson Kipketer, Moses Tanui, Pamela Chepchumba, Pamela Jelimo.

Marakwet: Moses Kiptanui, Ismael Kirui, Richard Chelimo, Catherine Kirui, Sally Kipyego.

Tugen: Matthew and Jonah Birir, Paul Tergat, Lydia Cheromei.

Kipsigis: Helen Chepngeno, William Sigei, William Kalya, Simeon Rono, Dominic Kirui, Wilson Kiprugut.

Keiyo: Rose Cheruiyot, Daniel Komen, Sally and Florence Barsosio, Brimin Kipruto.

Sabaot: Shem Kororia, Kipyego Kororia, Ben Jipcho, Samson Kimobwa, Andrew Masai.

Pokot: Tegla Loroupe, Wilson Musto, Simon Lopuyet.

GUSII (or KISII): Homeland in Nyanza Province, west of Rift Valley Province. Population about 1.6 million, 5 or 6 percent of national total, sixth largest tribe. Delilah Asiago, Josephat Machuka, Yobes Ondieki, Naftali Temu, Ondoro Osoro.

KAMBA: Homeland in Eastern Province, just east of Nairobi. Population about three million, .10–11 percent of national total, fourth or fifth largest tribe. Cosmas and Josephat Ndeti, William Musyoki, Benson Masya, Patrick Makau Musyoki.

KIKUYU: Homeland in Central Province, north of Nairobi. Population about 6.3 million, about 21 percent of national total. Kenya's largest tribe. Catherine Ndereba, John Ngugi, Douglas Wakiihuri, Joseph Kimani, Sammy Kamau Wanjru.

MAASAI: Homeland in Southern Rift Valley Province. Population about half a million, 1.5–2 percent of national total. Ninth largest tribe. Billy and Patrick Konchellah, John Litei, Gregory Konchellah (Youssef Saad Kamel), Gideon Ngatuny, David Lekuta Rudisha.

TURKANA: Homeland in Northern Rift Valley Province. Population about 400,000, 1–1.5 percent of national total. Tenth largest tribe. Paul Ereng, Joseph Ebuya, Peter Limoria.

In most years, about three-fourths of the members of the national cross-country team come from the Rift Valley Province.

Doing All to Be the Best

Personal choices make many Kenyan athletes stand out. Moses Tanui, a family man, had the steel discipline to leave the domestic comforts of Eldoret's finest neighborhood to live for three months at a training camp in a small hut with no electricity or running water without once returning home, despite the fact that home was as close as a twenty-minute drive. This attitude to do whatever it takes in the pursuit of excellence is commonplace in Kenya.

This absolute focus goes on twenty-four hours a day. All distractions are avoided during the daytime hours; the living standards are Spartan at best. Still, Dr. Mike Boit half-jokingly said, "Train Hard, Stay Relaxed. The Kenyan Way."

Kenyan coaches insist that the athlete sleeps, rests, and relaxes as much as possible during hard training. In the late 1990s, when the former Junior World 800-meter record holder, Benson Koech, started slipping out of the training camp to go home and attend to farming issues, it was clear that his days as a top athlete were numbered. Such traits are practiced not only by Kenyans, but by many of the world's leading runners. Paula Radcliffe gets ten hours of sleep per night, and two more in the afternoon, during her hard training phases. I thought, after a good night's sleep in Eldoret, that the high-altitude air might give the athletes a deeper, more restful sleep. But Dr. Valdi Sapira of Hoboken, New Jersey, responded, "I can't really think of any reason why that would be so. In fact, the opposite might be true, having less oxygen; you might get a less-restful sleep, as the body works harder to keep the oxygen up. [The feeling of waking more rested] might just be the cleaner air!" Nevertheless, many athletes visiting Kenya note their improved sleep patterns.

Geographically, the quiet running districts of Kenya do let one feel somewhat removed from the distractions of the "real" world. Everyday stress in the running camps is typically extremely low. The days amble by with little disturbance or noise. The most activity seen is usually athletes taking a stroll to break up the monotony of the day's sessions. Not much happens from dawn to dusk. But Kenyans are far from lazy. They are able to relax outside the demands of the workload—a factor that is instrumental in letting them bring a maximum effort to the next training session. One can imagine that the undisturbed and unhurried artisan makes the best masterpiece. Maybe the Kenyans have a greater understanding of which issues are really worth stressing about.

The rural life is beautifully simplistic in many ways. This is reflected in the philosophies of running the Kenyan way. Coaches in Kenya frequently think of Western methods as overcomplicating the art of running. New ideas and thoughts are welcomed, but the jargon is cut out and the explanations to the runners are simple. A lack of information can often be a good thing for an athlete Too many doubts and contrasting knowledge can shake belief in a training plan.

As this book illustrates, Kenyans do have a solid foundation of systematic training, and one general striking difference between Kenyan and Western training is the former's use of block work with nonactive rest periods. A good majority of the runners questioned for this book believe in using a three- to four-month block of training to reach a peak. After a series of races, the Kenyan then stops running completely from two to three weeks to one month or more. Not even cross-training is done to keep in shape.

Compare this to the American collegiate cycle in which the runner rolls from cross country straight to the indoor season, to the outdoor track season, to the summer camp, and then back into cross country. The term "active rest" (in which one goes to the gym to keep in shape on rest days) does not apply to Kenyans.

The environment of Kenya entails having to approach athletics in a basic fashion, and maybe that in itself is an explanation for Kenyan success. There are only two all-weather tracks, both in a bad state of repair, in the Nairobi area. Rural tracks, such as in Kamariny, are effectively cow fields. At Kapcherop, the coach, Boniface Tiren, laments that he doesn't have a flat 100 meter stretch of ground for training: "Everywhere is hills. I am asking the local MP to level a playing field for us. It really is not good for us that we don't have a 400 meter track, not even a grass one." That a league of World Championship Junior and Senior medalists and Olympic gold medalists have come from the results of training on Tiren's bumpy field seems to be a strong case for seeing Tiren's "negative" as a positive. As for footwear, no running stores in Kenya stock a supply of running shoes that athletes can pick from to select their choice of stability or overpronation shoes. When a young barefoot Kenyan was asked what his shoe size was, he replied, "My feet can easily fit into what you give me." When Philip Chirchir arrived in Iten, he did so shoeless, looking for facilities to begin training. There is not a single shoe shop in Iten, but Chirchir knew he would find a pair that would fit his feet. With an oversized pair of Mizunos, this man, who has run four 2:08 marathons in the last decade, resumed training.

Walk around Kapsabet town, and you will commonly see an Olympic runner yet not a gym or sports facility. In the next town, Tanui's gym has a solitary, antiquated, nonmotorized treadmill and other equipment from the 1960s. Moses Kiptanui says, "We used rocks and handmade equipment in a field for gym work."

In the village of Iten (population 4,000), Pieter Langerhorst and Lornah Kiplagat opened a large gym on December 19, 2005. Omulo Okoth, the sports editor for the *East African Standard*, who was present at the opening, noted that the facility was the best he had ever seen in Kenya. Although the gym is basic by American and European standards, Kenyans do not fret over the lack of facilities; they simply manage with the cards that are dealt.

Although Tanzania, Uganda, Somalia, and Ethiopia all border Kenya, the political makeup and histories of the five countries could not be more different. Certainly Kenya has had the most stable and progressive history of the five countries over the past century. Political stability has certainly played a role in helping develop athletics in Kenya.

Joseph Nzau recalls how in the 1960s, Uganda was the powerhouse in his event, the marathon. "That was till Idi Amin came and removed the programs. They went from number one, two, three, four, five in the events to number nowhere."

There is optimism in Kenyan that plays a role in the character of its citizens, a land where everyone is "always fine." It is the standard reply to every greeting in Swahili (*Mzuri*), even in cases when the individual is certainly not "fine." Visiting Samson Kitur shortly before he died, I found the man in visible pain, yet he refused to admit that he was anything less than fine. Kenyans simply do not complain. This ethic carries over to athletics. Never on a training run are words of objection heard. If the pace increases dramatically or if the 60-minute run becomes a 100-minute run, you will never hear Kenyans grumble, unless they have lived in the West too long. For example, on the way to the start of the Berlin Marathon from the elite hotel, the athletes' bus was overloaded by Eastern coaches and managers. They sat smoking cigarettes while the world's finest Kenyans, who were to showcase the event, stood in the aisle of the bus with their heads lost in thick clouds of foul smoke. Not a word of complaint was heard.

There will always be workouts in which targeted times are not met, but from an observer's point of view, the Kenyan athletes habitually will give their best shot. The Kenyan runners definitely question less and follow more; according to European coaches interviewed for this book. Naturally, a runner may comment about the training plan, but it is usually a well thought-out, pertinent remark.

Kenyan mental toughness flows into the ultimate goal of hard training, which is racing. For a Kenyan runner, the difference between first place and a non-money-earning position is huge. For a Western runner, it could mean an upgrade in home-entertainment equipment. Imagine two runners charging down the road to the finish line of an Italian 10K race. They have run together for 9,800 meters, and only 200 meters remain. Who do you think will make a harder effort to win?

Belief is the word in Kenyan athletics. Simply put, Kenyans do not hope to win a race; they take action to try to win that race. Perchance the hardships of life make wishes and fantasies redundant in Kenya. The true Kenyan spirit relies on self-belief.

John Ngugi was rejected by a man, not a system, for not having a runner's body and foot type. John, heavyset in comparison to his fellow Kenyans and a non-Kalenjin, did not feel self-pity or give up. He said, "Let me show them." He won five World Cross Country Championships. That is the Kenyan spirit.

Mike Boit tells a great story to illustrate of the power of the mind: "Remember I was a half-miler. I ran the Bolder Boulder 10K, and decided to do a long-distance tempo run of two miles at high speed. Therefore, I held the lead, but a man remained right on my shoulder. However, at two miles, the crowd was shouting so hard, 'Go Mike, go Mike!' I thought, how can I stop? So I continued. The crowd got wilder; how could I let them down? Imagine, I ended up winning the race! Then I found out that the man on my shoulder was also called Mike."

To excel at running, like most things in life, requires asking how badly you want the success. There is a cake out there, and the many slices constitute the key points discussed until now. With each slice that is missing, the chance of ultimate performance becomes diminished. For many Kenyans, running is a twenty-four-hour-a-day job. The first question athletes should ask is, "how many hours am I putting in?" As Paul Tergat once said, "Running is not a career you do with half your heart."

Training hard does not mean so much the quantity of miles, but rather an ethic of training with determination, dedication, and discipline. To sum up Kenyan training: Your success is what you do with your talent. Mental toughness is a commodity that cannot be bought; it is a decision you make. Go train like a Kenyan.

A *More Fire* view from Triple Gold Medalist Peter Snell

Peter Snell, the 1960 Olympic 800m champion who defended his title successfully in 1964 and won the 1500m that year as well now has a Ph.D. in exercise physiology. He gives his thoughts on the Kenyan success.

"Lifestyle is critical. When I grew up New Zealand, it was a lot like Kenya. Today, New Zealand is moving more toward being like the USA, and people aren't running well.

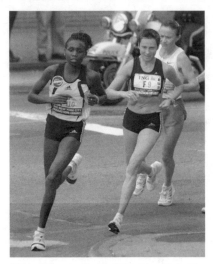

Hilda Kibet leads the ING New York City Marathon 2005. (*New York Road Runners*)

I was bloody poor when I was a runner. I would walk everywhere and cycle to work, but I had all I needed. I was doing quantity surveying for five years during the time I was the Olympic champion and setting world records. There is an erosion of the work ethic now. The Kenyans who really dominated, except for Rono and a few others, were the ones who did not accept college scholarships in the United States. It is too much competition. Also, take someone out of their environment, and bad things can happen—that is why I did not do a U.S. scholarship."

"The Kenyans do what I stress is most important; building an endurance base. I believe there are sociological reasons, too. I heard Kip [Keino]'s tribe was very proud of what he did, and he demonstrated to others what they could do. I am also aware of [Bengt] Saltin's work, where he discovered the Kenyans have a very economical running action. I sort of accepted that, because when you train to maximize your aerobic capacity, a superior aerobic capacity enables one to perform better."

"Is it altitude? I don't know. I mean, Nairobi is at the same level as Leadville, USA, but I don't see loads of good runners coming from there. The Rift Valley extends past Kenya, but you don't see Tanzania doing so well. Ethiopia has great runners, but not the masses like the Kenyans have. To be honest, I really don't know why Kenyans are so good!"

Training with the Kenyans from a Therapist's View

One of America's leading experts on techniques of body movement and athletic alignment is an Arizona resident named Phil Wharton. The author of the Wharton health books, an elite athlete, and a musculoskeletal therapist, Wharton not only went to Kenya to work on the athletes and teach his stretching techniques to the instructors at the Kaptagat and Kapsait camps, he also ran and trained with the athletes, which puts him in a unique position to talk about the Kenyans. His observations came from hours of sweat, both on the massage table and on the dirt roads of Kenya.

MORE FIRE: Lasting impressions of Kenya?

Phil Wharton: Firstly, it is a beautiful culture over there.

MF: What do you think we can learn from the Kenyans?

Phil Wharton: We need to get back to the simpler life.

MF: What body differences, if any, did you notice?

Phil Wharton: They have light, strong muscles, fluid, with a great range of motion.

MF: Could it be reasoned growing up on a farm leads to this body strength?

Phil Wharton: Yes, there is no better work than farm work; you are getting the trunk muscles worked. Kenyans run with the whole body. We [in the United States] get into bulk, and you can't run with bulk.

MF: What would you name as a major biomechanical difference?

Phil Wharton: There is a distinct difference in the height of the foot pad. The arch is like a spring in the body, and if it is not fully functioning, then the pain radiates up into the knees.

MF: And how can Westerners run more like Kenyans?

Phil Wharton: They [Kenyans] also always run on soft surfaces—we tend to forget that. Africans brought us back to running on the dirt.

MF: What are your thoughts on the dietary role?

Phil Wharton: The diet [factor] is huge; there seems often to be a three-week window where they [Kenyans] lose shape when over in America. Is that decompressing from high altitude? I tend to think not. The food over there is so fresh; the meat is just slaughtered and oozing with enzymes and energies. How old is the meat we eat, how much energy are we losing? The same with the fruits, how often do we eat seasonally and regionally fresh fruits? They fuel up at a much higher level compared to us. The whole key is to not break down in training, and nutrition plays a big part in this.

MF: Skeletal-wise?

Phil Wharton: Smaller pelvises; the frame is a lot lighter, making the muscle-to-weight ratio very dynamic.

MF: And the Kenyan mind?

Phil Wharton: I remember Chris Cheboiboch getting up at 3:30 a.m. for training, and he was saying, "For a man like me, it is nothing to suffer." That says it all. They mentally give it all. They are great believers.

A Brief History of Kenyan Running

Kenyan running, in the form of traveling from village to village to relay messages on foot and in the services of hunting and herding, had existed long before any European settler came to the country. However, the development of running as a sport began half a century ago in Kenya. Exercise of a noncompetitive kind was already deeply embedded in the East African culture. Joseph Nzau, a runner who grew up in an area untouched by the imperialists' influence, recalls playing traditional games involving running as a child.

Following the colonization by the British, after the protectorate was formed in 1895, British expatriates replicated sports they had enjoyed as students at universities and thus the emergence of Kenyan structured athletics began. The British introduced the modern Olympic disciplines to Kenya by holding small "socials" with a few track and field events.

Said former 400m hurdler ("I added the hurdles to stop the speed of Mike Boit from chasing me!") General Lazaro Sumbeiywo, who is credited for bringing peace to

Southern Sudan, in a recent conversation at the Baobab Hotel in Mombasa, "Patience, endurance, and determination. These are three attributes of Kenyan people, from warfare to athletics. I know, as I have partaken in both. Sport in Kenya has created a platform for communities. Sports are crucial, for character building."

As these sporting days grew bigger, small prizes, useful household items such as blankets and cooking utensils, were often offered as rewards. This must have been extremely attractive to locals living in Third-World conditions. This encouraged the British, looking to peacefully control the country, where sports were seen as character building and a means to create a social network. Barbara Arlaud (née Clarke), who spent her formative years in Kenya, recalls, "There were organized athletics at the schools back in the 1930s. But not much more than just the local inter-house school competition." Outside the schools, the meets were organized by district officers called "Area Championships" according to Arlaud.

"When we grew up, we chased after animals to hunt them, I would run after impalas, and we would catch them too!" recalls Moses Tanui, backing up what Ernest Hemingway so eloquently wrote in his nonfiction account *The Green Hills of Africa*, about how the Maasai chased after and caught a rabbit on foot.

Kenyan-British relations were fragile at best during colonial days. A Nandi warrior from Kapsimotwo, Koitalel arap Samoei, had fought the British rifles with spears and arrows successfully for ten years. He was tricked in 1905 after agreeing to meet with the British for supposed peace talks. A British officer, Colonel Richard Meinerzergen, ambushed the Nandi with a pistol. From then on, a taint of distrust enveloped any project the whites would initiate.

There was no justice practiced by the British colonists during this period of Kenyan history. Kenyans had welcomed the British thinking they were traders, like the Arabs, or traveling missionaries, who would merely pass through the country. Instead, the British confiscated the Kenyan land, dividing the country's rich pastoral areas between white settlers and instituted taxes for the landless Kenyans to pay.

The first Kenyan president, Jomo Kenyatta (he was elected prime minister in 1963 and was president from 1964 to 1978), said, "When the missionaries arrived, the Africans had the land and the missionaries had the Bible. They taught us how to pray with our eyes closed. When we opened them, they had the land and we had the Bible."

Kenya was declared a part of the British Empire in 1906. The news that only whites were to be allowed on the newly formed legislative council that would govern Kenya the following year probably was not met with joy by the Kenyan people. Neither was the first decree—that the native's occupation of land for cultivation, abodes, and grazing did not constitute a title of the land. Unheard-of 999-year leases were issued for the lands, only to the white settlers.

During the First World War, the 250,000 drafted Kenyans, used to defend British properties in East Africa against the Germans, soon saw many vulnerabilities among the white British. But more than one in five Kenyans died defending a country that was no longer their own. Realizing that the British were not invincible surely fueled the internal hopes for reunification of their lands.

Relations really took a downward spiral in 1922. All that was salable was confiscated and exported by the British for their own profit, so the Kenyans decided to form a protest. Outside the Kingsway Nairobi police station, an estimated 8,000 unarmed workers tried to voice an opinion. The police fired on the crowd, killing many Kenyans.

Politics aside, the introduction of sports and athletics to Kenya was a boon. From those small track meets, athletics unfolded into the culture. Soon the Armed Forces sent recruiters to the competitions looking for healthy bodies; hence the forces' domestic domination right up to the turn of the twentieth century in Kenya. The forces, in turn, introduced their own athletic meets to keep the troops in top physical shape. Schools began to add running to their curricula.

A stranger arriving in Kenya might have guessed that the Maasai tribe, over time, would produce the greatest runners in Kenya. Teddy Davis, of Manhattan, recalls a trip to East Africa: "I was on vacation in the 1950s staying near Nairobi. We drove two hours south and were standing on a hill. I was gazing down the valley and I saw four Maasai warriors. They were running very fast, paint on their faces and wearing colored beads. I distinctly remember the long strides they were using to cover the ground. They looked magnificent running with their spears in hand. I did not know anything about running, but looking at those specimens ... they ran in a fashion I had never seen before. The guide muttered they were out hunting. That was the only time I saw anyone running in Kenya, back in those days."

Yet, although the Maasai (*Maa-sai* translates to "my people") have produced many fine athletes, like the African Games 2004 800m champion William Yiampoy, two-time 800m world champion, Billy Konchellah (1987 and 1991), his brother Patrick, the Commonwealth Games 800m champion of 1994, and his son, the 2006 Asian Games 800m champion Gregory Meretei, who is now known as Youssef Saad Kamel of Bahrain, theirs is a minuscule success story compared to that of the Kalenjin tribe. This would hint that genes perhaps are not the biggest element of Kenyan running success.

It is interesting to note that the Maasai did not participate in the British structured sports as the Kalenjin did. The Maasai were known to be staunchly autonomous and self-governing. Kenyan Olympian Josephat Machuka, half-joking, notes, "The Maasai are plainly not interested in sports. If the British had put a lion near their cattle one hundred meters away, then the Maasai [with their spears] would have become champion javelin throwers. If they had put a side of beef on top of the high jump bar, the Maasai would have hopped up any height to collect it." The Maasai, who best fit the preconceived ideas of Western professors, with their long, thin, sinewy muscles, do not have a large number of runners when compared to neighboring tribes.

The Start of the Organizational Force

In 1947 Archie Evans, an English sports officer, was given a post by the British to develop sports and physical education in Kenya, with the objective of forming a competitive national team. He was based in at Jeans School, Kabete, Nairobi, also known as the Kenya Institute of Administration, and now as the African Union.

At this time, Kenyan athletes were typically affiliated with the Armed Forces, like the Nandi Kiptalem Keter, whose career extended from the 1940s through to the 1960s. Kiptalem was a corporal in the district officer's tribal police. According to Evans, nine times out of ten, the duties of these positions were similar in workload to those of the Kenyan forces' runners of the modern day. "If the D. C. knew they were talented athletes, they were given every facility to go and train, given every advantage."

In 1951 the Kenyan Amateur Athletics Association, today known as Athletics Kenya, was created by the late Sir Derek Erskine. Erskine, the son of a British politician, had been in Kenya since 1927. Evans, who had done the footwork, became the first secretary. He had enlisted in the British Army as an infantryman and had studied physical education at Loughborough University back in Britain.

Before Evans arrived in Kenya in this commissioned capacity, the Arab and African Sports Association, represented by district commissioners, or officers, controlled athletics in the country. This organization was entirely restricted for those ethnicities. Thus, Kenya had never competed outside Africa as a nation. Evans began building an infrastructure of committees that would not only change this but also open up all-inclusive championships and events in Kenya itself. "At that time we just had an annual match-up with Uganda," he recalls. "But I knew we had the talent to match up against whomever."

Success came quickly to the new team, as Kenya performed admirably, first at the Indian Ocean Games in 1952, held in Madagascar, and then at the 1953 Central African Games in Luanshya, Zambia. Gold medals were won at the latter competition in the men's 4 x 220-yard relay, timed in 1:31:2; the pole vault, by Chepkeitan, who cleared 3 meters and 20 centimeters, and the javelin, by Mamboria Tesot, who threw 60 meters and 45 centimeters.

As sports were heavily funded by the government and Kenya was under British rule, an invitation came next to compete in England. At the 1954 British Amateur Athletics Association championships, the Kenyans started to show the potential they would display at distance running in the future. Lazaro Chepkwony, barefoot on the White City cinder track, was an early leader in the six-mile event before he dropped out with cramps. He had been at the front for fifteen laps. Nyandika Maiyoro ran the three miles in 13:54.8. He led for most of the race before fading to fourth behind Chris Chataway, Fred Green, and Frank Sando. Chataway and Green knew all about Maiyoro; they had had to break the world record to defeat the gutsy Kisii tribesman from south Nyanza earlier that year at the AAA Championships. A man best qualified to talk about this era is the aforementioned Archie Evans.

Archie Evans MBE: The Father of Modern Kenyan Athletics

After the outbreak of the war, Archie, born in February 1922, signed up with the Royal Artillery. He then transferred to the infantry and was appointed to a post in Kenya. After a stint there, he made a quick trip back to Britain, where he married his wife Meryll. He then returned; only he left Kenya in 1966 when his position was handed over to a Kenyan and he found himself unemployed. "With a family of two boys, Rodney and Peter, and a girl, Kerrie, I had to do the sensible thing. Not that I did not enjoy coming back to England, but you can say I have a strong attachment to Kenya, and I am very proud of the role I played."

The first look at Kenyan athletics came in India. Shortly after the war, an officer approached Archie, as he was a physical education teacher and a keen sportsman, and said, "It's peacetime; why don't we send a team to Bangalore?" So they went on a ten-day trip. Archie competed in the 400m hurdles, and that was his introduction to seeing Africans compete in athletics.

When Archie began his task of developing sports, there was not a single running track in Kenya. "We used to use tribal spears as javelins, and sacks of sawdust for high jump and pole vault beds." Of course, all the athletes were barefoot. Evans, at once, had a "firm conviction" that the Kenyans would hold their own in international competitions. "There was an annual match each year against Uganda, and we were showing our ability, not just at track but also in the field events."

He immediately set about assembling a federation, then a British Commonwealth committee, then an Olympic Committee. At this time the local commissioners were in charge of athletics; that was adequate for domestic competitions but not acceptable for international championships.

Stationed at the Jeans School in Nairobi, Evans worked with the six established districts, bringing in athletes or traveling to their districts to teach and instruct athletics. Evans took a class in Swahili to better communicate with the athletes, as many understood but could not speak English. "The first week I was in Kenya, I got into trouble, as something I said was misinterpreted, so I studied hard to avoid any further confusions. However, I can say I never had any real problem communicating with the athletes."

There were no women running in Kenya at that time, and Evans reasoned that in his own position he was already overburdened developing the men's team as well as the national soccer team, thus it did not cross his mind to start a women's training group. Of the mentality of the athletes in the 1950s, Evans remembers, "They were totally subservient and trusted me 100 percent, following my instruction to the letter. It was not just athletics that I taught them. For example, many of the athletes had never used a knife or fork, and wearing the team uniforms would be the first time they had worn a suit. They were never any trouble. I was anxious we should present ourselves well, regardless of athletic ability."

"I discovered quickly that they needed more than coaching. If the athletes were left in the locker room, that was where they would stay. We were beginning from the absolute start—for example, Maiyoro, twenty-three at the time, was a character of note—in his first international performance in1953 in Madagascar, he completely missed the start of the race, caught the pack, and won the 3,000 meters."

Speaking about the lack of field athletes in Kenyan athletics today, Evans has this to say:"Yes, I was very concerned abut that. In 1954 when I started out, we had the high jump, the triple jump, and the pole vault. When I disappeared, every single team thereafter had no field-event athletes. I would feel a bit aggrieved if I was a Kenyan field event athlete. I mean one would not mind if the talent was not there, but the talent was, and is, there! Goodness, those javelin throwers and jumpers were world class. And hard working too. I recall Musembi ("Charles") Mbathi, a 400-meter runner. In Vancouver in 1954, we trained in the mornings, rested in the afternoons, and returned to the stadium for evening practice. Well, I saw a photo of Charles with a small child on his knee, and I asked, 'When was that taken, I don't remember seeing the child at the track.' He said, 'Well coach, I have been coming down here in the afternoons for some extra practice.' Yes, they were hard working!"

According to Evans, there was good media coverage in Kenya and keen interest from the public. The federation produced a magazine called *Athletics and Sports Review*, and the *East African Standard* (the second-largest Kenyan newspaper) had a paper called *Baraza* that had news about sports. Into the 1960s, a weekly program all about sports was produced for television. With this networking of media, Evans was able to start subcommittees in differing areas; thus his travel was reduced. "I thought it my position to build and educate a team of coaches in each area to fully develop the athletics in Kenya. For instance, we had a sprinter chap down in Mombassa—Seraphino—and I was able to keep in touch with his progress through one of the field officers, instead of traveling down there myself."

On the training, he says, "We all went out together often for the morning run. Typically forty-five to sixty minutes of running. No dangers of traffic, and if the runners went out on their own, there was no question that they would complete the training session. We built a track, four groundsmen and I, at Jeans School, out of Murram. In the afternoon, we would do sprints and faster running there. We trained seven days a week; there was no need to take a day off, as these chaps did nothing but train."

A typical session would be 10 x 400 meters with an ever-increasing pace over the session, though understandably Evans does not recall the splits today. He also used 800s frequently, and mile repeats were often used as time trials to gauge an athlete's fitness.

Slowly, pieces of equipment did start to trickle through for the athletes, and it took a while for the Africans to adjust to the gear. "I remember getting the athletes used to using shoes. Musembi Mbathi forgot his new track spikes once, so I leant him mine. After he finished, he told me they were OK but a little uncomfortable in the left shoe. When he removed the shoe, I found he had not taken out the fountain pen I had left in there." It has to be remembered that this man had never worn a pair of shoes in his life prior to that day.

Evans admits he was a "hard taskmaster," but he found that the athletes were up to the task and "well able to knuckle down to the workload."

In those days, there was no monetary reward for the team; at best, the athletes would be reimbursed the bus fare to travel from their home village to the training center. However, the Kenyans wanted to be a part of the team, which was a national pride.

Traveling with the national team was no luxury in that era. Evans recalls stories involving 500-mile trips when all the athletes use to travel in the back of a truck. Once, when the team picked up the uniforms in London for the Commonwealth Games, no transport was provided. "The box was so large it could not be placed inside a taxicab. Nyandika told me, 'no problems' and hoisted the box up onto his head. Then to everyone's utter amazement, he walked off and into the tube [subway] station and went down the escalators."

Evans thinks there is some substance to the theory of Kenyan athletic success deriving from the "footing" heritage. "Observing the Kenyans run, they are good to watch. I would say 95 percent of the athletes I saw seemed to have a quality that could be developed." Evans did note some strong personality traits. "I never, never came across anyone who bragged about their ability. All humble and soft-spoken." As for Kenyan talent, Archie likes to relate this story: "The buzz was the four-minute mile, and I was convinced there were Kenyans who could do it. A few years after Bannister had broken the barrier, I took Kip Keino to the track—and this was at 6,000 feet I should add—and on the mud he ran a couple of seconds outside the four-minute mark; that in a training run."

In 1954, the country entered its first team in the Empire Games (now called the Commonwealth Games); the country did not win a single medal. Nyandika Maiyoro, from the Nyamira region of Kenya, finished a notable fourth in the three-mile race, clocking a national record of 13:43.8.

Melbourne, Kenya's Track and Field Team Go to Its Olympic Games

Evans took the squad to its first Olympics in Melbourne, Australia, in November 1956. Along with the runners, Kenya sent a hockey team and a squad of boxers to the games. Against a higher-quality field than he had faced in Vancouver, Maiyoro ran splendidly to place seventh in the 5,000m event in 14:19.0 with Arere Anentia, Kenya's other 5,000m runner, knocked out in the heats (as Nyandika had been in the 1500 meters).

Evans had been preparing Arere for the 10,000 meters, the race that the coach-cum-captain-cum manager thought would be a showcase for Kenya. "I was checking on one athlete who was competing in another event, then helping another Kenyan in the warmups, and really I had to be in three places at once, because Arere was in the waiting room ready to be taken to the call-up. Well, nobody came for him, the Australians were supposed to, so when I arrived after finishing my duties, he was still waiting as all the athletes had been led out. We dashed to the stadium just as the gates were closing, and seconds later the gun fired for the race; it was a great shame." Due to budgetary factors, the Kenyan team's operation was a one-man show. Evans' responsibilities were overwhelming; following a brief hearing, he was exonerated of all responsibilities for Arere's misfortunes.

At that games, Arap Sum Kanuti, a Nandi, would have the distinction of becoming the first-ever Kenyan Olympic marathon runner. He finished thirty-first of thirty-three, recording 2:58.42. "We held a marathon in Nairobi, on the road out towards Mombasa, and Arap was clearly the best. He did some fairly extensive runs in preparations, and we were hoping at sea level he'd perform." Kanuti, who had good speed, gave Evans the impression that he did not really care too much about running but saw the rewards and the lure of international travel and so was enthusiastic to compete. In the field events, Joseph Leresae cleared six feet seven inches in the high jump, placing eighteenth.

By all accounts, running was strictly an activity one would see at institutions, schools, and universities. In the 1950s, according to some of his ex-pupils, F. H. Goldsmith, vice-principal of the Prince of Wales School in Nairobi, was an advocate of jogging for fitness and would be seen on campus exercising. Chris Greaves, who was a schoolboy at the time recalls, "My father worked for the Ministry of Community Development from 1957 to 1959. He worked at first in the Mau Mau detention camps, taking confessions and arranging activities for the non-'hard-core' detainees. Athletics was one of these activities. My dad was also involved in the activities leading up to the Kenya Championships held in Kisumu. As I remember it, there was a series of athletic meetings at the district level, then at the provincial level, to choose the athletes to go to the championships. I believe that Kipchoge Keino from Kiganjo might have been a teenage runner in these events. Definitely Seraphino Antao was a sprinter seen in the Kisumu games. Later on, we lived at the Jeans School, in Lower Kabete, where the Kenyan athletes grouped and trained before going on to the Commonwealth Games."

In 1958, at the Commonwealth Games in Cardiff, Wales, Kenya won hardware for the first time in a major international competition—a bronze in the six-mile race was won by Arere Anentia, and another bronze, in the 400m by Bartonjo Rotich. Earlier in the season, Nyandika had continued to chisel away at the Kenyan three-mile record, setting an international-class time of 13:34.8.

1958 heralded the arrival of another Englishman, who to this day has played a key role in Kenyan athletics. John Velzian, who was stationed at Nyeri, came to work with the police force at Kiganjo. That Velzian was a factor in Kenyan athletics is verified by the list of athletes he coached; Keino, Naftali Temu, and John Ngugi, to name a few. Like Evans, Velzian was struck by the raw talent he found in Kenya, and particularly by the ability of the East Africans to run cross country. "Cross-country running is a quintessential skill of mankind, and Kenyans were running, hunting on foot, until quite recently. This cardiovascular fitness was the backbone of Kenyan success. No other country has ever dominated a World Championship event in any sport in the way that Kenyans have in running in the IAAF World Cross Country Championships—a quite remarkable phenomena." In 2007 Velzian was a key figure at the IAAF World Cross Country Championships in Mombasa, Kenya.

Overseas Opportunities: Machooka, the First Running Student

Outside the championships, the Kenyan running development was continuing. In September 1960, Stephen Misati Machooka* became the first Kenyan to take an assisted academic grant, to Cornell University, in the United States. "It wasn't an athletic scholarship, so to speak, as the Ivy League does not offer athletic scholarships, but it was an educational program initiated by several Northeast universities designed to provide opportunities in the wake of Africa's decolonization," Said Brett Hoover, a director of the Ivy League in the United States.

Machooka, a smiling Kisii, was coached by his neighbor, 1956 Olympian Nyandika Maiyoro, and came to study in the school's agricultural program. "In those days such

---

*Although some sports archives have changed the spelling of "Machooka" to "Machuka," Stephen's son Musa assures us that the former is the correct spelling.

events were big news and the whole community was involved and celebrated in the sending off of one of their own," recalls Machooka's wife. He was the eldest in his family, and his travel to America was viewed as a window of opportunity for him to be more successful, and in turn to assist his younger siblings. He was the first man from the whole district known to travel to America. When he arrived on the East Coast, he made quite an impression.

Victor Zwolak, who was studying at Villanova, remembers the Kenyan well. "I was the favorite for the ICAAAA Championships. The race was in the fall of 1961 at Van Corlandt Park, New York. It was the worst weather, snow and rain, a mess of mud and slush." At this time the supermen of the running world were Eastern Europeans, and Zwolak, who would go on to win

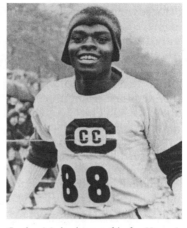

Stephen Machooka, one of the first Kenyan's to competitively run in the U.S. (*Ivy League Archives*)

this race the following year, had no reason to think that a tall willowy Kenyan would be a threat. "Kenyans didn't strike fear the way they do nowadays," he said.

Wearing mittens and a hat with earflaps, Machooka took off and won the race. "He ran away with it," Zwolak recalls. "I was striding and sloshing, and he was floating. A friend of mine who was spectating said he was 'Floating on top of all the ice and snow with his feet hardly touching the ground.' He had this beautiful long stride.

America is the most popular destination for immigrants. Following the 1968 Olympics, when many American coaches either watched or attended the games, opportunities appeared for Kenyans to migrate to the U.S. Two Olympians, Robert Ouko and Julius Sang, went to North Carolina Central University. News that universities and colleges would arrange visas and transport and pay living and tuition fees was greeted with joyful enthusiasm in Kenya. Former St. Patrick's high school student Jackson Kogo, who spent twenty-three years in the USA, choosing to stay after completing his studies, recalls, "I was the envy of my village. Everyone thought I was like a big man when I went to America. It was the wish of all." Not all Kenyans chose, as Kogo did, to stay in the USA. Many returned home with large amounts of saved cash. Stories developed that if you were in America, your lifestyle would be transformed into being one of the rich and famous. Kogo explained, "I would receive requests [for cash] with every correspondence I got from Kenya. People thought I was a millionaire just because I was living in America."

America, in turn, was getting world-class athletes (both Sang and Ouko medaled at the Munich Games) to sit in their classrooms. The development of Kenyan athletics moved Stateside.

Back in Nairobi, track and field was now a regular thriving sport at not only the schools and governmental bodies but also the universities. Barbara Mumford, a university librarian back then, recalls, "There were organized sports days where the students [main-ly African] competed in running, javelin throwing, etc." But Barbara points out that any activities outside of organized sports, like a Kenyan version of kayaking that her husband enjoyed, was not understood by the natives. "The local villagers were convinced that he was 'inspecting something'—they couldn't relate to someone doing that for pleasure." This ties in well with what Joseph Nzau says of starting to run: "You did not practice, or were not supposed to. You simply turned up to the race and ran. If you looked like a good sportsman, people would encourage you, 'Go for a race, and see what you can do.' There was nobody practicing in those days."

Certainly, the colonialists were promoting community involvement. Mumford remembers, "In the town [Enugu] we were in a multiracial club and played tennis with people of all races. Again, the school had a sports day with conventional sports [foot races, javelin, etc.]. Some would be barefoot."

All these activities, and this progression, did not add up to any one reason that Kenyans dominate the running world half a century later; this look at an East African country could be the development history of many African countries.

In the late 1950s and early 1960s in Kenya, as the struggle for independence took precedence over the country's internal matters, the British sports officers still tried to keep all sports programs running. However, postings were terminated, and jobs were lost. Native military officers were appointed as substitute coaches when positions needed fill-ing, yet these men lacked the schooling for the technical side of the sport, namely the short sprints and field events. The European Athletics Club, a resource for athletes, fold-ed when its leaders ventured to Britain.

The Steps to Independence, African Gold, and the Continent's Athletic Spirit

At the time of the 1960 Rome Olympics, Kenya was in the final throes of its struggle against the British. Concentration camps in Nairobi, killings, and political upheaval did little for the team's preparations. This was a step-through Games for Kenya. An estimat-ed 13,000 were killed fighting the imperialist British, with about 80,000 detained in prison camps.

The best result was again produced by Nyandika, who set a new African 5,000m record of 13:52.8.

However, the Games of this decade marked the rise of African running dominance. Twenty-eight-year-old Abebe Bikila of Jato, Ethiopia, became a legend in his lifetime. He stole the limelight by winning not only Africa's first Olympic gold medal, in the marathon event, but setting a world record of 2:15.16 in the process. For sports-minded people in Nairobi, the news of Abebe Bikila winning the Olympic marathon must have instilled bucket-loads of belief. Barefooted, Bikila visibly did not have any element they might have lacked in Kenya. When asked why he ran barefoot, Bikila was said to have replied, "I wanted the world to know that my country Ethiopia has always won with determina-tion and heroism."

Bikila was one of those rare characters whose win made more than sporting headlines; it remains one of the best-remembered moments of marathon running history. Bikila would successfully defend his title in 1964 a paltry six weeks after undergoing surgery to have his appendix removed; again he set a world record—2:12:11—in taking the gold.

Another Ethiopian, Demisse "Mamo" Wolde, would win in Mexico City in 1968, recording 2:20:26. However, the last person to finish that marathon, John Stephen Akhwari (in 3:25:17), like Bikila, captured the heads, hopes, and hearts of people worldwide.

Akhwari, from Endagikot, Mbulu district in Tanzania, demonstrated the African spirit that is embodied by the runners of that continent to this day. Bloodied and bandaged, he entered the Olympic Stadium well over an hour after the winner. He was the reigning African marathon champion, but he had taken a fall in the race and dislocated his knee, and he had limped to the finish.

Interview: John Stephen Akhwari

MORE FIRE: The statement you made following the marathon—"My country did not send me to Mexico City to start the race. They sent me to finish"—has become a motto for the "African runner" mentality, is this fair to say?

John Stephen Akhwari: Myself, I think yes, it is true. Because the explanation I gave, and the event in which I said that statement, made them bold words.

MF: What exactly happened on the course?

John Stephen Akhwari: I remember we started the race at 3 p.m., and the weather at that time in Mexico City was very cold. I was fine running with the first group until the 35K mark, soon after I suddenly realized that the legs could not move any further! Then I started feeling a headache, and finally, with muscle cramps, I fell down. The first-aid car came, and immediately they started to attend the wounds on my knees, putting bandages on the joints. The attendants told me to get into the car, but I answered that I am going to continue with the race till the end, and that is what I did. After the race they took me into the hospital, and I was hospitalized for a period of two weeks. I might have made a mistake training at sea level in Dar es Salaam for the Olympics that were held at altitude; I think that is why I got those muscle cramps.

MF: Coming to the finish line in the Olympic Stadium, what were your thoughts? Do you think your result inspired other Africans to have a fighting spirit?

John Stephen Akhwari: I remember I felt very happy, because finally I fulfilled my goals of starting the race and finishing regardless of all that had happened on the course. I think yes, I think the statement [of finishing against adversity] made a courageous testimonial for all athletes of the world.

MF: Did you ever think back in 1960s that Africa would dominate as it does today in the sport of running?

John Stephen Akhwari: Yes, because African runners have always been extremely talented; the only thing they lacked at that time was the basic running needs. For example, running gear and good coaches.

MF: How do you think people perceived African runners in 1968 before winning so many medals? (African men swept the 5,000 and 10,000m medals, won the 1500m and the marathon, and took the gold and silver in the steeplechase.)

John Stephen Akhwari: I think most of the people in those days did not have any expectations that African athletes were in the position to perform well, especially in 1968. This was because Africa, at that time, was performing quite poorly compared to other countries.

MF: What are your thoughts about African running today?

John Stephen Akhwari: I think African runners today are at a much higher standard compared to the athletes of my days. They are doing a great promotional job for Africa.

MF: As a champion marathon runner, and an ambassador for African running, what is your advice to runners?

John Stephen Akhwari: Make sure runners do not quit it [running] before reaching their goals. They should never lose hope. The important point for them to remember is when they start something; make sure they also finish it, regardless of any heavy odds against them in the process.

John Stephen Akhwari, today seventy years old, competed once more, at the Commonwealth Games in Edinburgh, 1970, where he placed fifth.

Seraphino Antao, the Golden Cheetah

The withdrawal of the European coaches, as earlier mentioned, arguably was the cause of the focused progress of Kenyan running moving toward the simplest exercise, long-distance running. There was one noticeable exception. One man decided if there was not a national specialized coach available, he would procure the services of a qualified expert himself find more information by talking to his international competitors. At this time, economic factors, discussed later, were yet to play their part, as there were no monetary awards in track and field.

Seraphino Antao, from the Makadara estate in Mombasa, was Kenya's first international gold medalist. "It has been said I started the medal rush, and when I retired I told a [relatively unknown] Kip Keino to keep the flag flying for Kenya. I think he did!" He says now.

In 1962 at the Perth Commonwealth Games in Perth, Australia, he won the 100-yards/200-yards sprint double. "The cheetah," or "the gazelle," as he was variously nicknamed, attended the Goan High School, and like most Kenyan boys, he preferred to play football than to run.

Antao, then eighteen, took up athletics in July 1956. As quickly as the following year he was on the Kenyan national team for the East African Championships, "The only time athletes [around Kenya] got together was during the local Provincial sports, and a week later the Kenya Championships, where the top two athletes in each event were selected to represent Kenya at the annual East African Championships between Kenya, Uganda, and Tanganyika [now Tanzania]. There certainly was not a big athletics circuit in Kenya."

Leaving school, Antao took a position as a supervisor with a shipping company and would train each day after finishing work in Mombasa. At the Rome Olympics, Antao was greatly inspired by reaching the semis in the 100m. Upon returning to Kenya, he found a professional trainer, Ray Batchelor, and took his workouts up a notch. In the Mombasa

Municipal Stadium, he would train for two to three hours per day, seven days a week. The results paid off with the two medals in Perth. Antao's times proved that his wins were no fluke; he clocked 9.5 for the 100 yards, and in the 220 yards final, he ran 21.1 (two-tenths slower than his time in the semifinal). A little-known athlete called Kip Keino finished eleventh in the three-mile event and was eliminated in the heats of the mile.

Assistance from the Sports Ministry only really materialized after Kenya gained its independence, but Antao does remember the Kenyan public being supportive and holding "various receptions in towns throughout Kenya." A benchmark of his global success was that throughout his career he was ranked in the top six in the world, never once losing a race in East Africa until his final year, 1964, when because of an illness he was defeated.

The local glory did not stop at Antao. Kimaru Songok, also of Mombasa, won the silver medal in 1962 in the 440-yard hurdles in 51.9, only four-tenths of a second away from the gold medal. Another Mombasa athlete, Peter Francis, went to the Olympics in 1964 to run the 800m.

The First Olympic Medal, World Record, and Women's International Medal

A milestone was reached in October 1964 when Wilson Kiprugut Chuma, trained by Archie Evans, earned a bronze medal at the Tokyo Olympics in the 800m. New Zealand's Peter Snell beat the Olympic record, equalled by Kiprugut in the qualifying rounds, to take the gold. As Kenya was in its first year of independence, it was a message to the world of the country's stability and sporting focus.

Wilson Kiprugut Chuma, who lives in Kericho, used to run 15K each day to school as a youngster. Following school, he enlisted as a driver in the Army in 1956, where he joined physical-fitness classes and discovered his running talent. He was selected to represent Kenya in the East African Championships in Nairobi, where he finished second in the 880 yards. The following year he won a trip to Tanzania, but the next two years he had to buckle down to Army duties and stop running. Resuming training in 1962, he was selected to travel to Australia for the Commonwealth Games. "But I didn't get anything there," he recalls. In 1964, he traveled to the Olympics. "I had one tactic, go to the front and run as fast as I could. I got an Olympic record in the heats! In the final, I should have got second but I was blocked by a Jamaican and had to go round him, causing me to lose a place. That silver was mine, but Snell [Gold] was too strong."

Upon returning to Kenya, Kiprugut became a national hero. "Oh yes, I remember it clearly—I was carried on the shoulders of men from inside the plane all the way to an open car, and paraded through the streets of Nairobi." Life in the Army, which included a promotion to Warrant Officer Two, got easier. In 1968, at the Mexico City Olympics, Kiprugut ran his last great race. "I was to win gold. I was leading the whole way. I was so so happy. Then an Australian took my medal, so close, right at the end!"

Following retirement from athletics in 1969, Kiprugut took to coaching in the military before leaving the armed forces and working for the Uniliver Tea Company for twenty-two years before retiring to his home farm. Today he has six acres of tea plantations

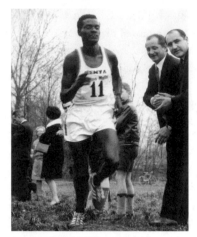

In 1970 Naftali Temu took first place at the Cinque Mulini cross-country race in Italy. (*Cinque Mulini archives*)

and thirty acres of pesticide plant growth crops. He leads a modest life and is interested only in the local district athletics. He hopes to start a team for them and continue with his passion for coaching.

In 1965 another high point was reached when Diana Monks won a silver medal at the All-Africa Games, Brazzaville, 80-meter hurdles in 11.8 seconds. It was Kenya's first-ever women's championship medal. Monks, born in Kenya but of British heritage, came through the ranks, competing annually at the Kenya AAA national championships.

On August 27 of that same year, Kenya got its first-ever track world record when Kipchoge Keino ran 7:39.6 for 3000 meters. In his initial attempt at the distance, Keino took a gargantuan six seconds off the record set by Siegfried Herrmann of the German Democratic Republic earlier the same month.

New Zealand's Peter Snell, OBE, who won two of his three gold medals at the Rome Games, reminisces about the Kenyan marvel in the 1960s. "The first Kenyan I heard about was a few years before Rome, in 1958. A guy named Nyandika did well enough to be noticed in the Commonwealth Games." The only reason Nyandika stuck in Snell's mind was that he was a non-European runner, as the Continent was dominant in the 1950s. "In 1964, Keino was around, but he was not quite ready; but by 1965, boy, he opened the floodgates. Flinging off his painter's cap on the last lap, he would crush people by running from the front. I wasn't studying him then; I was just aware that he was really good."

Snell recollects that Kiprugut's fast running in the Rome semifinals had not caused him any concern. "In those days, there was not much information about your competitors available like there is today. I thought he might not run fast in the final because of pushing it in the semis. I remember thinking 'Why are they so good?' I suppose I thought, like the popular consensus at the time, that they are good because of the altitude. Now I am not that sure."

In Kingston, Jamaica, in 1966, Kenyan runners continued the golden theme set by Seraphino Antao at the 1962 Commonwealth Games. Naftali Temu, an Army soldier from Sotik, who had run twelve miles to and from school each day, stunned the favorite, Ron Clarke of Australia, to take the gold in the six-mile race. Two gold medals were also won by the flying policeman Kipchoge Keino in the mile and the three-mile race.

It was a sneak preview of what would be seen at the Mexico City Olympics of 1968, the games in which Kenya would first become recognized as an athletic powerhouse. When the athletic experts were warning the world that race times would be slow in the distance events, the Kenyan runners were not listening! The first event for Kenya was the final of the 10,000m. Naftali Temu took the lead 700m from the finish and ended with a fine sprint to win in 29:27.4. He would also take a bronze in the 5000m. For good measure he led the marathon until 30K, before dropping back, to place nineteenth, in 2.32:36. Kipchoge Keino took silver in the 5000m and gold in the 1500m. Amos Biwott, just twenty-one years old, started the Kenyan steeplechase tradition with a gold medal. Kenya also took silvers, with Kiprugut in the 800m, Benjamin Kogo in the steeplechase, and in the 4 x 400m relay (Hezekiah Nyamu, Naftali Bon, Daniel Rudisha, and Charles Asati).

Kenya had arrived on the world's athletics stage in an unprecedented fashion. The young nation was second behind the might of the USA with a far smaller squad in the track and field medals count. The reputation of Kenyan running was cemented in Mexico. With American civil rights, the Vietnam War, the assassination of Martin Luther King Jr., and, ten days before the games, the terrible Tlatelolco Massacre, the world press was hungry for some human-interest chronicles. The incredible and enigmatic Kenyans made for cheerful headline news.

Some skeptics pointed to the high altitude of Mexico City and said, "It's a fluke; it'll never happen in 1972 at the Munich Games." This, of course, proved to be untrue, as Kenyans were on the podium for the 400m, 800m, 1500m, 3000m steeplechase, and 4 x 400m relay.

President Jomo Kenyatta began rewarding the golden athletes with gifts of large areas of land. Today the Kazi Mingi farm of Kip Keino stands on fields that Keino "inherited" with his sweat in 1975. A forty-acre farm at North Mugirango was given to Naftali Temu following the 1968 Olympics. This very visible form of compensation was more than enough incentive for a new generation of runners.

What followed was a phenomenal explosion of success for Kenyan runners. However, economics and social evolution contained the success within Kenyan borders. Track was very much an amateur sport until the 1980s. Certainly during the 1950s, living in a country with no social-security system, athletes were not lining up to sacrifice their careers and train three times a day to try to win a blanket or an iron medal.

Highlights of Kenyan Running Firsts After 1968

1970: Hezekiah Nyamau, Naftali Bon, Thomas Saisi, and Robert Ouko claim the men's 4 x 880 yards world record in Britain (7:11.6).

1972: Robert Ouko, Julius Sang, Charles Asati, and Hezekiah Nyamau win the 4 x 400m relay at the Munich Olympic Games.

1974: Ben Jipcho, world record holder in the steeplechase, wins that event, the 5000m, and misses the gold in the 1500m by half a second at the Commonwealth Games.

1977: Samson Kimobwa sets the world record at the 10,000m (27:30.5).

1978: Over a span of eighty-one days, Henry Rono sets four world records at the 10,000m, 5000m, 3000m, and the 3,000m steeplechase. For good measure, he wins the steeplechase and the 5000m at the Commonwealth Games.

1985: Kenya wins its first individual world title, the junior men's, at the World Cross-Country Championships.

1986: John Ngugi wins the first of his five World Cross-Country Championship titles. With three men in the top five spots, Kenya takes the first of its eighteen consecutive team titles.

1987: At the second World Track and Field Championships, Kenyans take their first gold medals: Billy Konchellah, 800m; Paul Kipkoech, 10,000m; and Douglas Wakiihuri, marathon. Ibrahim Hussein starts a trend—he is the first African to win a major city marathon, taking the New York City Marathon.

1991: Konchellah defends his title, despite suffering from chronic asthma, an affliction that rules him out of the following year's Olympics.

1992: Samson Kitur wins Kenya's first Olympic medal in a sprint event when he finishes third in the 400m in Barcelona. Kenya also completes a clean sweep of the steeplechase medals. It is a feat they will repeat in the 2004 Olympics. At the inaugural World Half-Marathon Championships, Benson Masya wins the men's race and leads Kenya to the team title.

1993: Moses Tanui becomes the first man to run under one hour for the half marathon in Stramilano, Italy. Kenya does not include Tanui in the World Half-Marathon Championship team later the same year, though Kenya still easily wins the world team title. As a 15-year-old, Sally Barsosio takes a bronze medal at the world 10,000m championships

1994: Helen Chepngeno becomes the first Kenyan woman to win the World Cross-Country Championships.

1994: In New York City, Tegla Loroupe becomes the first African woman to win a major marathon.

1995: Moses Kiptanui becomes the first man under 8:00 in the steeplechase (7:59:18).

1996: In Atlanta, Pauline Konga takes Kenya's first-ever women's Olympic medal with her second-place finish in the 5000m. Yet another unknown Kenyan confuses the journalists: Joseph Keter seemingly appears and disappears, stopping on the world's stage just long enough to pick up the sport's highest award by winning the Olympic steeplechase.

1997: Daniel Komen becomes the first man (and the only one to date) to run under 8:00 for two miles (7:58.61). Sally Barsosio wins Kenya's first-ever gold medal at the Track and Field World Championships.

1998: Hoping to add diversity to the sport of cross country, the IAAF introduces a 4K event to the World Cross-Country Championships, trying to attract European middle-distance runners. Kenyan men sweep the top five places, and for good measure they also take six of the top seven places in the long course. In Rotterdam, Tegla Loroupe becomes the first African woman to hold the world record in the marathon.

1999: In winning the London Marathon, Joyce Chepchumba claims the world record for a women's-only field. She earns the largest recorded first prize in marathon running, $230,000. Chepchumba's outstanding career saw her complete a record-breaking seventeen sub-2:28 marathons.

2000: At the World Junior Track and Field Championships, Kenya finishes first in the medal count, including seven golds, with a squad far smaller than those of many other nations.

2001: Kenyan policeman Charles Kamathi does the unthinkable: he ends Haile Gebrselassie's eight-year unbeaten record in the 10,000m races at the Edmonton World Championships.

2002: Another flying policeman, Rodgers Rop, wins both the Boston (2:09:02) and New York City (2:08:07) marathons. The remarkable double was last accomplished by Rop's countryman Joseph Chebet in 1999.

2003: Paul Tergat becomes the first Kenyan man to break the world record in the marathon.

2003: Catherine Ndereba wins the World Championship marathon in Paris. It is Kenya's first women's gold in the marathon.

2004: Margaret Okayo, Catherine Ndereba, and Salina Kosgei take the major spring marathon wins at London, Boston, and Paris, respectively. Kenyan women outdo the men, who "only" take London (Evans Rutto) and Boston (Timothy Cherigat), although Raymond Kipkoech Chemwelo places second in Paris.

2005: Catherine Ndereba becomes the first woman in Boston's illustrious history to win the event four times. Samuel Wanjiru becomes the first teenager to hold the world record at the half-marathon distance with a time of 59:16 in Rotterdam.

2006: Janeth Jepkosgei pulls a "Kamathi," beating Maria Mutola to take the Commonwealth Games gold at 800m. To prove it was no fluke, she then runs the world's leading time for the year, a Kenyan record, and beats Mutola again in Lausanne. (Twelve months later she would take the World Championships 800m gold.)

2007: At the Mombasa World Cross-Country Championships, Kenyans take twelve of the sixteen individual medals on offer, winning three of the four team titles. Had Lornah Kiplagat never switched citizenship to the Netherlands, the number of medals would have been thirteen and Kenya would have swept the team titles. The juniors in both divisions sweep the podium spots. In Osaka, Ndereba becomes the first woman ever to take two World Championship marathon titles.

2008: Teenage sensation Pamela Jelimo, 18, who ran her first 800m only five months earlier, wind the first-ever Olympic gold medal for a Kenyan woman. Five days later, Nancy Jebet Lagat takes Kenya's second gold in the 1500m. Samuel Kamau Wanjiru wins the first gold medal in the Olympic Men's marathon in Kenyan history.

Kenyan Management and Eldoret Town

Godfrey Kiprotich, of Kimwarer, Keiyo, is not at home, or at least at the home I think he should be at this morning. He said, "call for me around 10 o'clock," and I can see that his car is not in the compound of the Kimbia house number one, behind the Iten General Post Office. Kimbia, a running-management business, has three houses in Iten and is a faction of the Kim McDonald dynasty that split after Kim's premature death a few years ago. The other faction, Pace Sports, is doing very well, too.

Two young children come up as I hesitate outside the gate, "Can you give me your bicycle?" they ask. It costs nothing to ask, and as I shake my head, the next request is for my wristwatch.

I see that someone is home, as the front door is open, so I push the bike through the corrugated iron door that is cut into the compound gate, leave it on the grassy lawn, and walk up to the house. "Hodi!" I call, announcing my presence. A Tanzanian boy comes to the door. He looks no older than fifteen. I later find out he is the junior 5,000-meter champion of Tanzania. An old Puma tracksuit hangs from his shoulders like a loose sack on a coat hanger; I can see each bone in his face as it protrudes beneath his clean, thin, almost transparent skin. The Tanzanians generally have lighter skin color and different eye shape than do the Kenyans, and typically their English is not as proficient. Just my luck; Junior does not speak any English. I talk to him in my spare Swahili. Surprisingly, he understands and tells me, "Nyumba mbili." As I turn, James Kosgei enters the compound and says, "House Number Two!" Before I can tell James that I understand, ever-smiling Kosgei asks, "What about it?" I tell him I am meeting Godfrey Kiprotich. "He'll be sleeping, that man is not a runner." Although Iten is a drowsy village, everyone who is a runner is up before the crack of dawn.

Godfrey Chirchir Kiprotich used to be a runner, one of the very best. In fact, at the first race I ever ran in Central Park, New York, hoping to win a couple of airline tickets, I met Godfrey on the starting line. I knew him from previous races around the globe, and I was delighted to see that his stomach was a tad oversized. I had known him since the mid-1990s, and he definitely did not look in fighting shape. The first mile was uphill; despite every trick I threw, Godfrey refused to be dislodged from the leader's spot. 4:29 . . . the tickets were his. That was Kiprotich, a supreme competitor, who admitted after the race that he was *far* from his best shape.

I find House Number Two by walking along the lane back toward the post office and looking over the gates until I see a white Toyota truck. True enough, Godfrey, who used to be in the Kahawa (Coffee) Army division, is asleep when I enter. This is not his home—he lives in Eldoret Town—yet when business calls, he will sleep in Iten. The small house is empty except for a huge number of cooking utensils. It is a cool stone house, with blood-red concrete floors and whitewashed walls. Its shade is welcome after the hot sun that has already hit the sky. All the rooms are exceedingly simple: a plain foam mattress or two and scant bedding. Shiny stainless-steel draw bolts allow each room to be individually locked. A Westerner could be excused for thinking this house uninhabited.

I was spending the day with the Keiyo runner for old time's sake. Godfrey provides an interesting insight to the intricate business of running management. Before an athlete breaks the tape at the ING New York City Marathon, winning the richest prize in marathon running of $130,000; before the manager signs the deal for the athlete with Mary Wittenberg, the CEO of the New York Road Runners and race director of the ING New York City Marathon, the buck starts with the athlete finding a manager.

The first time I met Jos Hermens of Global Sports was in Kenya. He was the world record holder at 10 miles and a favorite for the Munich Olympic 10,000m. He had chosen to go home after the Palestinian terrorists murdered eleven Israeli athletes and one German police officer. "It's not a party any longer when people kill each other. Then the games should stop," said Hermens. He was in Nairobi, sitting in the shade of a green canvas table umbrella, at the Thorn Tree Café in the New Stanley Hotel, sipping a beverage and looking through his gold-rimmed specs. In the colonial days, this café was the meeting and mixing spot for the settlers, and to this day, it remains a traditional assembly spot for the capital. Hermens sat writing and signing contracts with a group of Kenyan athletes, who approached his table one by one. Today, with a team of assistants, Hermens still has about forty Kenyan athletes under his management, among more than 120 athletes.

The Kenyans had all performed admirably at the National Championships and caught Jos's eye. A couple of hours later, I had driven with Paul Tergat to a similar setup at another hotel in Nairobi, where Gianni DeMadonna, an amicable Italian manager and also a former world-class runner, was signing contracts with the likes of Tergat, Moses Tanui, and other Fila athletes. However, the literally hundreds of other Kenyans searching for a way out of Kenya and into the international circuit have to either write hopeful e-mail messages to foreign managers like Paul Kimugul or Richard Yatich or impress a local middleman like Kiprotich. Intermediaries have become more common, as they can give an overseas manager a true picture of the current form of the signed athlete. Lisa Buster, who is based on America's East Coast, uses a close-knit group of athletes who advise her on new prospects. Former Swedish manager Stig Eklund found that even after the successful recruitment, he had to be careful, as athletes can drop out of form. This makes a resident man like Godfrey invaluable. For Eklund (who had no Godfrey), a pair of scales sufficed; as Stig explained, "They would arrive in Sweden overweight. So when the runners got in shape. I weighed them. The next time I was in Nairobi, I left a pair of scales. Before any trips I would ask them, 'What do the scales read?'" Needless to say, Godfrey plays a role in getting the fit athletes to the starting line.

You need a great deal of patience to do business in Kenya. "Ten o'clock" can be ten, eleven, twelve, or even ten o'clock the following day! In my experience, ordering a bunch of T-shirts from a clothing store has proven to be a four-hour process, and that was just requesting the paperwork.

People in Kenya are perpetually not where they say they will be. For the first few days, trying to do business is frustrating. After a while, everyone slips into the "no rushing" mode, and in the end, everything that is needed is done. "I don't know how the days go by the way they do, you think you have free time, and then suddenly a cup of tea here, one there . . . the day is gone," says Brother Colm, gazing through his rose-tinted glasses one afternoon and looking at the upcoming week for a time to schedule afternoon tea.

The Kenyan side of athletics management begins like this: Godfrey, who works for Kimbia, pushes aside the *Eastern Standard* newspaper from the passenger seat of his truck. "We have to track down Cherigat [the Boston Marathon champion of 2004] because he is yet to sign with us. Let me just try to get him on the phone." He makes a hurried call as he reverses the truck out of the compound. We slowly bump and rock over the narrow dirt trail that will lead us to the tarmac road. A runner with yellow teeth approaches and raps on the window. He asks for running shoes from me and for the next few days' running program from Godfrey Kiprotich not only does sports management, he also coaches the runners. Willy Korir goes on his way with a recipe of 30K runs and 400m repeats for the next couple of days. This runner, who last year used to live with Christopher Kandie, would make a breakthrough in May 2007, when he would win the Eldoret Family Bank Half-Marathon. Incidentally, Helena Kirop, another Iten resident who lives 400 meters away from Kandie, would win the women's race.

We make a right turn and pass the village post office; another runner walks over. Godfrey's car is easily recognizable in Iten, and we are driving at five miles per hour, if that. This time, it is the talented Gilbert Koech. Koech has recently joined Kimbia after spells with a few other managers; he wants to know when his next race is going to be. He dropped out of the last one, the Chicago Marathon. Godfrey sighs and asks if Gilbert is training hard yet, to which Koech replies that he is just starting up again. "Let's see what Tom says," says Godfrey, referring to Tom Ratcliffe, the founder of Kimbia who lives back in Boston. It is a catchphrase that Kiprotich often uses that allows him to be the dismissive member of the team. Tom will be making an annual visit to Kenya the following month. Bwana Tom, as he is affectionately known when he arrives, started working with Kim McDonald many years ago, operating the U.S. base of the business that he founded in London; he and Godfrey go back donkey's years. Tom, a former elite distance runner, has done outstanding and sustained work in the philanthropic arm of Kenyan athletics. He is a manager who has proven time and again that money is not the reason for his vocation and that the athletes he manages are more than machines.

I ask Gilbert how his wife, Edna Ngeringwony Kiplagat, is doing. I knew Edna when she was a shy fourteen-year-old student at Kapkenda Girls School. She is now twenty-six, represents the police team, is a mother, and has just returned from a successful season on the U.S. road-racing circuit. "She is good. You must come for tea." I agree without asking the directions; that is the beauty of Iten. You do not need an address; you simply arrive in an area where you think the runner resides and ask around. It is a foolproof method.

We finally turn left onto the tarmac road. Now we will make progress as we drive to Eldoret. As we travel, Godfrey tells entertaining tales about runners who have come and gone throughout the years. He also tells of visits by foreigners and how he notes the different ways they perceive Kenya. After fifteen minutes on the main Eldoret road, we slow to make a right turn. The first athlete we have to hunt down is Abraham Chebii, a silver medalist in the World Cross-Country Championships. He lives a long way from the Eldoret tarmac road, and we drive over dirt roads that must be impassable after heavy rains. Finally, we reach Chebii's house. It is in an area called Kiplombe where many Marakwets, like Chebii, have settled. "This is because Moses Kiptanui owns a lot of land around here, and he rents it to his tribe's folk," Godfrey explains.

Chebii, who lives in a nice home with double-gated security is not around. Typical. The watchman tells us where we will find him in town. We pass an old colonial house. "That belongs to Kiptanui, too." As does the milk van that drives past us clanking over the bumps and ruts, overladen with old metal milk churns.

Back on the road to Eldoret, we swerve to avoid a mangy-looking sheep that wanders with a suicidal swagger across the road. The next swerve is for one of the many potholes. This road is actually one of the better in Kenya. Try driving to Kericho from Kapsabet; the road is so bad—rutted and pockmarked—that people literally abandon the tarmac for the bush on either side.

We pass a site where Ben Maiyo is constructing some buildings. Godfrey asks me if I want to stop and say hello, but my thirst is calling for a black currant Fanta soda, so we drive on. As we pull into Eldoret, Godfrey spies the small pickup of Laban Kipkemboi, another of Kimbia's athletes. He pulls over and whips out the cell phone as Kipkemboi drives off in the opposite direction. However, Laban is not picking up his phone, and Kenyans do not typically have voicemail. "Later," Godfrey mutters. We are going for coffee first, to the best place in Eldoret—a small, cheap café called the Picnic Basket in a building complex behind the Sirikwa Hotel, one of the most expensive hotels in Eldoret. If you want to spot the richer athletes, the Sirikwa is one of the favorite haunts for afternoon tea.

We give the yellow-jacketed parking man "ten bob" (twenty cents) for a space in the car lot and walk to the café, but for some reason it is closed. It is not that the café *should* be shut, as we are here during the operating hours; it is just because this is Kenya. The Kenya Electric and Power offices are next door in the same complex, and I see Pieter Langerhorst and Lornah Kiplagat's Land Rover parked outside. I know they are trying to get power lines in Iten to extend to their residence, which currently runs on solar power. "The only problem with solar is that my espresso machine doesn't work!" says Pieter, the man they call Starbucks.

We stand outside the Picnic Basket looking in. "No problems," says Godfrey, "we have to meet Peter Tanui, so let's go to another place." We walk into the town's main street, watching out for traffic. There used to be traffic lights, but too many people refused to obey the lights, especially old farmers coming into town on their tractors, and the lights caused more trouble than they were worth. Nowadays, he who pushes gets the right of way. Claudio Berardelli, from Team Rosa, with his ace Italian driving skills, is great at navigating the Eldoret roads. As for the rest of us, we suffer the dents and scrapes. Only a week ago, Starbucks and I were hit by a runaway driver that turned out to be the brother of Daniel Yego. I had to go first to the town prison, and then to the Eldoret courthouse to save him from getting a police record after he was arrested for the crime!

Upstairs in the cool and spacious Klique Hotel, owned by Nicholas Biwott, one of the richest and most powerful political men in Kenya, Godfrey sees Tanui. I have not seen Peter since we ran an 8K race together a dozen years ago in Iowa, of all places. One of the Kenyan athletes who was with us on that day has since been convicted of murder; we talk about what he, others, and we have been up to of late. Then I leave Godfrey and Peter to talk about the upcoming races and which athletes they will select to go where, and I spy Nixon Kiprotich in the café. He is lounging with his daughter, drinking a pot of Kenyan tea, at least twenty pounds heavier than the last time I saw him, which was not too long ago. Kiprotich, joking about his weight gain, asks how long I will be in Kenya. We used to run intervals together on the Eldoret airport landing strip, before it was opened up to planes, as Nixon had a bad back and could not run the bends on a traditional 400m running track without pain, so I enquire about his ailments and he tells me about the various operations that ended his running career. Nixon had been the Olympic 800-meter silver medalist in Barcelona in 1992.

When I return to Godfrey, he wants to order food. He tells me about the troubles of the spring races. "A lot of the runners are not in shape yet, and you know Kenyans believe in themselves. They want to go to Boston, but you saw K____, and he is fat; there is no way I can send him." There is a smaller race in Japan that the athletes are also interested in, but it is only two months away. "For that I'll have to send someone who is in form. Someone who was not resting over Christmas. I think maybe Laban." Laban did go, and he placed third in a new PR of 2:08:38. I ask who is going to Boston, and he tells me Ben Maiyo, who was the runner-up the previous year, and Stephen Kiagora, the ING New York City Marathon runner-up. Maiyo would finish sixth and Kiagora, third. "Those are serious guys, they will be ready," he tells me, and indeed they will be.

The Klique, due to its popularity, has a 200-shilling minimum-order policy to stop loitering. You pay 200 shillings at the door, and it is redeemed with your bill. Somehow I never get asked, probably because the staff know me from previous visits. As 200 shillings are above the daily wage, you usually meet many of the wealthier residents of Eldoret here, like Patrick Sang, who has just walked by. Sang had just delivered Eliud Kipchoge to the airport. "He is a top-shape man; he's going to run well in Spain at a 10K." (Eliud would be the first ever to run a 10K road race under 27 minutes a week later). Patrick is like a captain of Eldoret's running circle, involved in many things, and looking to start a new club. He mentions the name of it, something beginning with an M.

Godfrey continues to explain that Kenyans, disciples of block training, give him trouble as they often take a lengthy Christmas vacation. "When we open the camp, all the athletes have to report in and sign contracts for the year, and then we can see who is ready for what race. When we go out for a morning training run and someone cannot hang, we know the form. I am there in the vehicle watching. But at the moment I only want to get everyone's name on the contracts." He again speed dials Timothy Cherigat. I had seen Cherigat two days earlier at the Sirikwa hotel, and I knew that Timothy would need some time to get into shape; he would not be the man for the Japanese race.

Kiprotich, as Moses Kiptanui, had originally been from the KIM camp, was an ideal scout; he's a former world-class athlete and there is no fooling him. The waitress brings the food and about five scraps of small paper that seem to constitute a bill. I wonder why she has not totaled the bill, as there are only two of us. I ask and get a blank look for an answer, and she scurries away in embarrassment. Kiprotich, moments after sitting, leaves the table to talk to a Kenyan in a pink shirt who he notices a few tables away. The man lives in America and is visiting. "He was a star runner at St. Mary's in the 1980s," Godfrey tells me before he walks over. Left alone at the table, I whip out my cell phone to make some calls, but before I can, Christopher Cheboiboch, who is wandering past the table, stops to say hello. Boston is the hot topic; Cheboiboch wants to know if I can call the marathon on his behalf. "I ran second there, they know me, and I want to run again." I explain to Chris that firstly, I know his manager, and secondly, I am not a manager myself. That, it appears, is not an issue. He whips out his own cell phone and speed dials his manager, Volker Wagner in Germany, trying to put the wheels in motion.

Lunch was chicken sandwiches with violent-red tomato sauce for Godfrey, and I had two chapattis, folded into crescents, with a fried egg slapped inside of each; I learned this choice from the late Richard Chelimo. We now go out onto the main street because Godfrey has heard from another customer that Cherigat is in the next street. Laban, who saw on his phone that Godfrey had tried to call him, phoned and said he would meet us at the gas station in ten minutes. Ezekiel Kipkemboi, a deaf and dumb man who is a good 10,000m runner, comes up to us in the street. Godfrey shocks me with his fluent understanding of sign language, and we start plans for an Achilles Track Club branch for handicapped athletes in Kenya. Not fluent in sign language myself, I start talking to two people standing in the street; they saw a program about Shoe4Africa on KBC television and have questions. It amazes me how everyone knows everything in Kenya.

We are across the road from the Bata shoe store, the chain where seemingly every Kenyan kid gets school shoes. Mary, a cousin of Lornah, works here, and it has become the message center (along with Silas's Hotline Butchery) for the people of Kabiemit, Lornah's home district. That is a special place for me; it is close to where I got my Kalenjin name (Chebaibai, "Happyman") from the people of the area when I was visiting with Pieter and Lornah about five years ago. If you want a ride to their camp in Iten, then just go and hang out at the shoe store, and someone will drop by who can drive you there.

Kenyan towns are always lined with people standing along the streets like drawn curtains, just watching, always ready to talk, full of local knowledge. They do not look as if they are waiting for opportunities; merely as though they are watching the day roll by. One Christmas day I was trying to find Rita Jeptoo, and I drove into her town and asked the first street-stander I met, "Where's Rita?" And I got an answer; like a fishermen's wife at the harbor, the villagers know all the goings-on.

My conversation is interrupted as Mr. No Emergency changes tack. "Quick, quick, hurry, we must catch Laban," Godfrey says, while walking toward the Toyota. It is starting to rain gently, which is odd for this time of the year.

Eldoret, whose name is derived from the Maasai word *eldore*, meaning "stony river" became an official town in 1910. It is the fastest-growing town in Kenya, and the property prices are rising, due in large part to the wealth that runners have brought into the district. A textile and farming industry made the place survive before the runners' millions elevated the town's status until it began to be referred to as the district's "Beverly Hills." Today each luxury home and recent business venture appears to have a runner's money as the key driving force. The most successful Eldoret businessperson is Moses Kiptanui, who has an Indian business collaborator. His five-story building in Komora houses not only Moses' own office, but also a large supermarket (Tusker Mattress) on the first two floors and many other small businesses. Kiptanui is taking in 50 percent more revenue in rentals than he projected. Despite his wealth, he has both feet on the ground and has not changed a bit since he first came onto the European circuit in the early nineties: positive, friendly, and full of initiative. When he suggested that we go into partnership with a training camp in Kenya, I did not hesitate a second. Kiptanui's reliability, punctuality, and integrity are hallmarks of his name.

There is a lot of runner business in Eldoret; Yobes Ondieki, together with a partner, opened a small gym in town on the Uganda road, as did Moses Tanui, along with his Grand Prix restaurant and bar. Currently Tanui is installing security cameras over the bar till so he doesn't have to deal with ever-diminishing finances each night. Tanui is also building a row of shops to rent in the complex. A former Tanzanian runner hangs around Tanui's café each day asking for money to return home. Moses just gives him food. "Once an Australian came to me and cried that he could not get home; he begged me to lend him the airfare, so I did, and that was the last I ever heard of him. I won't make that mistake again!" Yet Moses cannot turn a soul away; it is his nature. Pieter Langerhorst and Lornah Kiplagat have a few plots of land where they are now building rentals. The same goes for Sammy Korir and Daniel Komen. Korir has a lot of property to rent in central Eldoret. Many athletes are now building schools, as these are proving to be extremely profitable ventures for those with disposable capital. Cheboiboch, who opened Salaba Academy, hopes that the venture will be his retirement nugget. The main problem with real estate in Eldoret is the 16 percent mortgage rate, but if you have cash, it is a buyers' dream right now.

Then there are the snappy housing estates where the rich athletes have virtual palaces. The two name-dropping hot spots are Elgon View—where Moses Tanui, Said Saaeed, Shaheen, Ondieki, and Joyce Chepchumba, among many others, have places—and Kenmosa Village, a gated community where Ismael Kirui, Patrick Sang, the Keinos, Wilson Kipketer, and Reuben Seroney Kosgei (the Sydney Olympic steeplechase champion) all have houses. On a side road, Tegla Loroupe has a gigantic house, the size of an embassy building. The rooms are huge and luxurious. It is one of her many properties, and Dr. Gabrielle Rosa currently rents the building for the Rosa Association business.

We drive to a small residential area called Kapsoya four kilometers away from the center, on the Kapsoya road that one would take to drive to Uganda. This is where Godfrey's home is. We are here to pick up some contracts, and this area is also a home to the runners Leah Malot, Esther Kiplagat, and Andrew Masai, among others. Masai, who was a founding member of the Fila team and raced extensively on the roads, once came back from a trip to Europe to find half of his possessions missing—it appeared that he had married into the wrong family. Once while running with a guitar strapped to my back, and in the company of the Irish Olympian Noel Berkeley, I stopped at Masai's house as he was about to venture into the masters' racing scene for forty year olds and older, and he was complaining that certain competitors were taking drugs, a claim I dismissed at the time but was later found to be correct. There is no fooling Masai these days.

I eat a small finger banana at Godfrey's house, talking to his three children while he looks for the papers. I try to find them wives and husbands in the small ads in the Kenyan *Daily Nation*, and they look at me like I am crazy and explain that they are way too young. I settle on a woman called Esther for Godfrey's eldest pre-teen. She is looking for a rich husband who has been "saved," and she writes that she has a generous-sized body.

As we drive back out of the estates to the main road there is a disabled beggar sitting on the side of the street, I give him all my small change. He cannot move an inch—clearly he has had a terrible accident—a street boy sits by his side collecting money.

Godfrey shouts out the amount of shillings, as the boy has been known to take a small commission for crossing the street. As we get back on the road, a battered, old, white car flashes its lights and Godfrey pulls over. It is Joseph Chesire, one of Kenya's best 1500m runners in the 1980s. When I ran my personal best at Kakamega track in the KAAA 1500m, I followed—upon the advice of Joseph—his brother Mike who ran within a second of what Joseph predicted he would run. Recently Joseph has had a string of bad luck concerning cars. His driver keeps on crashing them. Joseph, now a coach, and Godfrey are cousins, and as they start to talk business in the Kalenjin tongue, I wander down the road. As I stand on the street, a girl called Lilly comes up and asks me for my phone number, and in her next sentence she says she wants a white husband. I try to think of a polite way to tell her I don't want a 15- or 16-year old bride. (Only in Kenya.) Then Stella Keino, the daughter of Kip, and Kippy, her youngest brother, who is studying in the United States, walk by, and we talk. Stella has a house in Elgon View and each year throws a mean New Year's Eve party.

By the time Godfrey is finally finished talking with Chesire and we get to the gasoline station, Laban has left for the Marakwet district, his home. Understandably, he got bored waiting for us and disappeared. Kiprotich is annoyed that he did not wait for us; he asks the attendants when the gray pickup left the station, but they cannot remember. "I'll get him later!" Godfrey says. The cell phone rings and Cherigat tells Godfrey that he will be available in fifteen minutes. We decide to go to the Wagon Wheel for a coffee and to re-strategize. It is here that we meet Sammy Kipketer, known as "the smiling Kenyan." Whilst Godfrey talks to a local politician in the car park, I sit with Sammy in the restaurant. We are the only guests. The hotel is one of Eldoret's best and it was here that the international peace talks with the Somali warlords took place; it is another popular expat hangout. Not really my kind of place. I prefer Rose's tea shop—a shack on the street where Rose will hand-wash the cup in front of your very eyes with one grubby hand and a bowl of dirty water before pouring you a cup of steaming sweet tea for five bob. You get to sit on the curb as about one thousand black-fuming taxi buses blow billows of carbon monoxide in your face. There is an untouchable grace about taking tea at Rose's on the street in Eldoret.

The café trade in Eldoret is big business; the town has a thriving social scene. At first, the place to go was Sizzler's, a noisy place with pizza and Formica tables. The local athletes loved it and Kip Keino was a popular customer. Then the Klique "downstairs" became "the" place—till it closed and Freddie's Café took over. Freddie's is still very popular; it is on the Barclays Bank Road, but the new Klique, on the Kipchoge Keino Sports Store road, up the street from the old place, became a tad upmarket, and has lost some of its crowd. The Keino store, not a café, sells exercise books and school sports uniforms, not much in the way of a real sports store. Will's Pub on the corner of Sociani Street is the new popular place for the current crop of athletes; for those who do not want to be recognized, there is downstairs seating.

Godfrey taps his fingers on the table as the waitress brings another coffee, in fact a cup of hot water and a small sachet of Nescafé granules. We have now moved to a new café where Cherigat has since promised to appear. Godfrey looks at his watch "One day, and only one athlete—not good!" It's a good job; we aren't being paid by the hour. He tries Cherigat's number again; Cherigat is not picking up. He asks me to dial Cherigat on my phone. "He may be hiding from me," he reasons. At home in New York I don't use a mobile phone, and as I fumble with the numbers a portly gentleman with a familiar face passes the table. It is David Kiptoo, formerly a 1:43 800m runner, who used to be a regular pacemaker in the nineteen-nineties. He stops to talk; funnily enough, we had just been talking about him after bumping into a Canadian woman in the street, Lise Ellyin from Vancouver, who knew David when he was a coach at the Kip Keino training center. Kiptoo told us he now works for the Bishop of Kenya as his assistant. "The only Bishop in the whole of Kenya! Imagine, me, his assistant!" he says laughing and smiling as though disbelieving the fact.

Finally after more talk we give up on Cherigat and walk back to where the car is parked. Lo and behold, there he is waiting by the car.

As the rain is still spotting, Timothy jumps into the backseat and reads the contract. There are a few minor details he wants to talk about, but he signs the papers, making Godfrey happy. Cherigat promises to report to the camp in Iten tomorrow. He jumps out, and we turn the car around to head back to Iten. "You have to have patience to be a manager in Kenya!" Godfrey says, smiling. "And time," I mutter under my breath.

Up ahead, another white Toyota pickup is pulled off to the side of the road, and we see a runner talking to the driver. "Shaheen," says Godfrey with eagle eyes. Sure enough, as we approach, we see that it is the great steeplechaser, so we too pull over. I wind down the window for the greetings. It is good fortune, as Shaheen is talking to Benjamin Kimutai Kosgei, who is helping him with some advice concerning an injury that is bothering him. Kosgei starts up the conversation: "Hey, White Man, I am on my way to see you—remember you said three o'clock? Well, I know you white people are very punctual, so I am coming." I had completely forgotten I had arranged to meet him. I look at my watch; someone in Kenya is on time. No surprise, Kosgei also has a "managerial" request. "I was second at Boston, I want to go back there, yes, I know you are not a manager, but can you fix it?"

The Women Warriors: Kenyan Women Run the Country

"People think African women are subservient, it is not true. I did not meet a subservient woman until I left Kenya."—Professor Jepkorir Rose Chepyator Thomson

The question why Kenyan women have not been as dominant in numbers as the men have been is purely a question of circumstance; it has nothing to do with lesser of athletic ability.

"If you visit a home, and the man of the house is not there, they will say that nobody is home."—Lornah Kiplagat, on the role women play in the Kalenjin district.

It is a fact that there are as many girls running in the primary schools as there are boys. Around the age of sixteen, the equation changes. Arranged marriages are still common in Kenya, and families, eager to sell off their daughters, are quick to negotiate a marriage. Although Nicholas Twolongut did not marry his bride until she was sixteen years old, the respective families had arranged it four years prior to the ceremony.

As soon as the woman becomes married, there typically comes a progression of expectations: that she will bear children, help tend to the crops, cook for the family, and clean the home. That she will collect firewood from the nearby forest, and care for the kids when they arrive, and also for the cattle that roam around the *shamba*. A typical Kenyan woman just cannot fit training into her daily schedule. The Kenyan boy stands a far better chance of being given the rights to proceed from school into an athletics camp. A startling difference is seen in the numbers of postgraduate schoolchildren in Kenya—a junior men's event typically has tripled the number of entrants as its women's equivalent.

Kenyan junior women beat their elders to the post in attaining individual and team gold in the World Cross Country Championships. They have consistently out-medaled the senior team.

"It is hard to find the time for running if you leave school and get stuck with a husband early."—Sally Barsosio.

An escalating set of circumstances dramatically cuts the numbers of women who are able to train at the level to reach an international standard. Gladys Otero, a Kisii who won the Tuskermatt Wareng 6K Junior Cross Country in December 2006, is lucky; she comes from a changing generation. She explains, "We had no money for school fees, but because of sports, the government supported me. My parents realized that sporting was something. So they let me off doing chores at home, so I could train." Mr. and Mrs. Otero were especially happy when Gladys, now 20, used her winnings to add a cow to the family livestock. Not so fortunate was Nancy Chemeli, whose parents were not as supportive. As a 16-year old, barefooted Nancy ran a superlative 53.0 for 400m. She ran this off natural talent. Nancy explained that she could not pursue a career in athletics, as her parents wanted her to remain at home and help with the *shamba*. They did not wish for her to "gamble" with a running career, rather they preferred that she would stay at the farm and help them with the everyday chores. After an appearance at the Eastern Africa athletics championships in Kampala, Uganda, Nancy faded out of the running world.

"Was it hard to go out and train? Of course, yes. Boys teased you; men shouted at you as you passed by, society was not meant for us to be runners. It [society] was not ready at that time. We were doing something wrong and dirty in its eyes. And yes, everyone told you."—Esther Kiplagat

Slowly, expectations of women are changing, the deep-rooted traditions left behind, and Africa as a continent is moving toward a Western way of thinking. For instance, today it is less common to find a polygamous household. A couple of decades ago if a man was not satisfied with one woman, or wished to elevate his social standing, he would take a second or third wife. A 1992 Olympian, David Kibet had four wives, Susan Sirma being one of them. Nowadays, more men are supporting their spouses' endeavors to be bread-winning athletes.

In terms of economics, if a Kenyan woman and man are of similar running ability, it should be the woman who pursues a career in athletics. It is a less competitive field that the woman will have to face. At the 2006 ING New York City Marathon the time differ-ence between first and tenth place was three minutes and 15 seconds for the men, and seven minutes and 40 seconds for the women. These are extremely typical margins for a major city marathon. Women's sports rights campaigner Katherine Switzer agreed: "Oh, yeah, now it is not equal, the men have a much harder time [earning prize money]." It is common sense that, should a choice have to be made, the women should get the first tick-et and the hours to pursue the sport. But in most cases, they do not have an equal chance.

Kenyan coaches, for the most part, tend to be men. As Florence Gitau noted, "I live near the track outside of Iten, and there must be 100 men to three ladies being trained by the coaches, who are all male and volunteers. I ask why, and the coaches tell me, 'These ladies are too complicated; we don't want to handle them. One day they are strong, the next they are weak.' You see, they do not understand things like the menstrual cycle, they just focus on performance. When are we going to educate our coaches?" Peter Mathai admits to this: "You can rely on a man; he is more consistent, and of course then easier to work with."

Katherine Switzer, the first woman to try to officially run the Boston Marathon (she famously had to be defended by a male friend when the race director Jock Semple tried to pull her off the course) was asked if she sympathized with what the Kenyan ladies endured. She replied, "In many ways yes, but I had it easy compared to them. Firstly, male runners encouraged me even if society mocked me. But society did not make it almost impossible for me as the society did for those women. What those women had was sheer guts, determination, and desire. I am not sure I could ever have been so strong. I admire them more than I can say. The women today in particular are changing the social status of women in their country, and the way women are regarded by society. They are helping to eradicate myths, and also addressing the country's poverty issue with the philanthrop-ic drives you see the women of Kenya doing." Switzer herself is an ambassador of the Shoe4Africa foundation.

In 1996, Lydia Cheromei married Hosea Kogo. Cheromei had just run a World Junior and Kenyan national record of 14:53:44 for 5000m. Hosea, albeit a fine athlete, was not on the same level as Lydia. However, Hosea decided that Lydia should concentrate on the family home business and he would attend to the traveling abroad and running affairs. It did not work out, as each time Kogo would return from Europe, sans funds, he would need to send Lydia over to try to make some money. The following season he would revert to his original plan.

There was a distressing twist to the story. With a new boyfriend, Lydia decided to start a family. After taking the silver medal at the World Half-Marathon Championships, she closed the season with her third victory at the Sao Silvestre 15K in Brazil. She stopped running and, purposely, gained weight. In an out–of-competition random drug test, she tested positive for clompiphene, a fertility drug. In February 2006, she gave birth to Faith Chelagat. Again, a lack of information crippled Lydia; firstly, she did not realize that a fertility drug would ever be on the banned list, and secondly, the drug could have been legally administered had she known about it and informed the IAAF. Holding little Faith, Lydia has no regrets, but it is a sad turn in an amazing career.

The Men Take the Opportunities, by Right

If a pair of shoes is given to a family in Kenya, it is the man who will typically take them. So it goes with the traditions. A T-shirt was given to a Kenyan girl a few years ago; it read, "Ignore me, I am suffering from PMS." The following day the husband was wearing the T-shirt. Deep-rooted customs developed, in part, because of the dowry ritual, whereby a man as good as purchases a wife.

Patrick Boiyo, of the Mount Elgon region, explains, "It is about ten cows for a good wife. When I was younger it was less, and often a gift of land. Now land is getting scarce, but cows are still plentiful. Then the woman is yours. She cannot leave, or there will be problems between the two families."

There are many instances of Kenyan women's careers being cut short by unsupportive boyfriends/husbands, and numerous stories of the man spending all the finances, insisting the wife stays home, and then later realizing his folly only when it is too late.

A Kenyan woman does not inherit family lands which would allow her the chance of living from the estate. That is the position of the males in the family. However, with earned wealth, a Kenyan woman can buy lands and establish wealth, and independence, something that is happening in modern-day Kenya with more frequency.

Societal coercing in small villages can be extreme, and in a country where, for a married woman, it is taboo to show bare legs and highly irregular to exercise in public, it is easy to understand why so many Kenyan men do not appreciate their women becoming objects of ridicule. As Twolongut delicately put it, "It is something I don't want my wife to do, but I hope my daughters will have chances. It is not for me to change traditions."

There have, however, been many notable exceptions where the husbands have been more than supportive, often sacrificing their own professional careers. Yet there is a growing number of single mothers' and other women in Kenya unable to find that harmonious situation. Looking at the development of Kenyan women it appears that the trait is "train hard but marry well." Catherine Ndereba, with the support of Anthony Maina, her husband for more than a decade, dispels the notion that marriage and childbirth should impede Kenyan female athletes. Yet a single mother, Helen Chepngeno, blames the opposite sex as being non supportive and disruptive to an athletic career. Both women are world champions, but have two differing perspectives.

Kenyan women with sound and supportive relationships have records of great longevity. Examples are Catherine Ndereba (married to Anthony Maina), Joyce Chepchumba (Aron Kitur), Salina Kosgei (Barnabas Kinyor), Lornah Kiplagat (Pieter Langerhorst), Esther Kiplagat (Solomon Tanui), Helen Kimaiyo-Kipkoskei (Charles Kipkosgei), and Leah Malot (Simon Ruto). The last three women competed at an international level from the mid-eighties up until a couple of years ago! An obvious factor is that these husbands are relaxed, confident men who are obviously not threatened by the successes of their wives.

"A woman's place is not to be running!" yelled a man as Sally Barsosio ran across the Iten Location field a decade ago. I questioned the man, who gave the name Lagat from the Army Rifle temporary barracks, and he explained, "Why, if she is not at home, who will be seeing that the children are moving in the right direction? She will be too much concerned with her own doings. Running is like that, it takes lots of energies. It is a man's game."

The Kenyan Junior Women's Powerhouse: Kapkenda Girls School

The women's equivalent, along with Sing'ore Girls, of famed St. Patrick's Boys High School today is probably Kapkenda Girls. This is largely due to the legacy left by Headmistress Ank De Vlas, who, sadly, passed away in 2001.

The Dutch headmistress of Kapkenda was very motivated and a strict disciplinarian. She adored athletics, especially running. When I visited the school in 1995, unwittingly outside the hours permitted by the school, Ank De Vlas would not allow any special privileges to her star athletes: "No, in school hours I will not take them from a classroom for anything to do with sports." They had to be "A" students in and out of the classroom to stay at Kapkenda.

She voiced her opinion on why the Kenyan Senior women performed on par with the men. "It is society, the Kenyan customs. Of course it will take time, but it will change, it will develop. When Kenyan women get the liberty the men enjoy, then you will see the full development of Kenya's female athletes."

Joanna Vincenti, an American physical education teacher, lived and taught at Kapkenda from 1984 to 1985. Vincenti was recruited by DeVlas, who was very keen on upholding the school's tremendous running tradition. "She was a forceful woman who usually got her way. The school was one of the best in Kenya for running, no doubt, along with Sing'ore Girls, that is," Vicenti says.

Vincenti was speaking of the era when Kenyan schoolgirls were starting to run world-class performances. "It was very different from the U.S., and first of all we had no facilities. I remember standing out at the school gate sending them to run, telling them to remove their flip-flops." Because none of the girls had running shoes, Vincenti made them run barefoot. She also made them remove their skirts. "They had these bloomers, games

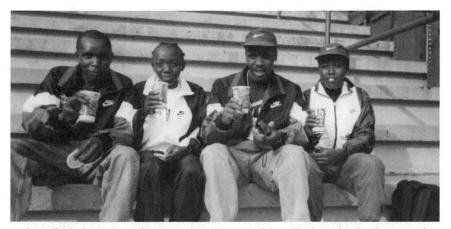

A change for the better: Bernard Barmasai, Rose Cheruiyot, Gideon Chirchir, and Lydia Cheromei—four world-class Kenyans who travel the globe as equals. (*Author*)

kits, but they would always try to run covered up, in a skirt." Kenyan culture still makes young women try to cover up their legs when out training. With the introduction of running tights, very few of the junior women at the renowned running schools now train in skirts.

The training prescribed at Kapkenda was more often than not a 10K run, out and back. "The girls knew the distances," says Vicente. It was not like in the U.S. when we would hide in the bushes. They were well motivated, and they loved to run." She recalled the daily gym classes from 4 to 6 p.m. On other days, they would do 400m repeats on a grass track. Every weekend there would be cross country meets, and Vincenti would drive the athletes round the country. The girls would always qualify from the districts, to the provincials, to the Nationals. "They were great kids, good obedient students; they worked and worked, obviously with a strong drive to succeed," she says. She notes that the athletes, although with standouts like Susan Sirma and Esther Kiplagat ("I loved Esther, she took my cat when I left Kenya"), were very focused on their lessons and learning: "They didn't know what would happen when they left school. There were no guarantees of anything in sports. I mean, then, if you did not get a scholarship, you simply did not get out." Vincenti pauses, as if remembering that distinctive time in her life. "Yes. There was something about them. Something very different. In a way you almost knew they were chosen individuals."

Her lasting impression of the girls of Kapkenda was that, "They were expected to do very well when they joined the athletics team, as the school had a great reputation, and so they did do well. . . surprise, surprise, doesn't that say something."

As early as 1985, Esther Kiplagat, running the 5000m in Nairobi, in 16:35.1, was a national senior champion of Kenya. She won a scholarship to Jackson State University where, amongst other great performances, she ran a meet record in 1990 at the Texas Relays (1500m, 4:15.71) that stands to this day. Thus it was no big surprise, a decade after

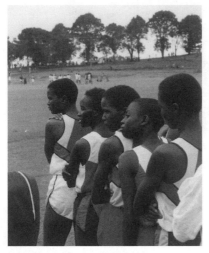

Virtually every girl at Kapkenda has earned her Kenyan national team uniform. (*Author*)

she began running when she ran a PR for the 5000m of 15:07.87 in 1992. What *was* a shock was that a further decade down the road she was setting a personal record (PR) at the Paris Marathon of 2:25:32, finishing third.

"It was not easy, not easy, to be running back in those days. I don't know how I survived!" she half-jokes about her early running career. "At school the support was there, but elsewhere? Forget it. You could be hearing some very negative things when you were trying, trying your hardest to be the best. I always wanted to be a runner, and I suppose that is what gave me the strength to keep on persevering when it was the difficult times." She recalls that she was very motivated by two clear paths: to get a scholarship and to be a famous name like Kipchoge Keino: "At that time there was a song in school that everyone sang about him." Kiplagat remembers that her best Kenyan running moments came whilst training at the Kapkenda school, where she could run with other girls "Then it was okay, in numbers, but training [back at her village] outside was hard, hard I tell you. You cannot imagine that time. Even me now, I don't know."

Leah Malot, an athlete from Chebyemat village who came to Kapkenda, was another example of the school's ability to produce athletes who were able to successfully balance parenthood, athletics, and longevity. When in New York, after pacemaking the city's marathon in 2002, she relaxed at a table in Pasta D'Oro on Seventh Avenue with a glass of wine. Her schoolmate Esther Kiplagat, who had finished third in the race, joined her at the table. Both of the runners, who are mothers (Leah's daughter Sheila Jerop was born in 1995) and are considered "old" by Kenyan measures for running, spoke of their surprise at their lengthy careers. They suggested that perhaps it was due to the work ethic instilled in Kenyan school-children: that you have to work hard in life to get any chances or opportunities, and that if you are not diligent and hard-working as a schoolchild your life will be unproductive and fruitless.

The year before, 2001, Kiplagat and Malot had made nearly $100,000 between them ($52,595 and $41,860, respectively) in prize monies alone, not counting appearance fees. Both admitted that back at Kapkenda Girls' they never dreamed that nearly twenty years after they first started running they would be still earning a veritable king's ransom.

Malot, a middle-distance runner at school who had started running in Chepkero primary Class Six, became known and shot to stardom when, in front of a home crowd, she won the 1987 All-African Games 10,000m Championships in Nairobi in 33:58.15 whilst a student of Kapkenda. It was her debut race at the distance! The same year, she had qualified for the Kenyan Senior cross country team for the World Championships although only 14 years old. In those days, there was no junior competition. Barefooted, in cold weather, she ran to a respectable eightieth position. Nobody could have guessed that in 2005 she would win the highly competitive Discovery Kenya cross country race in Eldoret.

Today, Malot, who works for Kenyan Telekom, has begun yet another comeback finishing in the top eight at a highly competitive cross-country race in Eldoret. Kiplagat has just given birth to her third child.

De Vlas would be proud today. In December 2006, a team from Kapkenda Girls' (Maureen Kipchumba, Eulita Tanui, Sally Kirui, Leonida Mosop and Sharon Kipsang) won a trip to the Nike Team National Championships Open races in Portland, Oregon in an initiative organized by Martin Keino, a former top Kenyan runner who today works in sports marketing. Leonida Mosop, 15, a Form Two student, ran the legs off everyone, the Kapkenda way.

World-Champion Mothers

Edith Chewangel Masai was born on April 4, 1967, in Chepkoya in the Bungoma district. Today a Senior Sergeant in the Kenya Prisons, she is based mainly in Nairobi Prisons housing, but she has a house in Kitale and an apartment in N'gong. She has a fine collection of running PRs: 3000m—8:23.23, 5000m—14:42.64, 5K road—14:50, 10,000m—30:30.26, 10K road—31:13, half marathon—67:16, Marathon—2:27:06. Her honors include: 4K World Cross Country champion 2002–2004; bronze 2001; silver medalist, 2002 Commonwealth Games 5000m; 2006 African Games 10,000m champion.

An abnormality in the sport Masai ran in school back in the 1980s and had success in the 800m and 1500m. Upon leaving secondary school, she signed up for the Prisons in 1990, had a son, Griffin, and promptly disappeared from the running scene except for competing for the Prison's team. Nearly a decade later, she returned to the running stage. Now divorced, she was living on the Prisons compound in a small wooden hut close to a main road on the outskirts of Nairobi. She needed funds, so she asked Jacob Losian, a cousin to Tegla Loroupe, who had been to Europe a few times and was based with Volker Wagner, a German manager, if he could find her a manager. Losian lived in the next row of huts to Masai and knew she was in good form. "She was killing every one in training," he recalls, "I found her one, and she went and did good." Masai points out that she realized nobody was going to help her; she would have to orchestrate her own luck. She trained with determination knowing that now that she had a break, she needed to cultivate the opportunity.

In 2001, Masai had her international breakthrough, placing third in the World Cross Country Championships 4K, an event that she won for the next three years. She was also dominant on the track, running at both Olympic and World Championship level, before she turned to the marathon. In 2005, she won her debut at the Hamburg Marathon, her only problem being a muscle spasm at the 41st kilometer.

The results and achievements Masai has accrued are outstanding, and to do this as a single mother in Kenya is mind-boggling. Masai waves off the compliment in her ever-cheerful manner: "Women in Kenya often need to be married at an early age, or their families are arranging these things—it is often not the best situation. In life you have to do your best and work for everything. Everyone has difficulties." In 2007, Edith Masai, 40, won a silver medal at the All-Africa Championships and set a masters 10,000m world record of 31:31.18 in Algiers. In 2008, Masai, 42, won the Kenyan national 10,000m championship.

A woman who did not fair so well is another World Cross Country Champion, Helen Chepng'eno, an Inspector in Kenya Prisons Service, she now lives in Bomet. In 1994, she became the first Kenyan to win the World Cross Country Championships. It was a tough ride to get to the starting line. In 1993, at the World Road Relays she fell out with officials when they failed to provide food after a plane delay. Money was not forthcoming either in Beijing, and Tegla Loroupe (who was on the team) helped out by buying dry bread.

After winning the race, the women divided prize money equally, annoying the team officials, who had probably hoped to take a cut of the $7,000. Although Helen Kimaiyo was the team captain, Chepng'eno was singled out as a troublemaker. At the Embu World Cross Country Championships training camp, Chepng'eno trained hard and ran well in all the training runs. When the team was named, somehow Helen was not included in the squad, despite her beating nearly all the other women in the trials races. (In fairness to the Kenyan selectors, the team did end up winning the race that year.)

The following year, Helen started training at the Embu camp with Paul Tergat and William Sigei. She already had her own ticket to the World Championships, paid for by her manager, Kim McDonald, as a backup to being left behind. "I was tense, always alone or with the men. I was seething with anger at what had happened the previous year. Even when on the plane I was not talking to anyone for fear of something happening," she says now.

Furious Helen pushed straight from the gun. "I ran like a mad person and won," she says with a steel conviction. Chepng'eno then flew to America for some road races, and ran with success before dislocating her knee in New Orleans. Back in Kenya, McDonald arranged for Helen to fly to the UK for treatment. However, her employers refused to let Helen travel saying she could as well be healed in Kenya. This did not happen. "Women were second class, all the federation was interested in were the men," she says. Nobody helped Helen, the federation was not interested, and the injury remained. Finally, years later, a visiting Canadian doctor who was in the country found Helen: "He came to Kenya to help poor people, and he corrected the knee." With the help of her old teammate Tegla, Helen made a brief return to the athletics world to win some European 10K road races in 2000 and 2001, albeit years past what should have been her halcyon era.

Chepng'eno harbors acrimony today against the officials of the federation: "Yes, I am bitter with officials. I was the first women to win a World Cross Country title, yet I am completely left out. Can't they appreciate and involve me even with the World Cross Country Championships coming to Kenya for the first time? I sacrificed a lot for this country, but nobody wants to acknowledge me. Only a certificate and a plaque were given to me last year. I am so angry with them that I don't step in any stadium to watch athletes. In fact, I switch off my television whenever athletics competitions pop on the screen."

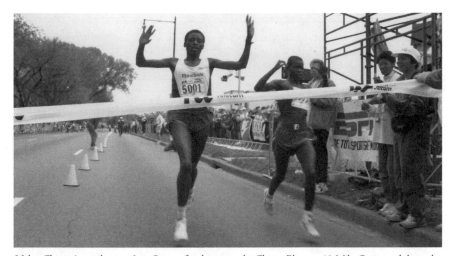

Helen Chepng'eno edges out Jane Omoro for the win at the Cherry Blossom 10-Mile. One month later, she was crowned World Cross Country Champion. (*Bob Burgess*)

As a single mother of two sons (15 and six years old), Chepng'eno has a good perspective on a female athletes and motherhood. "Men, in life, are the real problem for us. When we win races and earn some money, then men want to sweet-talk us to cheat us out of our hard-earned money. They promise marriage and everything, but with their eyes just on our earnings. When you get married, another problem emerges—control. They want children, and we can't say no. The big conflict between career and family can't make an athlete continue. He is your husband, he wants a child, and he wants to bring up a family. You can't say no. This has caused many problems for us women athletes."

Finally, to the story of Jackline Bonareri Maranga. In 1992, she took second place at the World Juniors 1500m, a position she took again two years later in the 800m. Two more years later, she again took silver in the World Juniors 1500 meters. In 1998, she won both the Commonwealth Games and the African Championships at 1500 meters. The following year, she won the World 4K Cross Country Championships. In 2002, she won the African Championships 1500m before leaving athletics to mother her first of two daughters, Sheila. In 2005, she had her second child, Eugenia. Jackline, a Kisii tribeswoman, is married to World Championship 5000m bronze medalist Tom Nyariki.

It is a tight-knit family that has had its fair share of traumas (the diminutive Maranga was attacked at gunpoint and robbed of her car in 1998 in Nakuru near her home in a church compound, and Tom lost an eye when escaping car-jackers in Nairobi). "I am lucky because I am married to Tom and he is understanding," says Maranga. Tom wishes for Jackline to return to professional running: "It is only that after the childbirth of our second born Jackline was suffering from some back pains. As soon as they are fixed she will make a comeback." When asked why more Kenyan men were not supportive of their wives participating in sports, Tom cites tradition: "It is not in the culture, but we are changing and improving. I mean, why not? I will help, and support her, all I can. You know my career is nearly over. Maybe she can take over now; she is still young." For those women married to non-athletes, Maranga has one piece of advice: "Just retire. You will never make it with a non-understanding man."

The Forerunners

Tecla Chemabwai Sang, from the Mosombor village in the Nandi Hills, Rift Valley, is a friend and advisor to most of the women who are involved in competitive running today around the Rift Valley, first as a woman who had experienced the pains of being a pioneer in a male-oriented society, then also as a commissioned chaperone and a coach for the athletics federation of Kenya. She had began running at the Chepkunyuk ("handle of a sword") Primary School, starting a career that would see her win the first-ever Gold for a Kenyan woman at a championship event.

The training for Tecla was running to school. "The language of training came later on. In games I did everything, the 100m, the 200m, the jumps, the whatevers!" She was great-ly encouraged by her teachers, who saw her talent, but not by her parents who feared that troubles might affect her at this young age; competitions often meant traveling a day before the event, and Tecla was very young. She would leave home at 5:00 a.m. to reach school on time, "I remember once I woke and thought I had overslept, so I set off to school, running very fast as it was dark and the route took me through the bush. On arriv-ing at school, I realized instead I was way too early, it was around midnight. So I climbed under my desk and went to sleep." Athletics was an exciting game to Tecla, and the actu-al trip to the Olympics in 1968 was more enthralling than the actual competition, "All I thought about was the airplane ride! The thrill of going to Mexico was far greater than anything to do with running. I did not even know what the Olympics were. It was later I developed an attitude of winning, at this time I was running for fun."

Tecla was at Kapsabet High School with two other girls who would travel to Mexico, Elisabeth Chesire and Lydia Stephens-Okech. She looks back on school competitions with fondness: "I was winning a lot, and I remember there were quite a few girls compet-ing in those early days. I did not know I was an athlete; that is what helped me [against preconceived notions that women could not run] in Kenya." She was spurred on by the incentives offered as prizes "We got useful lasting things like cooking pots and knives. These things meant a great deal to a family who did not have much, so I was really encouraged."

In 1971, she gave birth to her first child. At the 1972 Olympics she ran the 400m in 53.38 to advance to the second round, but then she was eliminated. Five years later, she took the gold at the Commonwealth Games, this time running the 800m. She was mar-ried to Julius Sang, who was a member of the victorious 400m relay team at the Munich Olympics, until he passed away in April 2004 in Eldoret. Tecla credits the lifetime full support of Julius as the force behind her success: "Julius was my neighbor, we were influ-enced by the USA lifestyle, and he also was a coach for me at one time."

Tecla took a track scholarship to the States in 1980 after missing both the 1976 and 1980 Olympics through boycotts when in her prime shape. "It was in America that I learned about coaching."

Tecla has done a lot of soul-searching about why Kenyan women were not perform-ing as well as the men, and she concluded that the focal reason was that Kenyan women have such a hard domestic workload that allocating time for athletics was simply not pos-sible: "Even as children, the boys go out and play, have fun, but the girls are doing house-hold chores." She explains that after marriage things do not get better. "Most men are jeal-ous and don't like the women to be more successful than them, they feel they have no con-trol. The culture of the dowry has to change. The way athletes succeed today is only when their husbands allow them to train." She cites the classic case of Cherono, who married the steeplechaser Amos Biwott. "She was a very talented lady who could have done many great things, but he insisted she stop.

Promoting change, Tecla has become involved in Shoe4Africa, where she will use her influence to try to keep young women from getting married before leaving school, and from leaving school for a running career. "A lot in running has changed. The running mode is now financial. It has of course helped, but it has exploited, too." Tecla grew up racing for Kenya as an honor, but she sees today's athletes trying to race often for dollars. She notes that these days the turnover of athletes is very fast: "The body is not iron. We don't have spare parts, you have to be careful."

Three Kenyan women competed at the 1968 Mexico City Olympics. The defending East and Central African Championships 800m champion, Elizabeth Chesire, placed sixth, and last in Heat One of the 800m in 2:10.9. Lydia Stephens-Okech, the eldest of the three and the only one to have graduated high school, ran the 100m but did not score, and Tecla Chemabwai finished fifth in the third heat of the 400m in 54.0. The victory was that Kenyan women were running at an Olympic Games at all.

Professor Jepkorir Rose Chepyator Thomson, of Kapkon'ga village, was born in 1954 at a time when there were few female Kenyans runners, to say the least. The small village sits three miles west of Sing'ore, and as a schoolgirl Thomson ran 12 miles a day—to and from the school in the morning, at lunch, and in the afternoon. The eldest of eleven, she had her hands full with chores ranging from cattle tending, to water fetching, to farming. She began running at Kapkon'ga primary, "Really because of the influence of the enthusi-astic teachers, maybe because of the influence of the Catholic schools." At school one day, when attending Sing'ore, the whole class, as punishment for not understanding an assign-ment, had to run a three-mile race. Whilst flying along the Kapsowar road, Rose found her talent: she won. The teacher, Steve Murilla, specialized in geography. He started a running program in the school. "Yes, you can say he was my first coach," says Rose, who went from those humble beginning to being one of the top 1500/3000m runners in Africa.

Role models were scarce. When pushed, Rose remembers only one female athlete that she had heard of at this time, "It was a Marakwet, from Chepkoria—she was a shot-put-ter called Lillian Jerotich. Then much later I remember in 1972 I did meet Tecla Chemabwai; she was encouraging. However, she was a 400m runner. We were pioneers at that time."

Thomson recalls the early training, "We ran on the [dirt] road, or in this field that was 400m from the Sing'ore School on the road to Iten. It is not there now, it is a cornfield. We would run three laps, or a fast 200m then you run and then again. Mainly I remember running on the road. We would run 30 minutes out and then back, with pickups. The emphasis was always on 'run hard' from our teachers."

The following year, Thomson was representing the Rift Valley at the middle-distance events. She received little support from her peers, yet she persevered, believing that what she was doing was right, making a statement by running. In 1974, she made another bold statement by marrying a Caucasian American, Norman Thomson, who was in Africa as a Peace Corps volunteer. In the next couple of years, she and Norman started a family. After the births of Patrick and Kip she started training again, an unprecedented move by a married Kenyan woman at the time. Thomson resumed competing. "I was running the Brooke Bond [a tea company] Kenya three A's meetings against primary school girls. It was really tough, absolutely brutal, because there was no support. People were asking, 'Why are you taking the prizes from the girls? You should be home with your children!'"

The criticism was because of the role that women were supposed to play in the 1970s. "There was a division of duties, and the woman's role was to look after the children, which is a very powerful position. I was proving that you could do both—be a successful mother and have a running career."

Thomson's ambition was never to run for fitness or health. "I was trying to be a good performer and get a scholarship. I had heard about Philip Ndoo, who used to write about me in the *Daily Nation*. He had gone to America for a scholarship in New Mexico. I wanted to see, if guys can go, then maybe. . ." she trails off.

The couple decided to move to the States, where Rose did get a scholarship and became a twelve-time All-American at the University of Wisconsin from 1979 to 1983. Rose set Kenyan and African records during this period, and she would have been at the Moscow Olympics had it not been for the boycott.

America was not smooth sailing for Rose. "It was tough. Because I was older, I now got criticized not for running after marriage and childbirth as in Kenya, but for beating younger girls, 19-year-olds. Again, absolutely brutal, but you have to survive or else go home and take care of the goats!"

Today, with another edition to the family, 12-year old Kipruto, she is a professor at the University of Georgia. "I was the first Kalenjin to get a PhD, imagine. I did it; I was a successful mother, a scholar and a good runner. I proved it possible. I do not think the [female] runners in Kenya realize what it was like for me. They take it for granted [Kenyan society accepting post-marital mothers as runners], like the civil rights here in the States."

The Kenyan women who were running in the 1960s and 1970s were fearless. It is hard to imagine the social pressures, abuse, and lack of support they received. One can only reflect that today, half a century later, with economic change, multimedia, and increasing education, many Kenyan women continue to struggle against their male-oriented society. In 2001, Christina Chepkon'ga, Ruth Chebii, Jane Kiptoo, and Florence Komen sat on the short grass at Kamariny braiding one another's hair. They were between 18 and 22 years old, fast runners capable of earning scholarships or prize money in virtually any road race worldwide. None of them felt comfortable training unless in the company of the other's, and none would consider running through a village center, unless at home in Iten (and then only as a group).

Other notable names from that era, names that few of today's heroes can recall:

After Diana Monk's silver medal in the 1965 All-Africa Games 80m hurdles, Sabina Chebici became the second Kenyan-born woman to win a medal at an international competition, when she placed third at the Commonwealth Games 800m (2:02.61) in 1974. She also placed fifth in the 1500m (4:18.56) and was a member of the 4 x 400m relay team at those Championships. Soon after that, the teenaged Chebici retired from athletics to start a family. According to friends, her husband asked her to stop running and become a homemaker. "This is a typical story where some tribes pressure you to be married with children by a certain age. You could not be seen running," says Chemabwai.

Mary Chemweno was the first prolific medal winner for Kenya; in 1977 she took the East African Championships 800m (2:06.5), and two years later she retained her title. Another two years down the road she won the 400 meter at the same Games, clocking 54.3, and the 800m (2:06.5). At the 1980 Commonwealth Games, she placed second in the 800 meters, clocking a Kenyan-record 1:59.94, and won the 1500m in 4:08.76. And in 1987, running in front of a partisan crowd, Mary took the 800m bronze (2:04.34) at the All-Africa Games in Nairobi.

Today, with five children, Chemweno lives on a large farm outside Iten. She has always been affiliated with the Prisons team, and today she continues to coach a team from the Prisons. Chemweno emphatically states that she was helped by a savvy marriage. "I took a man who was not from the usual thinking of a Kenyan man at that time. He was the reason I was able to continue running."

She wed Nandi veteran Kipsubai Kosgei, who won gold in the 10,000m and bronze in the 5000m at the 1984 African Championships, then silver in the 10,000m the following year. Age 42, Kosgei took the bronze in the 1988 World Cross Country Championships in a year when the Kenyan team had one of its podium clean sweeps. Simply put, Kosgei was a Kenyan legend. Sadly, Kosgei, who was competing well up until the age of 46, died of malaria a few years ago in his fifties. He began running in 1962 and had a worldly attitude. Kenyan Wilson Musto remembered him as a father figure to all overseas Kenyans, "He was fast for a mzee [old man], and whenever we did intervals he would be leading them." Kosgei had run 3:38 for the 1500m in Mombassa, albeit in 1977, yet he kept his speed, like his enlightened views, into the 1990's.

Salina Chirchir from the village of Iten ran at the 1984 Los Angeles Olympics in the 800m heats. In 1986 she won the World Junior 800m, and whilst a schoolgirl at Sing'ore she won a 800m/1500 double at the 1987 All-Africa Games in Nairobi. In the same year, she ran her 800m PR, 2:02.90, at the heats of the World Championships. A decade later, after turning to the marathon, she ran a 2:32:35 at Houston that qualified her to represent Kenya at the 1996 Summer Olympic Games. Living in Albuquerque during the nineties, she had little desire to return to her native Kenya, despite owning prime land near the Kamariny Stadium. She says, "When you are an athlete, you cannot be a mother at the same time, unless you have a very understanding man. When I go home people

do not understand: they say to me, 'Are you barren, is there something wrong with you?'"
Today, after running a slew of minor marathons and winning most of them, Chirchir lives
in Mexico and no longer runs.

Rose Tata-Muya, from the village of Kapteren, twelve kilometers from Iten, has the
honor of being the first Kenyan woman to represent Kenya at the IAAF World Track
And Field Championships. She is also the youngest athlete to compete at the
Commonwealth Games.

In 1983, at the inaugural World Championships, she ran a heat of the 400m hurdles.
The same year, at the All-Africa Games, she won the gold in that event. At the African
Games in 1979, running the 800m she took silver in 2:10.9, about nine seconds slower
than her PR of 2:01.32. Her best for the 400m hurdles, 55.6, set in 1988, remains a
national record to this day. She was awarded the Order of the Golden Heart of Kenya for
her services to the country. Today she lives for six months of each year in the north of
England. "I have a foundation called the Kenya Sports Development Organization. We
deal with youths, orphans, vulnerable street children, and women groups." and Rose is
trying to develop a piece of land given to her near Iten to build a sports ground. She is
also an ambassador for the Shoe4Africa foundation.

Rose began running in school in the physical education classes, where she surprised
her teachers by giving the boys a run for their money. Rose cited a lack of funds, poor
facilities, and problems arranging to travel to competitions as some of the struggles that
she faced in her early career. She added, "My school was extremely supportive, and my
friends, but lastly were my family; they thought that I might be exploited by not finishing my education, or get married, or in a relationship under age."

At the age of just thirteen Rose finished eighth in the finals of the 1974
Commonwealth Games 800m (2:13.26) and was a member of Kenya's 4 x 400m squad,
which finished in the same position. Her international career would continue until 1996,
when she became an athletics coach. "Women really supported each other because the
participation in sports was so low," she says. "Nowadays, with Kenyan women being recognized as being the best in the world, it is different." In 2007, at the age of 47, Rose
decided to make a comeback to compete at the World Masters' Games. Taking an uncon-
ventional path, she planned to "put up at Kasarani for two months" and train for the 400m
hurdles. This meant leaving her job in Manchester, renting a room near a running stadium in Nairobi, and training the Kenyan way.

Susan Sirma, of the Keiyo tribe, a distant cousin to Lornah Kiplagat, was the first
Kenyan woman to take a medal at the IAAF Track and Field World Championships. The
year was 1991 and Sirma took a bronze in the 3000m in Tokyo, recording 8:39.41. The
same year at the All-Africa Games in Cairo, she won the 1500m in a championship
record of 4:10.68, improving on the silver she had won in 1987, and successfully defended her 3000m title from 1987 in another championship record of 8:49.33. 1991 was
Sirma's stellar year: She set PRs at 1500m (4:04.94), 3000m at Tokyo, and 5000m,
15:03.52)—superb times, even by today's standards. Her 12K road best of 38:27, set
when winning in San Francisco in 1991, is still the second-fastest time ever recorded at

the distance and only four seconds slower than Kenya's Dellilah Asiago's world best of 38:23. She was also the inaugural IAAF World Cross Country series winner for the 1990-1991 season. Today Susan is an ambassador for the Shoe4Africa foundation.

Professor, author and authoritarian Gina Oboler was the primary investigator in a Kenyan study of women's roles and status, and socio-economic change, in the running-rich Nandi district, of Kenya in the 1970s. Now based in London, she gives a great insight to the life and role of Kenyan women during that era, fully why the Kenyan running explosion was principally a masculine phenomenon.

Oboler was based in Kaptel, North Nandi; she noted that the key roles of women were childbearing, child-rearing, and domestic labor. Furthermore, the women helped

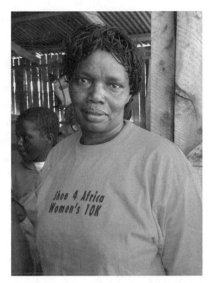

Susan Sirma, Kenya's first medalist at the IAAF World Track and Field Championships. (*Author*)

with the agricultural chores. "It is very common, across the world, for new opportunities of all kinds to become available to men first, and only later spread to women," she says.

Oboler says she never saw any woman out running. "In a word, no—unless to get out of the rain." She observed that the main career focus of the time was to earn be qualified to a salary: "What people wanted [more than sports] was to get credentials and qualifications that they believed would lead to good salaried employment. It gradually became clear to some that another avenue of opportunity was to go to a college in the U.S. on a track scholarship. At that time, there were interscholastic track and field competitions that involved both boys and girls, but it seems to me they were seen as recreational. Those who were very good at this began to realize that it could open other doors. Higher education was seen as mainly for males, which is not to say that a girl who did extremely well in school could not also be encouraged in that direction. However, higher-level professions were also seen as primarily for males, and most people saw giftedness in running primarily as a means to the end of higher education, and that avenue was seen as mostly for males.

"Running at this point in time was clearly symbolically associated with men of the warrior age-grade. At women's initiation, girls wear garb that symbolically mimics the male role that they are repudiating any claim to. In the old days, they wore bells and colubus monkey-fur leg ornaments of the kind worn by warriors. In the 1970s, their outfits included a men's white shirt with a tie, knee socks, and 'track' shoes. The kind of shoes desired were described to me (in English) as 'track' shoes, or something that could pass for them. This is clearly a statement that track shoes are men's shoes. Is it too much of a stretch to say this is an encoding of 'track' as a male activity?"

Oboler's suggestion backs up the views of most of the Kenyan pioneers from the 1960s, that men ran, women stayed home. With a very few exceptions.

Pamela Jelimo Captures Kenya's First Women's Olympic Gold

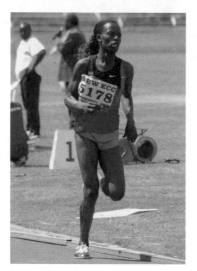

Pamela Jelimo clocks a 2:01:02 in the 800m on April 19, 2008, to qualify for the the African Championships. (*Jeroen Deen*)

In 1989, in the village of Kiptamok, Koyo district, Pamela was born to a single mother Rodah Jeptoo Keter. Rodah had been an athlete when younger competing in the 100/200m and placing fourth in the latter event at the provincial level in Nakuru town. Living in poverty Rodah prayed that one of her nine children (Pamela is the third born) would "do something special in life" and help a family that struggled from day to day for the bare necessities like food. "We had to help Rodah, the local schools accepted her children as she never had any funds for school fees," explained a teacher from Koyo Secondary. "I cannot tell you how hard I prayed for successes, and how many times I have prayed for Pamela to do something at running," said Rodah.

Rodah's dream came true. On August 18, 2008 Pamela made history by being the first woman from Kenya to win an Olympic gold medal— forty years after Naftali Temu took Kenya's very first Olympic medal in the 10,000m back at the 1968 Mexico Olympics.

High up in the Nandi Hills in a small wooden two-roomed house with an ill-fitting corrugated iron roof and newspaper pages of Pamela glued to act as wall paper, Rodah and a roomful of well wishers roared their approval while watching on a small battery-powered black & white TV, the Nandi goddess stride unchallenged to a new Women's 800m Olympic record of 1:54:87.

Pamela Jelimo, who graduated from the police academy on 24 March 2008, had been coached by Elijah Langat since 2005 and he takes up the story, "She started running without success in 2003 and was running distance races. Her mother came to me in the marketplace asking for a kit and some shoes for Pamela so she could train. A school in Canada was offering some kits, but only for form two and younger students; you see Pamela was in form three," he remembers drawing her name into three distinct syllables, Pam- Eh- La. "I lied for her so she could get the equipment." he smiles.

Langat had a small group of athletes and they competed in the school races, "I put her in long races, but she always struggled. Then one day at a cross country race I was waiting for all my runners to finish and I saw her, as usual, at the back running in, but then when she was about 400m away from the finish line she began to sprint, and how she

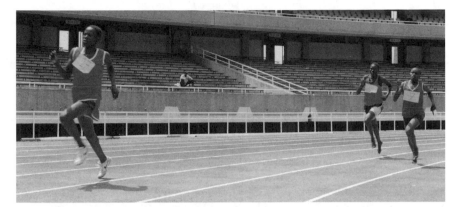

The first-known running photo of Pamela Jelimo, then 14, as she sprints to victory, in what has become her signature style. (*Author*)

moved! I saw her talent—she was a true sprinter, what power! I entered her in some 100m and 200m races, and from then on she ran, how she ran!"

In that summer she won both the 400m flat and 400m hurdles national junior championships. "She ran a 24-second 200m that was exceptional for Kenya," recalls the 60-year old Langat.

In 2007 she won the 400m African junior championships, and in April 2008 she ran her first 800m in a trials meet for the African Championships. A renowned coach for the Kenyan team takes up the story, "We saw the result and presumed that the clock was wrong, but as she won the race we sent her anyway, not expecting anything special. Then nobody was interested in her."

She made her senior national team debut in Addis Ababa, Ethiopia, where at 2800m altitude, on an old worn out tartan track she won a gold medal and set an African Championships record of 1:58:70 beating the legendary Maria 'Maputo Express' Mutola en route! Returning to Kenya she was approached by a new coach and a manager, and rising public interest. Soon, her international life would explode into the biggest middle distance running talent seen this decade, male or female.

At her first race in Europe at Hengelo, Holland, she ran 1:55:76, setting a new junior world record. Going into the 2008 Olympics, with an improved 1:54:97 African record, she was the favorite. She did not disappoint, running a commanding powerful second lap to destroy the field, and leave the reigning world champion, Janeth Jepkosgei, trailing for a silver medal, albeit for Jepkosgei in a personal best time. The two train in Kapsabet town, but with different coaches. Wilfred Bungei who won the men's 800, also comes from the small town, thus Kapsabet, with a population of 64,000, claimed three Olympic medals in one discipline in Beijing!

A sweet ending came to Jelimo's first, and undefeated, international season when she won the IAAF's one million dollar jackpot in Brussels on September 5, 2008, the first teenager to win the series. With less than 12-minutes of performance Jelimo had made her mother's wildest dreams come true.

Langat, a Kipsigei's tribesman who once ran 10.6 seconds for the 100m explains the training that took Jelimo to 800m success, "Never were my intervals longer than 600m for her. I trained her to have speed, for me the 800m is a sprint event and speed is what is needed. Sundays was the hard day of intervals that we would do at Kipletito primary school (a grass track). More than often 4 x 400m, with 2-minutes rest, then a ten minutes rest, then 4 x 200m, with 2-minutes rest, then ten minutes again before 3 x 100m. All very fast. This from October till June. Wednesday would be a tempo run of 40-minutes, but most other days would be steady runs of between 40-60 minutes. Always with 20-30 minutes of strength/flexibility exercises. The area is full of hills so she built very good strength from her daily routine."

Andrea Kipterer Koros, Pamela's grandfather was a runner. In 1964 he placed third in a three-mile trials race at Marsabit behind Kip Keino, and Kipsoi Sigira, but was not selected for the Olympics, thus retired from the sport in 1965. As his granddaughter broke the tape the smile on his face wiped away 44-years of Olympic musings, a star was born, a star of his own blood.

The Stars and Stripes of Kenyan Running

What is a road race without a Kenyan runner? A general answer would be, one without prestige or prize money.

America can claim to having laid huge foundation stones in the development of Kenyan running. The opportunity America offers, with schools, scholarships, and prize money for road racing, makes it the go-to place on the globe for Kenyans. Talking to the young athletes at an Athletics Kenya cross country race in Kericho, I found that there was just one place everyone wished to go: America.

America was the first country to offer large amounts of prize money at road races, and given the fact that a moderately successful season could provide a lifetime's security in Kenya, the runners gravitated toward the United States. It made a logical case; English is the national language of Kenya, and with England offering neither prize money to match America's, nor sports scholarships, as the States did, and it was a natural progression.

Kenyans have long been blamed for a relatively poor championship record in marathon running—"only five" Olympic marathon medals since 1988 in no way mirrors the success Kenyans have in the money-making non-championship marathons. Economics has played a huge role in this medal count. The German marathoner Uta Pippig's sponsorship money was probably ten times that of Catherine Ndereba. African runners do not generate large amounts of sponsorship money, outside shoe contracts. Domestically Paul Tergat has recently become an advertising option for Kenyan companies, but prior to Paul it would have been unheard of to see, for example, John Ngugi endorsing a cell-phone company. Thus with the ING New York City, The LaSalle Chicago, and the Boston marathons, America has always been the place for the opportunity to make one's fortune and fame. In 1996, Moses Tanui's main goal was to win the centennial Boston Marathon, not the centennial Olympic marathon in Atlanta. It is a reality that the overwhelming majority of Kenyans, because of their financial state of affairs, run for money over medals.

The economic implications of America's involvement cannot be underplayed. When Paul Bitok made the Kenyan cross country team for Boston in 1992, before the ticket was taken from him for lacking international experience, after years of scraping by living on a base army salary, his village did not celebrate the fact that Bitok would now be wearing the national colors of Kenya. Instead, they rejoiced at his good fortune of being able to race on the American circuit and make dollars.

To get an American scholarship, or a visa to go to America and race, has not been easy at any period of Kenyan running history, as is the case for any immigrant. One of the first to get a scholarship and race successfully was Joseph Nzau in the 1970s. Unlike Philip Ndoo (who, sadly, passed away at age 58 in 2005), or Mike Boit, two Kenyans who had gone to New Mexico, Nzau stepped from school onto the American road racing stage, and he made his living that way for well over a decade thereafter.

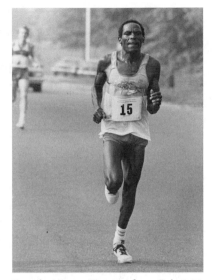

Joseph Nzau, Kenya's first Sub-2:10 marathon runner and a prolific road racer, here at New Haven road race. (*Leo Kulinski, Jr.*)

Joseph Nzau, The USA scholarship with the Kenyan mind.

Joseph Nzau, from Nguluni, of the Kamba tribe, was a standout at the University of Wyoming, where he won the Most Valuable Track award in each of the four years he attended the college. Following graduation, with an engineering degree, he became the first Kenyan to win a major city marathon when he out-leaned Hugh Jones of Britain by a half-second to take first place in Chicago in 2:09.44.3. (Recalled Jones, "That was a very expensive half-second of my life").

The following summer, in Los Angeles, Nzau would finish seventh in the Olympic marathon and tenth in the 10,000m. He has been a mentor to many Kenyans, one of whom who was Cosmas Ndeti, whose grandmother is Joseph's aunt.

Joe started racing in high school, in 1970. He says that in those days athletes did not train, but merely turned up at a race and performed. "There were very few people running, it was not a highly recommended thing, like it is today. Now they [Kenyans] see people making a good living from it, so it has become popular. No, people did not train. Also we thought running was bad because you would die, we knew the story of Pheidippides and how he died after running."

Nzau turned up at the Tala High School for his first race, and, in his words, "Just like that I jumped in and 'go,' and I won the race." He did not get support from anyone at this time; even his parents were not interested in watching him compete. It was on a whim that he entered his first marathon, in April, 1972. "The principal of the school was running, it was in Nairobi and he wanted a water carrier. So I volunteered." Joseph decided to run until he got to the water stations and then stop to help his friend. He was given a pair of field-hockey boots for footwear. "After some miles I met a friend who asked why I was so far behind in the field, this was not usual as I was winning everything in Kenya now. I told him my job and he said, 'No, go, I will do it. You run.' So Joe did, and although there were not enough miles left for him to make any impression on the leaders, he finished feeling fresh in ninth place with a time of 2:56. The next try was at Kahawa Army station, again in the capital. After finishing fourth, Joseph made a vow: "I swore next time we meet no one will see me not win." True to his word, and with an increase in training, in October of 1973 Joe won the Mombasa Marathon. "I cleaned everyone by two minutes, my friend, and I was only a high school kid," he says now.

Joseph was dominating the Kenyan distance-running scene, yet he could not get a break to leave the country. "The man they selected for the Commonwealth Games 1974, I was cleaning him by two minutes when we met!" he recalls. He had now begun marathon training, running fourteen miles after school each day. Each time he was invited to a race, as his name was seen by meet promoters around the world in the newspapers, the ticket would be retracted at the eleventh hour, "I was told, 'You are a student, and you don't have experience.' And they would send people who never beat me." Following graduation, Nzau joined the Prisons team in the hopes of receiving support, but it was not to be. A trip to San Blas for the Half–Marathon in Puerto Rico arrived for Nzau in 1976, but someone else managed to procure the ticket. Close to quitting, Nzau went to see the Commissioner of the Prisons to complain. Unbeknowned to Joseph she was a close neighbor, and he agreed to stay for a year while she looked into the case. "I got morality and pushed hard in training," he says. The results paid off, as Nzau "cleaned them" in the National Cross Country Championships. He then went to the track and lapped the entire field to win there, too, but again, when an overseas chance arose, he was left at home: "I was supposed to be taken to the African Championships that year. But the head of the federation said to me, 'I have not seen your running.' How was it possible when I was winning the Nationals?"

Frustrated at being the "forgotten man" Nzau decided to take one of the scholarships that were offered to him. He turned down Washington State and El Paso and accepted a ride to Wyoming, as he was very impressed with the outlook of the coach. "When I arrived, the coach, Ron Richardson, was like a father to me. There was a lot of cramming for schoolwork, and I didn't know how I would find time to train, but the coach said to me, 'Your education is what is important, Joe, this is a time in your life when that comes first. While you are Wyoming if you run and score points for us that is great, but first and foremost, I want you to get a good education.'" At this time Nzau was the best distance runner in Kenya. He was the first Kenyan to run a sub 2:15 marathon on home soil and was undefeated at the marathon distance since making his vow to be such in the fall of 1972. "There were other Kenyans in America at the time who took a different route, putting running first, but I decided to study," he says.

Nevertheless, despite experiencing cold weather for the first time and running in well-below-freezing conditions, Nzau, a six-time All-American, was the school's best runner for every year he attended the university. Adapting to the climate and conditions, from baking hot Kenya to Wyoming, was not as dire as one could imagine: "I didn't know cold, a professor looked at me in a T-shirt and brought me a big jacket. I remember I did not like it wearing it for the first time, I felt like my hands were hanging somewhere, like they were not attached to my body. As the cold did not exist in my mind, it did not bother me." Joseph reverted to wearing the heavy sweatshirts the track team had given him.

It was a true learning experience. "I came to know intervals, hill climbing, and how to train instead of just going out to run miles. These things I had never done in Kenya, never." Nzau's career came during the period of the Kenyan Olympic boycotts, but he harbors no bitterness. "I am a Christian, and if it had been God's will for me to have been there, then I would have been. Don't blame the situation; things are always how they are meant to be."

In many ways Joe's achievements could be overlooked if one didn't know how he tenaciously struggled for that initial first break, how he raced at a world-class level whilst finding the schooling demanding. "When I became the first Kenyan to run a sub-2:10, I was at a school studying hard," he says. Thirteen days later he ran at Tulsa and won a big race there, running 43:55 for 9.3 miles. "People asked, 'How can you do this? You are not even spending time training properly.' You must remember sub 2:10 was not common in those days, 35 years ago, and for a student who was busy with his studies. Well I told them—and this has been the help for my life—you have to have faith, to know that you can do what you want to do." Belief in himself, and faith in his religion was behind Joseph's success.

Dr. Tim Maggs and the First USA/Kenyan Running Camp

At the Boulder 10K, a major race in Colorado, Tim got into a conversation with Joseph Nzau, who was suffering from a back ailment. As Nzau was going to the Boilermaker race in Utica, in Maggs' home state of New York, he invited the Kenyan to come and stay for treatment.

Within a year, Dr. Maggs had 17 runners living with him. Maggs makes some very interesting observations about the Kenyan runners.

"They have such a different psyche. I remember when we drove back from Cherry Blossom [a ten-mile race in Washington, D.C.] in 1994 when William Sigei broke the world's best, well, Josephat Machuka and Thomas Osano had also run under that world's best for 10 miles. You know how 'we' are, talking for hours about a race? Not them, they were silent. They did not say a thing about the race!

It appears it is a lower level of consciousness, but the irony is it is an internal, not external stimulus—a higher level. People talk about going to live with the Kenyans to adopt their secrets, but how can you? We had a runner called Phillip; his job on the farm was to keep the lions away with a spear. What a major change of culture! You know how kids are today; if they do not have the latest Playstation, they are all bored. I remember coming down to the living room and twelve of the runners were huddled round a torn-up shoebox they had made into a checkers game.

To run like a Kenyan, you have to reduce the level of stimulation and spend more time on the things that are needed to be done. We are overindulged here in America. The way this society is set up, you will never get the droves like Kenya, you may get one or two, but we'll never compete unless there is a dramatic culture change.

Everyone did the actual training, together as a group. They were very structured and organized. They socialized well together. Ran, rested, read the Bible, ran, all helped with the cooking. Spending a lot of time together, doing stuff together, so different from what we are used to. Yes, and they did train hard. I remember going out on the bike when they'd do 25-mile runs at six-minute mile pace. I would be in awe!"

Washington State University at Kenya

John Ng'eno, who was the USATF cross country champion in 1974, was the first successful Kenyan in the NCAA's Division I. He had an outstanding record for Washington State University, winning the following seven titles: Indoor 3-mile, 1974-1976; outdoor 5000m, 1975; outdoor 10,000m 1974-1976.

Other titles won by Kenyans for Washington State: Outdoor 5000m 1975-1976 Joshua Kimeto and 1984, Julius Korir; Steeplechase 1976-1977, James Munyala; 1978-1979, Henry Rono; 1982, Richard Tuwei, and 1985 Peter Koech; 10,000m 1977, Samson Kimobwa; cross country, 1976, 1977, and 1979, Henry Rono.

The man who brought all these Kenyans to Washington State was John Chaplin. "I first heard from Dr. Jonathan Ng'eno, the brother to John. He was an advisor to President Moi, held a PhD from Southern Illinois, and was at the University of Puget Sound in Washington. He came to my office and told me a story about John that he ran 13:45 back in Kenya, and I thought, 'Yeah sure.' He had contacted about four other colleges and they had thought the same thing."

At this time Mal Whitfield, the 1948 and 1952 Olympic 800m champion was over in Africa, so John sent him a telegram to ask whether he could check this story out. It turned out to be true. "So I called Jonathan back and said that I could not pay for travel, under the NCAA rules, but if they were to turn up on my doorstep, I would give them a full scholarship."

In the fall of 1972, Ng'eno showed up, in a large suit with great big lapels, on Chaplin's doorstep! As a freshman, Chaplin had him run the 3-mile, and in the finals he finished fourth in 13:12. "Not a bad time!" laughs Chaplin.

For three years John was undefeated in the NCAA's 3-mile indoor and 6-mile outdoor. In the Montreal pre-Olympic 5000m Ng'eno defeated Lasse Viren (who would win the Olympic gold) clocking 13:20.6. He would have been one of the clear favorites had it not been for the Kenyan Olympic boycott. "He had great track form. The year after he arrived I had him run cross country, he had a real short step, not great for country, but he won the AAU. His stride was much better for the track."

Ng'eno, like most Kenyans, was a very religious man, and Chaplin recalls one time when Ng'eno set his indoor PR at three miles, "It was a devil-take-the-hindmost race in Seattle in 1974, and Ng'eno keeps passing people, looking back, and eventually ends up running 13:08! All because he was not 100 percent sure this guy was not really connected to the Devil!" A superb indoor runner Ng'eno also clocked 13:34.6 for 5000m distance in Portland. "Oh yeah, he had great speed, he ran a 4:01 mile," says Chaplin.

Today Ng'eno, a pioneer who quit running on returning to Kenya with an education, works in Nairobi for the Ministry of Education.

Another student at WSU who would play a very instrumental role in Kenyan athletics was Coach Mike Kosgei, a Social Sciences grad in 1979.

As opportunities outside the armed forces opened up for athletes in Kenya, the standard of athletes searching for U.S. scholarships dropped dramatically. From the six U.S. scholarship athletes making the Olympic finals in 1988, only one made it to the 1992 Olympics.

The Will to Win Means Nothing Without the Way to Get Out

To paraphrase Juma Ikangaa, the truth in Kenya is that sometimes running qualifying times, or placing correctly in selection races, is not a guarantee of even leaving the country once an athlete has done the physical work. "If you have no money or connections, you will not make it in Kenya nowadays, these days and all the days. Talent alone is not enough," says Joseph Nzau.

At the Kericho Athletics Kenya cross country meet in December 2006, ten junior athletes (men and women), who had finished in the top fifteen places, were asked some simple questions. When asked, "What is your motivation for running?" fourteen answered that it was for financial reasons. One wished for a scholarship. "What is the biggest hurdle facing an up-and-coming athlete in Kenya?" Thirteen answered facilities, and two answered money, which amounts to the same thing. Every single athlete questioned would prefer to be given a race entry in a $5000 prize road race in America rather than a slot on the Kenyan national team for the African Championships. Asked why money was such a key reason for running, apart from the obvious, the athletes were all in agreement that if they had money they could secure their own means of leaving Kenya, and not have to rely on waiting for a selection committee's approval.

The stories of Kenyan athletes riding the waves from poverty to stardom are many, yet the numbers of talented runners who never progressed past the provincial levels of domestic competitions are far, far greater. The high concentration of world-class runners in Kenya makes a domination of the local scene nigh on impossible. As a coach from 1981 to the present day, John Macharia has seen an awful lot of Kenyan races. "Every week, someone new! A new face ready to take on, and beat, he who won last week. If you want to be noticed, you better do something very special. Winning a race is not enough. Then they [selectors] will ask, 'Do you have the experience to win in Europe?' and that of course can not be answered!"

Even finishing in the top three places for a national trials race does not guarantee a Kenyan a ticket to Europe. The medal count for Kenya in World Championship events could often be higher.

Kenya traditionally sends small teams to the events due to the budgetary factor. At the Barcelona World Indoor Championships in 1995, Benson Koech was the only Kenyan to run on the track; he won the 800m silver. By 2006, believing the chances of medaling were good, Kenya sent two runners in the 800m, (Wilfred Bungei won gold), two runners in the 1500m, (Daniel Kipchirchir Komen took silver and Elkanah Onkware Angwenyi took the bronze, and two runners in the 3000m (Eliud Kipchoge took bronze). However, athletes reaching qualifying standards by either time or place often do not travel.

At the World Junior Track Championships, where Kenya is always at or near the top of the medal table, the team is usually outnumbered by the American squad ten to one. "If you don't stand a chance of taking a gold medal, we will not send you," says Coach John Macharia, underling the lofty level athletes must reach to gain national-team selection. As an example, in the 2006 World Track & Field Junior Championship in Beijing, Kenya headed the table with six gold medals to Russia's and the USA's four a piece. In 1996, a group of 19 athletes were seen off at the Jomo Kenyatta airport to compete in the World Junior Championships in Sydney. They returned with nine medals. The U.S., with a team of 110, won 12 medals.

A runner by the name of Nelson Otieno, was on the Navy team. Nelson trained religiously, three times a day, to try to be the best. In a bout of heavy training, he caught pneumonia; he had no finances to go to a doctor. He had no money to travel to his home village and solicit his family for help. He died trying, alone and shivering. Kenyan running is not a glorified story of wealth, happiness, and medals. There is a theme of struggling that most of the accomplished runners have faced to reach success, and there is an unbelievable seam of optimism in a part of the world that is ravaged by disease, drought, and deficiency. It is no wonder the Kenyans who do break through are world beaters.

Kenyans believe in themselves as being the best. They have a grain far deeper than the marrow of their bones that says, "I can be the best."

In December of 1995, a trial race was held on the roads of Iten. The federation, then called the KAAA, was looking to see who should be sent to the famous S?o Silvestre New Year's Eve race in Brazil. A host of world running stars attended the event. Ezekiel Bitok, who a few months later would place second at the centennial Boston Marathon, had just been dropped by his manager and was looking to prove himself. Simon Chemoiywo, a perennial top place finisher in the World 12K Cross Country Championships and a former winner of Sao Silvestre, was also at the event.

The distance would be that of the Brazilian race, 15K. It was the top race of the month in the world's hotbed of distance running. As the event drew to its conclusion, the spectators, such as Moses Kiptanui, strained their eyes and did not recognize the race leader, who had clearly run away with a win at this high-status road race. He was bare-foot on the tarmac road and wore no brand name athletic clothing. Following the prize ceremony, it became clear that no other competitor had ever even seen this athlete before, yet he had decimated the field by over a minute. Would this happen anywhere outside of Eastern Africa? That is speculation.

The runner's name was Mark Wendot Yatich, and he came from Marigat Centre. In the first race he was sent to (no, he did not make the selection for Brazil), the Stramilano Half Harathon, he ran 61:27. He would progress to winning the Los Angeles Marathon, Falmouth Road Race, and many more prestigious events. Yatich was asked how an unknown, coming literally out of the forest, could defeat a world-class field in his first race.

"They [the other runners] are just human, like me. Why should they be any better than me? We have the same color blood. I knew I could win from the start. I wanted the way out [to South America]." He said this without a trace of brashness in his tone.

He was asked why he had not surfaced at any earlier race. "My family have no money. This was the first race that I could travel to with little expense, otherwise I would have run other races." It was no exaggeration; the family ate bread once a year, at Christmas, and ate meat exceedingly sparingly. If Yatich had not believed so strongly in himself, he would not have taken the road that day, back in Iten, to being discovered.

A Typical Kenyan Training Run: On the Roads of Iten

The chilly pitch-black darkness that spreads around the high-altitude training center like a watchman's cloak will soon disappear; the sun rises with the speed of a juggler's hand on the equator. There are no street lights in Kamariny, and there is little noise to be heard save one noisy rooster cleaning his throat. Although it is barely 6:00 a.m., a group of well-trained athletes, with hardly an ounce of fat apiece, silently mill around the camp. Sharp eyes pick out their own pair of training shoes from a pile of thirty or so pairs spread on the concrete floor by the corridor entrance to the dormitories. Most shoes are discolored with a dark russet stain from the glutinous mud that clings to not only the footwear but also the socks.

No words are spoken, as some athletes are still sleeping in the camp. There is a group of visiting European runners, and they will wait until after breakfast for their run. Another group of runners who usually leave at 7:00 will still be sleeping now. The Kenyans, however, typically all run together on non-specific training days. They leave in a group and then the tempo and distance are worked out literally on the run.

The camp has 24-hour security and the guard, Julius, who likes to eat grasshoppers and is dressed like a Second World War trench man, unlocks the gate with a bunch of keys befitting a bank. The village is peaceful and virtually crime-free, but precautions should always be taken. As one leaves the camp, there is a short walk up a stony driveway to the morning's meeting place. To the right is the ramshackle old Impala Inn, a haunt of a favored few retired athletes. It was here that I first met the legend Vincent Malakwen,

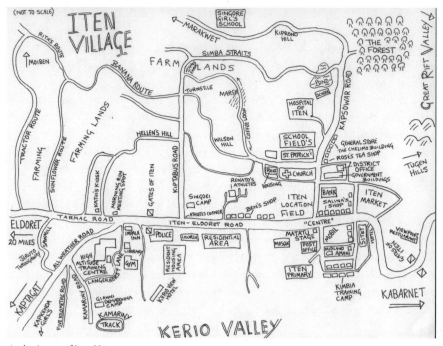

Author's map of Iten, Kenya.

who used to have the record for the fastest 800m run on Kenyan soil, 1:44.1. That was before Iten resident Japheth Kimutai ran 1:43.71. I was leaving for a morning run as Vincent was stumbling home.

Now the talk begins, a light susurrus of the lyrical Kalenjin tongue, interrupted by a slight giggle or a cough. Hilda Kibet and Doris Changeiywo, who room together and are matching in identical Adidas uniforms, talk to a man we know only as Samson who had been waiting outside at the camp's gate. Pieter and Lornah, the camp owners, pay his rent and board in a nearby house so he can try to make it as a professional runner.

There is a sweet smell of burning charcoal drifting in the air, as distinctive as salt and sand to the beach. It is the local villagers lighting their fires, making the milky morning tea that, for many poorer families, is the meal's complete menu. As the well-tuned athletes reach the top of the path, their number can be seen to be around a dozen. There is a loose arrangement that the runs begin at 6:15 most mornings, unless otherwise planned the night before. This is a good-sized group; typically the starting number is less.

Yet a few more are arriving from the left and right. Nearly every runner is wearing Lycra tights and a looser-fitting running jacket. The eye of Zeus, with shafts of orange and gold, is now breaking over the Kerio Valley. Suddenly the landscape has light and depth. A line of ruffle trees runs to our left, the type you would see in the English countryside. If you strain your eyes to the right, you can see the area on the other side of the Rift where Paul Tergat was born and raised. This morning he could be waking at his country residence, near his birthplace, to go for his morning run. Although busy, Tergat is a man who never misses his morning run.

Helena Loshanyang Kirop and Peter Limoria skip across the road. She is a Pokwot, and he is a Turkana. They rent a single room in a concrete two-story apartment building with twenty or so small rooms. Thin cheesecloth divides their one room, no bigger than a typical kitchen, into two halves. Living quarters and a bed. On the floor of the living room, between the TV and the sofa, are a Jiko (paraffin stove) and a pile of aluminum sufurias (pots) for preparing the food and making chai. Next

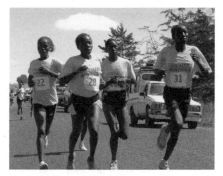

Doris Changeiywo (#1), Sharon Cherop (#2), Caroline Kiptoo (#3), and Edna Kiplagat (#4) on the Iten-Eldoret road in the first annual Shoe4Africa Iten Road Race. (*Jeroen Deen*)

to the TV are the trophies that Helena has won in the past year. Running clothes are strewn haphazardly over the furnishings; there has been rain, and to dry clothes that are in continual use is not easy when the sun does not shine. There is not a single tumble dryer in the entire town of Iten, let alone in a one-room apartment.

Standing by the side of the road, the group begins the usual ritual of stretching the sleep-weary muscles and double-tying the shoelaces. Caroline Kiptoo's arms reach to the sky, and she arches her back before letting the arms fall. Someone stretches her hamstring by hoisting the leg onto the serving ledge of a roadside kiosk that in the daylight hours sells local fruits. Unfortunately, the weight causes the awning of the shack to fall down. Nails are sparse in the construction of many of these huts. Another athlete pulls his heel to his buttock and stands like a heron in perfect balance. Doris is holding her hands behind her back and pulling back on her shoulders, whilst Peter skips on the spot, lifting his knees alarmingly high, seemingly to his teeth.

A diesel Land Rover pulls up; it is painted royal blue with a white roof, the exact color of the Kenyan police force. It is Pieter Langerhorst and Lornah Kiplagat, the aforementioned owners of the camp. Last year, after living in the camp for five years, they moved into a modest New Mexico-style house perched on the ledge of the Kerio Valley. It is self-contained, with solar panels and a nourishing vegetable garden with a wide variety of produce. The expansive glass in the living room gives to-die-for views, and a sweet hint of coffee perfumes the house. Athletics memorabilia and trinkets from their constant global trotting adorn the rooms.

I feel incredibly fortunate to know Pieter and Lornah. I met Pieter when he became my boss, back in 1995. I ran for Saucony Europe, and he was the European team manager. All the athletes liked him; he was approachable, charismatic, and effective—one of the most unselfish people, in a sport swamped with egotism, that you will ever meet. I met

Lornah the same year, in Kenya, when she was a shy, unknown athlete wearing Reebok hand-me-down clothes, and before she met Pieter. Diffident and doubtful, she backed away at first when I tried to talk to her at the Armed Forces Championships, maybe the first race she ever won as a senior. Even then, I knew she was going to be a world star; she has that aura about her that transcends us mortals.

Pieter, who is known as "Starbucks," is the coach of the local assembly. After a group of his athletes ran 2:07 and 2:08 marathons, and his wife, Lornah, ran a few world records, the belief in his methods spread throughout the town like wildfire over a thatched roof. Each day it is not uncommon that a new athlete will come to the camp asking for Pieter's guidance. Lornah is the boss of the group; what she says goes. She pulls back her thick braids and walks back to look on the dashboard of the Land Rover for a hair band. "Today we do past St. Patrick's, then the hill to the banana, then the tractor, eh? But easy, right?" she says, referring to some well-known routes. She smells of soap and her tracksuit is spotless. Not like mine; Kenyans, unlike most Europeans, are very skilled at hand-washing. Years ago, when Lydia Cheromei was my neighbor, she looked at my forlorn efforts and offered to rewash my entire wardrobe and shoes. I was horrified at the thought of a World Champion doing such a deed and resolved to be a tad grubby instead.

For a woman to lead the group in not normal in Kenya, but Lornah is no ordinary woman. Daniel Mukche is an example of an athlete who was at first mocked for training with Lornah. "She's using you, if you train with her you'll run like a woman!" he'd be told. Talk settled down a little when Daniel received sought-after training facilities. Then everyone stopped chiding the likeable Keiyo runner when he placed sixth at the Nairobi Half-Marathon in an unbelievable 62:09, at altitude, on a road that looks like it was involved in some Gaza Strip bombings, and beating more than 2,800 seasoned senior athletes.

The training run begins heading toward the village center. The camp is two kilometers away from Iten. The pace begins as a stumble; this is the Kenyan way. We pass the police station to the right, and visions of Richard Chelimo, who as a 17-year-old finished fourth in the World Cross Country Championship spring to mind. When Chelimo's pick-up truck was stolen in town he sprinted to the police station faster than the thieves could drive (albeit across fields) to halt the astonished crooks. Lantana shrubs skirt the roads, the pretty pink-and-butter yellow flowers on the bush coloring the landscape. The locals, to repel the annoying mosquitoes, burn the leaves; it works remarkably well.

The path where we run is red clay that is molded by the weather and hardened by the sun. Its ruts and runnels play havoc with the Western ankle, yet the Kenyans dance over the grooves as if the road was as smooth as a billiard table. The sweet smell of chapattis now tinges the air as the fires are warmed up. Made with *unga* (flour), *magi* (water), *sukari* (sugar), *chumvi* (salt), and a little *mafuta* (fat), these flat round fried breads are delicious. A former world record-holder in the road 5K and 10 miles, Rose Cheruiyot, who used to live in Iten, would make the best chapattis, kneading the dough for hours before using an empty soda bottle as a rolling pin to shape the breads.

The runners, now numbering fifteen, come to the corner where Philip Singoei has a small camp of a dozen or so runners. Singoei, who is the course record-holder at the

Eindhoven Marathon with his 2:07:57, supports his group by offering free accommodation in a house with Spartan living conditions whose rooms he typically rents. Lornah's camp is a paradise compared to every other running camp in Kenya as far as living conditions. There are cooks, hot showers, and a full-time staff who clean and run the place like a Western motel.

Singoei's group has left and is 100 meters farther up the road. Four or five of the runners are wearing old blue Fila tracksuits; they were probably part of the now defunct Fila training camp that used to be based in Iten. It was disbanded when

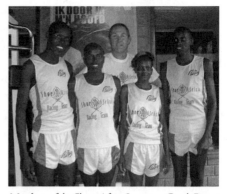

Members of the Shoe4Africa Iten team. Coach Pieter stands with (L to R) John Kiptoo (cousin to Josephat Kiprono), Justus Mebur, Gladys Otero, and Daniel Mukche. (*Author*)

as the company moved from the running world, supplying athletes like Paul Tergat and Margaret Okayo, to the fashion market, with the likes of Paris Hilton. The runners ahead stride in unison; no music plays although they appear to be moving in a rhythmic trance.

The word "camp" can be misinterpreted; a camp is often a solitary house rented by a manager affiliated with a sports company, nothing fancy, just a bare residence with wooden bed frames and, if you were lucky, mattresses. Food is often a problem. Many times when visiting a camp one can find that athletes have been missing meals. Robert Cheruiyot tells some illuminating stories about food rationing at the Kaptagat "Fila" camp, where one loaf of bread was to be split between eleven runners for a meal. I remember the first time I visited the camp where Felix Limo trained, shortly after his world-record run in Holland. Dedication and desire were all that replaced the material objects we in the West need.

In these places, two athletes share one mattress, and there are four to a room that would be offered as a single in European conditions. All these thoughts and more fill my head as I glide on. Four hundred meters into the run, the pace has picked up slightly.

Nobody who visits Kenya ever fails to remember the experience, and as small and insignificant as the village of Iten is, you simply cannot dislodge it from your mind. This mesmeric place has a numinous aura that I cannot quite understand myself. It has been fourteen years since I first set foot here, and I have sent a lot of visitors here since. Not one has been disappointed. I thought it was perhaps the running factor, yet non-runners share my thoughts. Amber Robbins has been there a couple of years now as a Peace Corps worker; she's not a runner but she loves the place. It is a paradox I ponder as we run. How can a place of such little apparent activity be so very inspirational and exhilarating?

As we run uphill, the talk dies down. Although the pace is still slow, the 2400-meter lung-shrinking altitude makes climbing a challenge at any speed. On our left we pass

Ben's Shop. Ben owns a fleet of matatus (communal taxis). His brother-in-law, Josephat Kiprono, is the first ever man to run two sub-2:07 marathons. Kiprono retired at the age of thirty and today is a farmer. Although rake thin, he does not run a step these days, not even for fun or fitness. Strange for a man who used to run more than 120 miles per week.

Ben has a couple of his vehicles' engines warming up and the fumes are an unpleasant smudge on the fresh air. The houses and buildings are now lining the sides of the road as we approach Iten center. A white Muslim mosque sits up to the right proudly on the top of the hill. Prayers in the early-morning hours resound from this building through an antiquated PA system.

The road now descends on a stretch that leads into Iten center. To the left is a big location field before the turn that we will make toward Sing'ore on the Kapsowar road. The location field is where Wilson Kipketer, his skin pulled taut against his high cheekbones and his open mouth gulping down the air, often used to be seen moving with celerity, perfecting his elegant stride, galloping over the grassland. He would stretch out his stride over the soft ground, extending his limbs through differing gaits, his heels coming up to his shorts when he sprinted. He owns the current world record at 800m—1:41.11.

We will climb Wilson Hill on this run, named in Kipketer's honor by a group of local athletes. In the early nineties, I would play darts sometimes with Kipketer, whiling away the hours before the evening Swedish Grand Prix meets. Wilson played darts only a little better than I did, except his technique was more warrior-like, making for prolonged games. Time has now proven that he was the world's best 800m runner ever; at this writing he has run seven of the ten fastest times ever recorded and his world record has stood untouched for more than a decade.

It is across this same location field that Bernard Barmasai of Timboroa, then a world record-holder, helped cart my iron trunk on his shoulder from St. Patrick's to the Iten stage. Kenyans, even when they become world stars, never fail to retain their humble assisting nature.

The center of this small village is a junction of roads from three directions. To the right is a smattering of shops, including the bluest blue and pearly-white post office, where Mrs. Koila will sell you stamps and persuade you not to take part in any business that requires undue paperwork, like express mail. "Why not send it normal? It will still get there. It costs you less and you don't need to do anything except buy a stamp."

The post office used to have internet access until the computers broke down and left Iten without a public Internet connection. There are many little shops, such as the one that develops photos, or "washes your snaps" as they quaintly put it. Cassette tapes are more popular than CDs, and it is easy to imagine that this Kenyan village is put in a time warp. Respect is given, and kindness is an expected token that the villagers take for granted. Times are changing, though, and many signs around this center remind me that we are in the twenty-first century. Large lime-green signage for Safaricom, the big Kenyan cell-phone company, is everywhere. Any direction you look, you can see Safaricom. In a country with few land lines, the cell-phone business has flourished; it amazes me that everyone in Kenya seems to own a cell phone—they lead East Africa in this respect.

There is a system that lets you "flash" some-one's cell if your credit has run out. An instant message appears asking the receiver to call the sender. This way even the penni-less stay in touch. Incoming calls, unlike in America, are free for cell–phone owners. It was quite a surprise when a week earlier, a Maasai warrior in full regalia had visited the camp and somewhere under a multitude of tribal beads his phone started ringing.

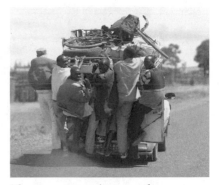

The trusty matatu—always room for one more on board! (*Giuliano De Portu*)

It is in front of this post office that the *matatus* gather to collect customers. At this early hour, a few are already parked at the stage and blowing their horns, trying to attract trade. For a dollar, you can ride twen-ty miles to Eldoret. The government recently clamped down on the condition of the *mata-tus* making the modern version much safer to ride than that of a decade ago. I remember hanging onto the outside of the swinging back door with another gentleman, William Koila, who was then the under-18 world record-holder for the 1500m (3:37:95), traveling to see William Mutwol, the former world 5k record-holder. The inside of the vehicle, built for 12 but carrying more than twenty, was stuffed to the seams. Each pothole on the dirt road was a near-death experience as the driver raced along with bald tires and poor brakes; he was eager to offload and begin the return trip. Unfortunately for me, Mutwol lived a long way down the road. When you wish to alight, you use a coin to tap on the metal roof, alerting the driver who sits in the front with at least two others, invariably he can't operate the gears, as someone's legs are jammed against the stick shift.

A *matatus* begins its run when it is stuffed full. The meaning of the word refers to the Swahili word for the number three (tato) and '[Always] room for one more." The conduc-tor packs everyone inside, then hangs on the outside of the vehicle. When a police officer is spied, the conductor somehow pushes himself inside, albeit further squashing the pas-sengers, and slides the side door shut.

One of my very first rides in a *matatu* was when I visited Olympic bronze medalist Joyce Chepchumba in Nakuru, the town of the pink flamingos. A green foreigner, I was bundled into a decrepit vehicle with blaring Christian music, wooden benches that had replaced the original seats, and three fat Kenyan women and one child on my bench squashing me next to a window that had a waxy coat of what looked like grime and grease, and smelt no better than a pint of old sweat. We happened to be driving over a railway crossing just as an officer was spotted. The conductor struggled to climb over the mass of passengers and into the matatu, and the jolt of the rails and the force of his body-weight suddenly caused the large sliding door to fall off. The conductor and one passen-ger fell out. The door was then tied back onto the body of the minibus, the passenger was shoved back in, and we were off again.

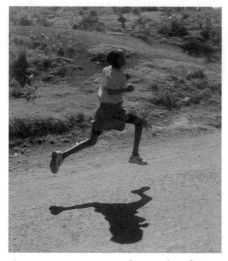

A young runner on the roads of Iten. (*Author*)

Each day the local radio news would begin with how many people had died on the local roads. "Today two buses collided on the road to Kisumu, more than seventy people dead." Then boom, next piece of news.

I had run with Joyce in Europe, traveled with her in America, had gone to the famous San Blas Half-marathon in Puerto Rico with her, and it never ceased to amaze me how attentive, caring, and unassuming she remained despite year after year of being one of the greatest marathon runners in the world. You could talk to Joyce for a week and not even know she was a runner, another week and you might find out she did actually run, but you would never hear her mention a victory or the slightest boast, never. Once she was in an elevator with Magic Johnson, and he asked, "Do you run? Did you run the marathon?" Instead of replying that she had just won the city's marathon that morning, she smiled and replied, "I am one of many who love to run, yes." A typical Kenyan response with humility and honesty, not a bragging bone in their bodies. We invited Magic for a run the following morning.

Joyce trained hard and smart. She had discipline but also responded to warning signs of over training; it was no surprise that she had such a long and successful career. And it is not over. After recently giving birth to a child, she will make a comeback.

To the right is another a stony dirt path that leads up to the Kimbia camp. It is from this base that Matt Taylor of Boston made his inimitable documentary, *Chasing Kimbia*. With great camera-work he exposed and captured both the beauty of the village and the essence of the Kenyan runner. The dirt path also leads up to the Iten primary school. In December the school had over more than 380 participants in the Shoe4Africa race, and the kids won a school computer system for their efforts.

The group silently swoops left, the legs in unison moving like swinging pendulums, the upper bodies upright yet relaxed, the elbows at right angles and the hands never clenched. I observe that all the faces have a tranquil expression. Something looks incredibly right about Kenyans when they run. There is a feeling of power, but also grace; the essence of kinetic energy. We skip over small piles of garbage on the ground. There are no street cleaners in Iten, no recycling programs, and a lot of trash. It is not uncommon to see people throw garbage onto the street or out of a car window; no one blinks an eye. Occasionally a group of Peace Corps workers holds a cleanup project, but the next week there is a new carpet of refuse on the paths. I notice how, at this section, the athletes hop over the trash without even seeming to look down. Thankfully, once we are past the village center, the waste disappears and nature again rules the landscape.

If we were to have continued straight down the road, instead of bearing left, we would pass the village of Kessup, then Tambach, where there is a 400m dirt running track at the teacher-training college. The road drops steeply and makes for a great hill-climbing session. Further down the road you reach the bed of the Rift Valley. It is extremely hot down there, so hot that sharp-toothed crocodiles come out into the open and bathe in the shade, hiding from the sun's rays which are blocked by sandy brown rocks. River trickles from thirst, rarely gushing even in the rainy season. Last year, Benjamin Limo, whose son Tony

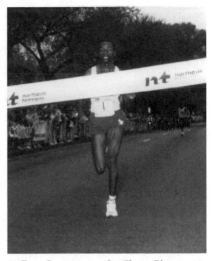

William Sigei winning the Cherry Blossom 10-miler, in a then–world-best time of 46:01. (*Bob Burgess*)

Helsinki, named after British Prime Minister Tony Blair and the World Championship city where he took the 5000m gold in 2005, helped me look for crocs when we returned from a visit to Kabarnet. Kenya was experiencing a deadly drought at this time, and the three rivers Kessup, Kimwarer, and Mong, which feed the valley, had literally dried up. The river we stood by had shriveled beyond recognition and only a cracked dry bed remained. There was not a leaf left on any tree or bush nearby. Rotting carcasses of cows and goats were a too common sight. Giant cracks spread the earth, and the throbbing sun made standing still uncomfortable. We saw no crocodiles.

Back in 1995, on Christmas day, I happened to be staying in a village close to the Masai Mara. Fresh from driving in to visit William Sigei, who was then the 10,000m world record-holder, at his large property in Bomet Town (named Oslo after the city where the record was set), I was touring around and checking out the local Kenyan countryside.

Sigei, from Kapsimotwo, was a Kenyan legend. He arrived on the scene by beating "King" John Ngugi at the nationals by a wide margin, running barefoot, as a newcomer at the Nyayo stadium ("footsteps stadium") in 1992. By the following year he was the champion of the world. At this time, he was at the dull end of his brilliant yet short career. He had bought a property in Teddington, England, and was talking about how he now had pressures beyond those of competition, how the business world was too confusing for him.

His best friend, neighbor, and training partner, Dominic Kirui, who was recovering from an Achilles tendon problem, reckoned that if Sigei would spend more time training and less time on other matters, he would break 26:30 for the 10,000m. A preposterous notion at the time, but looking back, his two-year stint was excessively short for a talent like Sigei to fully develop. We left Sigei's and drove to toward Ngorengore. Then the travel became a hike as the roads ended.

The village where I was staying consisted of a cluster of small mud huts and little else, just one kiosk that sold everyday necessities. It was an hour's walk into the bush from where the last matatu had dropped us. I was there for a number of days. I wanted Christmas to stand out from the other days that were quickly blurring into one another. So, on Christmas morning, I slipped out of the village very early from my little hut without waking my hosts, and ran/walked, exploring the area. I met a Maasai dressed in his traditional red-and-black blanket (*shuka*). He asked me what I was doing and then suggested that he show me some crocodiles. After greeting his wife, a strikingly attractive woman who was at least six feet tall and decorated in a kaleidoscopic rainbow of colored beads with jet-black skin and the most ivory-white teeth I had ever seen, we set off. "What luck," I thought, especially when an hour later we perched above the riverbank watching hippos wallow in the water, their piggish eyes protruding from the muddy water. I found a jawbone and skull of what looked like a hippo in the bush. There were two rows of fat teeth, and as hard as I tried I could not prise a tooth out to keep for a souvenir. (Looking back years later at a photograph I took I noticed there were two tusk holes, so it may not have been a hippo skull at all.) This was turning out to be a good Christmas.

I was not able to spy any crocodiles at first from high up on the bank, but my friend quickly pointed some out , luckily at some distance. They looked prehistoric, clumsy and disagreeable. It was hard to believe they could run as fast as I had seen them do on nature programs. I was sorely tempted to lob a stick at one to see if I could get it to scuttle away. Then my friend asked, "Would you like to see a herd of elephants?" I was enticed; this was a true safari. In order to reach the Elephants, I was told; we had to traverse the river. I started to reconsider, but my friend convinced me, "I have been crossing this river every day of my life. It is safe, I know, if you do it by quickly walking across down there. The crocodiles wait for pauses, so we don't stop." I inspected his legs for tooth marks before succumbing to his indigenous, but dubious, logic. This was Kenyan life, the real stuff you could not find offered by tour guides. He would offer further gems; "In the morning when you run through the field, make some noise and stamp your feet. Then stop and look at the grass, watch if the blades move against the grain. Then you know that snakes are moving around. Wait a few minutes before crossing."

With the highest knee-lift possible, I made it to the other side of the river. Then, after my friend selected a large thick stick, we set off walking. "The stick is just in case we meet any lions," he explained as if we were discussing the price of sugar at the market. "You see, the lion is very short-sighted. But he can see heights. So I wave the stick up high, he thinks we are giraffes, then leaves us alone." As we hiked on, following foliage that looked like it might have been trampled on the trail of the great Tembo, I tried my hardest to clear my throat for any giraffe impressions I might have to give. I was beginning to think the venture a bad idea when we saw, in the distance, a small herd of elephants uprooting some shrubs with their trunks. They were smaller in size than I had expected them to be.

It was a moment of danger and delight. The distance was far, but I really did not want too much of a closer look. It reminded me of the time I went to see a volcanic eruption in Iceland. Close is not always better. I asked if elephants were short-sighted, too. They seemed very engrossed in a group activity that appeared to be gang warfare against one bush, pulling hunks of flora from its branches with their wriggly trunks.

It was now well past noon and I was as hungry as a marching soldier. There was obviously no place to get food, so I suggested that we return for supplies. I had had my fill of the wildlife. My friend became annoyed when I asked him to point out the direction back to the river. He put his hand inside his blanket and brought out a small, dirty black cloth that was folded into an improvised bag. Opening the bag, he produced, amongst other things, a chapatti. He tore the bread in half and offered me a portion. Suddenly I was not so hungry.

He then froze, put his finger to his lips, and started to crouch down on his knees. His eyes opened wide and I quickly looked over my shoulder, expecting to see a lion approaching. Far off up a tree was what appeared to be an animal; looking through the zoom lens of my camera, I saw something like a leopard. "Very rare, lucky day," he said, eyes as round as saucers. I now had an amazing set of photos, and a strong urge to be back at the uneventful village.

Back in N'gong, whilst a group of us were running through the forest, one of the runners told me about a training run when they had met a leopard. Two soldiers nipped back to the camp, got a weapon, and returned to kill the beast. This was illegal, but when the police arrived, the soldiers remained tight-lipped. My friend, who had been one of the blood stained duo, mentioned the day as fortuitous. One more reason to keep pace with the pack of runners when out on a Kenyan training run in the wild!

The sighting of the cat creature decided it; I was definitely going back, and this person was certifiable. Just then, the animal slid out of sight into the foliage, and a second later, we heard the engine of a car approach. What luck—a Land Rover painted like a zebra was not 300 meters away. I yelped, screamed, and ran toward the vehicle with my friend following. The vehicle slowed. Through the windows, tourists pointed cameras at us, and then, to my utter amazement, simply drove off, leaving us stranded—on Christmas day no less. My friend snuffed. "White men, what do you expect!" It seemed pointless to mention that his big stick might have had something to do with the flighty reaction of the tourists.

To cut a long story short, we jogged for hours in subdued silence until the evening time when we, or should I say he, finally found the way back to where we had come from. As a teenager I had lived on the streets of Amsterdam for a while, often going without food for a day or more, and this day brought back lucid memories. I was famished and knew I was close to collapsing. We had been footing for over twelve hours. My shirt was torn to rags from clambering through the thorns and pins of the bush. I was sweaty, dirty, and exhausted. I could not have cared if a crocodile had eaten me this time when I waded back over the river. In fact, I waded across the stretch of water in no hurry at all.

However, what was to come next changed my way of thinking from that day to this. When I was alone again, I decided to take a short-cut over the hill to get back to my village as fast as possible. As I cut through the low bush, a lantern flickered in the dark ahead like a blond moth, then another, and to the right two more dim yellow kerosene lamps appeared from the darkness. Suddenly someone called out, "Jesus, Jesus is coming. It is Christmas, and He has arrived!" I should add that my hair was long and blond, past my shoulders. My shirt was shredded and I was as thin as the man that hangs on a cross in so many portraits across the globe, and in most Christian African homes. Whilst trying to explain that I was not Jesus, but would not say no to 500 loaves, I was virtually dragged inside the first of many huts. Although furnishing was lacking in the majority of the huts, virtually every hut you visit in rural Kenya had a portrait of Christ pinned to the wall. Considering that many of the Kenyans in Eldoret mistook me for other white men who actually had dark hair and coloring, I could understand that perhaps they saw a resemblance. "Oh my Lord," the women were crying, asking me to bless their children. Young children were being pushed into my arms. Apparently, as I later discovered, no white person had ever set foot in this village, and the commotion of an unexpected arrival on Christmas night was too much of a coincidence to be dismissed. It is a tradition that you have to drink a cup of tea in each house you visit. At first, I eagerly gulped down the liquid like a starving sailor, but after about seven huts, my stomach began to churn.

Finally, I reached the last hut on the edge of the village. Two parents and a child. I was given the solitary three-legged stool to sit on and told to wait. The parents left the child with me as they went, presumably, to the cooking hut. The child lasted two seconds before screaming and running after her parents. The strange thing was that in between huts I was mobbed, but once inside a particular family's hut I was alone, except for the host family. You went from pandemonium to silence in a few steps.

I looked around the room; one bed, two blankets on the mud floor, and that was it. I was expecting yet another cup of tea when it was announced by the mother of the hut that the last family hen had been killed in my honor and now was being boiled in the cooking hut. They, who had utterly nothing, gave me a not only their last possession but a big lesson. Beaming as I left their hut, they insisted how blessed they were to have a visitor on that night. I felt two feet tall leaving that village—insisting that I must leave, as they wished me to stay. I thought of all my shortcomings and walked home in a vortex of shame, convinced I would go home, metamorphose into something resembling a religious person, and give all my possessions to the nearest church. Of course, none of this happened. That is the Kenyan spirit that lives within its people.

I snap back to the moment. Three runners now join our group; I recognize one to be tall Daniel Kosgei. The other two men look familiar but I do not know their names. What first made me notice Daniel in Iten was his sun-bleached tracksuit. The black tights had become gray and threadbare like an old man's beard; the blue jacket was ashen white complete with naturally-worn ventilation holes and a scuffed collar that looked like a moth's nest. You could tell this young man had not yet been to Europe. He was a typical athlete resident, having come to Iten to make it to the professional world. Runners flock to Iten, both established and newcomers, from all areas of Kenya. They know the stories, they know that here they can find the ideal training conditions, and there is a certain abstruse air to the village that simply can not be explained in words, but is talked about and accepted. The Kenyans say *azima anga* (magic air) when talking about Iten's mystical properties.

As Daniel runs, I wonder if he will ever make it. I hope so. He seems to be very resolute and is consistent with his training. In 1996, I was running with Simon Biwott wondering the exact same thing. What had caught my eye first about Simon was not his running talent, but that he had a voracious appetite and always looked too chubby to make it to the world of elite running. Then a year or two later, I was walking through the Antaris Hotel breakfast room in Monterrey with the 1997 Boston Marathon winner, Lameck Aguta. We had just eaten a light breakfast of toast before a half-marathon race that we were to run. I noticed a plate piled high with cakes and buns on one of the tables where a group of Africans sat. I scoffed, thinking how the unlucky runner would be painting the roads a few miles along the course; we barely had an hour before the starting gun. A head looked up,

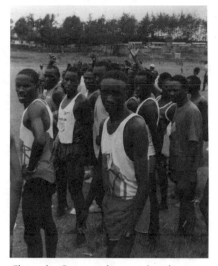

Christopher Sogot was the most talented junior in the Iten region in 1995, yet Japheth Kimutai (far left) and Abraham Cherono (barefoot in between the two) were the athletes who "made it." (*Author*)

and a voice called out; it was Simon! Not only did he win the race that day, but he set a Mexican all-comer's record of 61:27 as well. He had made it.

A similar thing happened to Ronald Mogaka. When I first arrived in Kenya in 1995, my luggage did not. Neither had my training partner, the Irish Olympian Noel Berkeley, who had all the Kenyan contacts. "Brother Colm, he'll look after us, I know him well," Noel had said

I sat in my hot and small hotel room for an hour thinking what a mistake I had made to come to Kenya—I had nothing but jeans and a T-shirt, and no address book of contacts. I knew a few Kenyans from races in Europe, but none well enough to turn up on their doorsteps. I decided that I would go for a run anyway, as it was what I always did. I stepped outside and decided to run to the right; I had asked the taxi driver the night before to drive me to a cheap hotel on the outskirts of Nairobi, as I did not wish to be in the crime-ridden city center. I started to jog along the side of the road. People shouted at me, "Hey, white man! Are you too stingy to take a taxi to where you are going?" How they laughed. My jeans flapped; at least I was wearing sneakers as traveling shoes, but I was not moving comfortably in my street clothes. It was very hot, and I feared that a malaria-ridden mosquito would come and bite me (yes, my pills were in my luggage). Just by luck I saw a runner up ahead; as I caught him he started to talk to me as we ran. "Are you a manager? Will you take me to Europe? I am very good; I have run 1:41 for 800 meters." Right, I thought. This scruffy kid, who was not much better dressed than I was for running, had clearly *not* run a world record for the 800m.

The run became like a TV commercial. Suddenly from a side road came one runner, then two, then twenty, followed by twenty more. A coach on a bicycle kept the pace. I followed the runners and within ten minutes, we arrived at a running camp. *The* running camp.

"Sit down, have some rice, have some tea and food. Come and stay here." Sitting amongst Paul Tergat, Paul Koech, Simon Chemwoiyo, William Kiptum, Ismail Kirui and more, I knew I had arrived. It was a royal introduction. With a flip of fate, I was the happiest man in Kenya.

Back to my young friend whom I had run with first on the road: As we parted, he told me his name. I thought it would be the last time I heard it. Years later, I was in Litchfield, Connecticut, competing in a road race. There was a post-race competition to see if you could hit the race director's chimney with a champagne cork, and I was trying hard to achieve this impossible task when a runner tapped me on the shoulder. "Excuse me, Mr. 'Tobby'. Do you remember a man called Ronald Mogaka? I am him." He had "arrived" and soon after that would set the course record of 46 minutes for The Broad Street 10-mile run in Philadelphia. Therefore, my friend Daniel, do not give up, because I think you are going to make it too. Daniel, I could give you ten more examples like the ones I have just remembered, but it is important for you to know that belief is golden in Kenya. Run and believe. I am talking to myself, because I am certain that Daniel knows, is convinced, he is going to make it.

Of course, succeeding athletically is only half the battle. I had been sharing a cup of Lipton's tea with Brother Colm, eating sugar-coated biscuits, and asking the learned Professor of Kenyan running about what had happened to various Kenyans who had disappeared from the loop. Colm, never at a loss for explanations, pointed out that how a Kenyan handles success can be extremely different to how a Westerner does. "They grow up with absolutely no money. Does the athlete have the ability to handle suddenly getting an abundance of wealth? Suddenly someone is giving him thousands of dollars. It is more than a lifestyle change." True enough I think of Martin Ojuko, a Kisii runner. Martin was virtually unbeatable in Scandinavia during one period in the 1990s. We briefly shared the same manager and traveled around together. When he won the Stockholm Marathon, I was his roommate. I recall how fastidious he was about good health and nutrition. Drinking fresh juices and eating many fruits. Martin won a lot of money in a very short time. He returned to Kenya, hooked up with the wrong people, and was last heard of living in a back room of a bar trying to sell trophies that he had won in his glory days. I look at Kosgei; I cannot imagine him drunk.

Nobody ever appears to be working in Iten, not just at this early hour, but even at mid-day. There is little industry to be seen except in the kiosks and necessity shops. Of course, that is not true; there is a hive of industry taking place, but little that disturbs the notion that this is the perfect runner's village. During the daytime hours people are "around" as the popular phrase puts it, but Iten is best described as residential. It has a sleepy quality; time remains neither still nor moving, hours just slide along. There are only slight bumps that pass you from day to day.

As we round the bend, I glance back to see if more runners will join us from the village center. A *matatu* is being pushed out of the Mobil station that is owned by Chris Cheboiboch. Obviously, gasoline was not the answer. The station is the center stage of the village. When Chris took over the business, I asked him how he thought the production would be better than the couple of other gas pumps in the village, and he insisted that the service there, with his eight-man staff, is unbeatable in the area. "I am teaching them to be like *wazungos*, efficient and fast in service!" He grinned. "I am keeping time for the customers, because I know *wazungos* like that and they make good money." Well, if the story is true that Mexico gets things done *mañana*, then Kenyans shoot for Manana afternoon. Regardless, Chris does good business in the sleepy village, and all the runners support him in town by buying their gasoline from his pumps. He also sells cell-phone credit top-ups.

A couple of days ago I had driven 5km along this very road in the Eldoret direction to the Salaba Academy, a school Chris started in 2005 with his winnings. The school is virtually complete and already has 250 students. He showed me round the dormitories, built so the school could accommodate borders in the future; the headmaster's office; the newly built classrooms; and of course the sports field. Poor Chris had just been in an automobile accident in which his passenger broke both his legs. This time we drove very slowly. The first time I came to Iten, Chris was a steeplechaser. Now he wins marathons and has been the runner-up at both Boston and the ING New York City Marathon. I know we will not meet Chris running this morning, because the bruises from the accident are still bothering him. At the school, he had offered to loan me a motorcycle to ride around Iten on. I did a quick test of the bike's roadworthiness and said, "Chris, no wonder you have accidents—there are no brakes!" That bike takes some getting used to!

We are on tarmac now, albeit only for 100 yards. Salina Chirchir, one of the first women to get a scholarship to the United States, in Mississippi, has a family kiosk near this corner. There were days in America when Salina, a 1996 Olympian, would not eat at mealtimes after hearing news about famines or droughts in Kenya. "This food would choke me," she would say in tears. "How can I eat when I don't know if my family have enough to eat?" She was one of countless Kenyans who made their living competing on the smaller circuit of road races, running back–to-back minor marathons in far-off places like Tahiti and Trinidad. She had gone to Jackson State and had been entangled in some payment rumors, illegal at colleges. Nowadays she is apparently lost down in Mexico; her contact letters have dried up. Relatives crashed Salina's pride, a gold-colored 3-series BMW that she imported to Kenya, and the money she sent home is long gone.

This morning we will bear left and run by the famous gates of the St. Patrick's school. However, if we were to carry on straight, we would come to my favorite road, the one that drops to Sing'ore. The majestic Nandi flame tree, locally known as the *kifabakazi*, or internationally as the African tulip tree, colors the valley with effervescent orange trimmings along the roadside farther down the hill, together with the unusual acacia trees, or umbrella trees, as they are locally known. They stalk the edge of the Great Rift Valley as though they were hang gliders ready for launch. At sunriser, the valley is a gorgeous expanse of dramatic pinks, oranges, reds, and yellows—a sight beyond inspiring, indescribable and unrivaled in beauty. The enormity of the valley holding up the equatorial skies gives the impression that the whole world is opening before you to be explored with your gathering momentum, as you stride with speed down the valley. It was on this road that I first met up again with the great Richard Chelimo, after having run a warm-up jog with him in Lilljans-skogen before that auspicious evening in 1993 when he set the 10,000m world record in Stockholm. I had raced in an earlier event, with another man, then an unknown who would become a legend; the great Wilson Kipketer.

Richard had graciously invited me to run with him, on my cool-down, and his warm-up. It was on this road that I trained with the likes of Japheth Kimutai; with Wilson Boit Kipketer, another St. Patrick's man; with Sally Barsosio, whom I think of as a Kenyan sister; with Rose Cheruiyot and Lydia Cheromei. With the unfathomable Christopher Kosgei, and the hardworking William Mutwol, whose stride length belies his small body. It is on this road that I remember freedom is a gift.

Many with great names have run on this eminent road. Today it is no different; it is the road of legends, sacred yet open for us mortals to tread upon and feel the enchantment of its gloried history. No matter what speed you run on this hill, friendly runners will join you, and as you glide by their side, it is oh so easy to imagine you are wherever you want to be as you run with your head in the clouds. Peter Duncan, from Australia, came to stay at the camp in Iten a few years ago for this very reason: "You go crazy, suddenly I was tripling my mileage, setting out with guys you see on the television!" And, the most wonderful thing is that the Kenyans make you feel you truly belong.

The road snakes down to the Sing'ore girl's school, which once fielded its own team that, by itself, won the Junior Women's World Cross Country Championships, all the scorers finishing in the top ten places! Has that ever been repeated? Never. A security guard at the school is the brother to Anthony Kiprono, who lives close by with his wife Tabitha. Kiprono was a Sing'ore legend from Kobil village who could race, and sometimes beat, the legends like Tergat when he was a young and hungry junior. Just one of many legends that decorate the valley from the right to the left of the Kapsowar road. For instance, to the left is the cornfield that Rose Chepyator talks about in this book.

Back to the moment. To the right is the district office, but we take a ninety degree turn to the left past a "Drive Fresh, Coca-Cola" sign that, instead of coke-red, is now washed-out orange from the burning sun's daily beating. Underneath are the words "St Patrick's" with a directional arrow. It must be a couple of decades old, and I muse that the Coke people should use it for a running commercial and change the word "drive" to "run" and have a stream of St. Patrick's alumni running round the bend. Coca-Cola has a monopoly on the soda business in Kenya, and the best-seller in their line is Orange Fanta. My personal favorite is the Blackcurrant Fanta that I have been unable to find outside Kenya.

I notice the way Lornah controls the group from her random position. The pack moves like a stealthy pride of lions. If she accelerates slightly, even when at the back of the pack, the whole group steps up a gear. Her ponytail bobs with each landing foot but her head remains flawlessly horizontal. I look across to see into her eyes, but her mirrored

Adidas sunglasses reveal nothing but he glare of the rising sun.

I slide next to Doris. She is from the Mount Elgon region, a long way from here, but an area equally densely populated with world-class runners. They say Doris breathes through her ears. Sure enough, when I look across her mouth is tightly shut and there is no movement of her nostrils as we run. She is the defending East African cross country champion, and to get that title she went against the Ethiopians in her first year as a senior. I run most mornings with Doris and Hilda; they are both punctual and reliable training partners.

We now pass the large grounds of St. Patrick's, the school that has put Iten on the global map. It is here that Matthew Birir, Peter Rono, Benson Koech, Mike Boit, and Ibrahim Hussein all went to school, to name a thimbleful of star athletes. It is here,

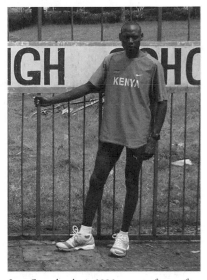

Isaac Songok, who in 2006 was one of a very few runners to beat the best Ethiopian, Kenenisa Bekele, stands outside St. Patrick's High School, where he lives. (*Author*)

Brother Colm tells me, that athletes like double world champion Ismael Kirui and Olympic 800m champion Paul Ereng were turned away from the doors as juniors as there was simply no space (and to many faster runners) in the dorms.

Following his victory at the Goteborg IAAF World Championships 5000m, Kirui visited St. Patrick's on his way back to the Marakwet district. As he left, he tossed someone a pair of running spikes saying, "Please give these to one of the needy athletes here." When asked if these were the very shoes that he had worn to win the Championships, he turned and nodded his head. "Why?" he asked.

Like Sing'ore, the school could field a World Championships–standard squad from its alumni. Today, Isaac Songok, Augustine Choge, and Mang'ata Ndiwa are a few of the residents (not students) on the grounds who wear Kenya's national colors. Coincidentally, Choge and Songok are on the road ahead of us, jogging slowly. This must be the biggest difference in training methods between Kenyans and Americans. Often in America it is hard to tell whether athletes are on a tempo run or an easy run. In Kenya there is never any second-guessing. The differential is vast. The first time I ran "easy" with Tegla Loroupe I remember thinking how someone could easily have walked past us as we jogged slowly along. However, when Kenyans do speed work very few runners can keep them within eyesight.

I remember a day back in Hofors, Sweden. I was at a training camp, and William Musyoki (a world-class marathon runner) and Benson Masya were there. We went for a 30K run, and the coach drove out to give us water. He knew the pedigree of Musyoki and

Masya and expected them to be passing 5K in about 16 minutes. When we did not show up by 21 minutes he drove off thinking he must have missed us somehow. William set the pace of about 22 minutes for that 5K; it was the final 5K that was run in 15 minutes. That is the Kenyan way.

I have a special affinity for the St. Patrick's school. I lived for many months on the school grounds, in an old priests' house that was deserted because of structural issues. I remember moving in and sorting through the rubble to clear a space to make a bed. I came across a basket of hockey sticks with the boarding-school attendees' names written on the handles, including Peter Chumba's, who had won the 5000/10,000m double in the world junior's and Wilson Kipketer's. I saw the old broken black–and-white TV on which the teachers from the school had watched their former student, Peter Rono, win an Olympic 1500m gold medal, back in 1988. The TV was now a screen with a web of old wires protruding from the rear. For me it was more alive than if it had worked. The place, for others, may have been a dump, but for me it was a paradise. All right, the bricks were crumbling, the staircase was rotten (hey, I didn't need two floors), and half the windows were smashed, but it was a home. My neighbors were world-class runners living in similar dwellings, a simple room with a door—that was all that was needed. If the electricity came we used it, if rain fell we washed, and if not, we used sodas to dampen the brushes and clean our teeth with. Each night we would light the paraffin stove, or the charcoal burners (the *jiko*) and cook *ugali* and vegetables for the evening meal. The night's entertainment was talking about running, about life, and living, as we surely were. Once a week, on Friday nights, we would all go to Brother Colm's house (forty yards away) and watch videos of classic films or athletic meets.

I still remember one night when we watched a rerun of the 1992 Barcelona Olympics 5000m. Not surprisingly, Kenyans—especially those who have not yet ventured abroad—do not hold much stock in the success of *wazungo* (white) runners. On this night, there was a group of up–and-coming athletes there. I informed them that they would see a white man beat the Kenyans. "It is not possible," they roared with laughter. I told them it had already happened. They did not believe it, and bets were placed, though of course never collected, as Germany's Dieter Baumann convincingly out-kicked Kenyan Paul Bitok for the Gold. A dozen years later, I visited the house, which was still in the same state of dilapidated disrepair and still inhabited by athletes.

To the left is the police compound, a small field with about twenty small bungalows. Very plain basic housing, where the police officers and recruits live. Benson Koech used to stay here when training with the St. Patrick's team, and I would often take morning tea with the police officers, as I was good friends with Sergeant Kiprono, who was the highest-ranking police officer on campus at the time. It was here that Stephen Biwott stayed in Iten, and here that Robert Cheruiyot walked to, back in the 1990s, half-starved.

Descending a hill just past St. Patrick's, I see Sylvia Kibet, Hilda's sister, waiting for us. She lives near there, next door to Solomon Busendich. Sylvia's positive attitude is welcomed on any day; she is always upbeat and cheerful. Her neighbor Busendich is another of those remarkable Iten characters. I met him first when he was an unknown junior Pieter was training him, and today as a world marathon star he remains unchanged, indisputably himself.

In the same row of houses you can find Gregory Konchellah when he visits Iten. He is the son of Billy Konchellah, and you can find John Litei, a Maasai world-class 800m runner like Gregory. Sylvia slips into the group and shouts back, "*Kwambai uii,*" calling to Irene, her regular training partner, to join us. Irene waves, but does not join the group; this morning she wants to run alone.

We swiftly pass Choge and Songok. They are jogging very slowly, merely warming up the body for a heart thumping session of fartlek when they will be straining to keep in front of Brother Colm's white Subaru. Colm, an Irish priest, has lived in Iten for thirty years. He drives his car over the dirt roads plucking up athletes for training, and following them in his car during training sessions, all for the goodness of helping others. If ever a man embodied the term "for the love of the sport," it is Colm.

I swear Choge and Songok are running nine-minute miles. Both men have run under thirteen minutes for the 5000m, their specialty distance in the past year. I look at Songok's new Adidas shoes and recall stories he told me of running barefoot and how his first pair of shoes had come from a friend of his called Lagat, none other than Bernard, who is the second-fastest man in history over the metric mile and has helped a number of Kenyans with his winnings. Choge nods his head in a friendly manner as we go by.

We now come to a Y junction. A week ago I had run to the right with Lornah and, following her light footsteps over a path, had sunk into deep mud. It pays to be a lightweight on the Kenyan trails. She told me to run in her footsteps, which I did, but she hadn't accounted for me weighing 30 pounds more than she does. Today we choose the left road. Both lead to the same place. The loop can be a good 2K interval route; Pieter has christened it the coffee loop. You can often find James Koskei running this loop, as his farm is close by.

Running on this red dirt, I never feel the aches and pains in my hips that I normally do when running back home. You have a floating sensation that invites the body to run farther more miles, more training. Silently we pass Cheboiboch's house. I wonder if his wife Rebecca is boiling eggs, as she likes to do in the morning hours. She is a schoolteacher, but not at the Salaba Academy. Running up the hill, I notice that the Kenyans are running *over* the ground, not *into* it, as I feel my legs are forced to do. Hilda's legs barely seem to touch the ground before she lifts her foot for another light step. It is a series of heel flicks.

Last night, at the Midlands Café, owned by the Counselor of Iten, Julius Kiprop, who is the field manager of the Shoe4Africa races, Marcel Hooiveld of Holland talked about the Kenyans' biomechanics when they run. An engineer by trade, Marcel had noted that the Kenyan heel lift was naturally higher than the Western runners' lift. He reasoned with graphs, diagrams and numbers, that it was a significant part of why the Kenyan running style is so efficient. Having run behind a vast number of Kenyans, I can attest to this biomechanical feature of their stride, but I do not know how I would explain it.

I look around and am pleased to see that people are breaking a sweat, though on reflection it probably has more to do with the sun which has now warmed the morning— and everyone, except me, is covered in layers. A long time ago I visited Paul Bitok, at a time when he had won the first of his two Olympic silver medals in the 5000m. I went to Lessos, near his home village of Kilibwoni. I fell asleep under a tree, the sun moved, and it caused a big blister on my heal that burst. In short, it was extremely hot. Bitok wore two complete tracksuits to go for the run, those on top of a long-sleeved T-shirt. "Don't think I am cold, my friend. This is the Kenyan way, so we sweat and it is hard for training. I am suffering in all these clothes!" He smiled with relish. "And then when the race comes, you throw off the heavy suits and you fly."

A similar method was used by Joseph Nzau who would run in size-13 shoes saying, "Imagine how light my feet feel when I climb into the race shoes!" Nzau typically wears a U.S. size 8-1/2. Although the outcome does not always match the desire, knowing these stories of trying one's hardest to suffer in training makes me understand better the success of Kenyan runners.

We swing to the right, and to our sides the scrub bush is fertile and emerald-green. A group of barefoot children suddenly come running from a mud hut across the field, and even from a distance their high-pitched screams of "Mzungo, Mzungo, how are you, how are you?" can be heard. None of these round, single-roomed constructions has gas or electricity. TVs are as scarce as hen's teeth in the rural country, and a passing foreigner is free entertainment, and the big event of the morning. Although Iten now has a consistent influx of foreigners training on its roads year round, the yells are far more popular than they were a dozen years ago, when a *mzungo* was rarely seen.

Looking only as tall as grasshoppers, the children navigate the overgrown field faster than we are running on the beaten path, despite dodging and hurdling giant clods of ploughed earth. Their thin sparrow's legs, so strong, yet without any trace of defined muscle, make a mockery of the general Western conception that weight training alone builds powerful legs. One boy, who leads the others, hurdles the old wooden fence, albeit at its lowest broken point, with the grace of a thoroughbred and comes chasing after us, catching us without breaking a sweat. Hilda says something to the boy in Kalenjin, and he beams and starts running alongside.

When I lived in Sweden, a physiology study had been led in Kenya by Bengt Saltin. The researcher told me about a pre-teen who refused to be dropped on the morning runs and would always inquire, "What are we doing tomorrow? Can we do more?"

I am so glad to see the radiant sun; the pouring rain that fell in sheets has caused very difficult running conditions. Yesterday we had had to abandon a speed session and run easy distance instead on the all-weather road; even that was a challenge, as we found ourselves skating over slick mud. We pass to our left yet another running camp, this one owned by a runner who now represents Qatar, James Kwalia, who is, however, generously supporting a group of runners from Mt. Elgon who will be tomorrow's national heroes. I had been sitting talking to him about how ironic it was that he finally now had funds to be able to support this venture, albeit with dollars from Qatar. Felix Kibore is his latest protégé.

A sharp downhill dip, then we surge up Wilson Hill, and now I can hear labored breathing from some runners; not Doris, I am sure. Helena's head is tilted down toward the hill; there is a deep frown in her forehead that shades her hazel eyes. I wonder if she is thinking about her children; she has left them at her hometown of Kapenguria so she can concentrate fully on her athletics career. She told me it is not easy, but that there is no other way. A week later, she would receive a payment of 4,000 euros in cash for having finished second at the Amsterdam Marathon, a couple of months earlier. She would say, "Running is the way I can secure their future, and it is for them I must struggle each day."

We pass a small brick house to our right that was flooded in the heavy rains. Water swallows the doorstep, and the inner field is a bog of puddles. I read in the *Daily Nation* that the heavy floods in Kenya had played havoc in the slums, particularly in Nairobi's largest, Kibera. A huge mudslide had rendered thousands homeless. Why it is that often the poorest areas of the world are hit by nature's harshest assaults?

Kibera is a shantytown with a population of well over one million.
The rains washed away the ramshackle huts and left Kenya's poorest even poorer, if it is possible to have less than nothing.

The first time I came to Kenya, I met a friendly runner in N'gong called Titus Muturi. He pleaded that I visit his family. "We never get visitors from abroad. Once a white man promised to come and visit. We made tea, cooked chapattis, but he never showed up. My mother was so disappointed. She blamed me, of course, she said I must have said something to put him off coming." How could I refuse? I agreed to go and stay with Titus for a week and train in his area. Unlike every Kenyan, I did not know that Kibera was the largest slum in Africa. Put it down to insubstantial geography lessons.

In an area of roughly 800 acres, scores upon scores of cardboard and wooden huts, with corrugated iron roofs, are thatched together like domino hovels. Little muddy paths run between the shacks, strewn with litter, foul-smelling garbage, and lumps of human excrement. A stream of what looked like urine flowed down a muddy, hand-dug, six-inch deep canal to the left and right of most paths. That was the plumbing. Walking down the little paths, you constantly dodge and duck under the washing lines that add some color to the village.

Every few huts there is a hand-painted sign nailed to the door offering some kind of service, like Kibera Barbers, or the Happy Chapel, or Baba's Tea Shop. AIDS, cholera, and typhoid are all rampant, although I did not know this at the time. As you carefully try to walk while avoiding the sewage, mud, and filthy water, the rancid smell makes you feel nauseous and weak. Going into Titus's family home, probably 12-foot by 12-foot, I found a dark area reeking of paraffin oil. Old newspapers sufficed as wallpaper. For once, I gladly gulped in the fumes, trying to drown out the smell of human waste. The good news was that once inside, you were clear of the flying toilets! As no one had a latrine in Kibera, one would use a plastic bag, tie the bag, then throw it out of a window.

I have a vision of Shoe4Africa collecting shoes at the ING New York City Marathon, handing out flip-flops in return, at the finishing line, and for the city of New York, in one swoop, to significantly cut down the spread of disease in Kibera by shoeing the people. To see people walk barefoot through this mire churns the mind. Shoes would be a start to helping Kibera.

That night it rained as if a thousand storms had been loosed from the heavens. The noise of the rain falling on the tin roof sounded as though a Jamaican steel-drum band was in the hut. It made sleeping impossible—but, I noticed, not for the residents. I lay on a thin bare mattress with four other people, as two others had been parceled off to visit friends to make space for the visitor. I lay awake dreading the next night, and wondering how on earth people survived in this environment.

Nowadays I go to social benefits in America raising funds for Africa. The good thing about these parties is that you meet fascinating people, like George Bush's daughter, Barbara, who most kindly offered to collect running shoes for Shoe4Africa and has done volunteer work over in Africa. However, I find that many of these benefits overlook, or perhaps purposely convey wrongly, the disposition of African people. We sit there being informed about supposedly disheartened and dejected souls living in these appalling conditions. To the contrary, the majority of Kibera seemed in better mental health than Manhattan's pill-popping socialites.

As we climbed up Wilson Hill, I thought of the family at Kibera. Titus had never made it as a runner, as far as I knew. I had searched magazines and newspaper results for years afterward always hoping to see his name. I wondered if they were still in Kibera, as optimistic as I had found them a decade ago, owning so little, yet so happy and appreciative of little things in life that I never noticed. I decided that the next time I went to Nairobi I would try to locate Titus.

The hill is short but steep. When an Australian news crew came to film a documentary on Kenyan running prior to the Atlanta Olympics, they used this climb for filming the hill work. The reason was probably that you simply cannot run up this hill fast even if you try—no chance of blurring a frame. Sylvia defies the hill's grade, she pulls the group, and we are forced to follow. Her acceleration is honed by racing the Dibabas and the Defars of the world.

The agricultural field that we now run over is often the breaking point for the group, or at least it was when I used to run with the St. Patrick's team. Some runners feel strong after the hill and push, others relax, and breaks are often made—always without a word being said. The slight downhill entices the runner to open up the stride. A couple of days ago I had done this, and had encountered string of barbed wire that had fallen across the path. My only option was to gracefully slide into the wire as another guy slid into my back. Luckily, Jeroen Deen, a physiotherapist in Iten, is used to these things: "You have to be very careful in Kenya—something can turn up very quickly here." Deen oversees more athletes that he logistically can, and his are the hands behind many a fine Iten performance.

Having crossed the field, we come head-on to the Kiptabus road. We slide through the wooden turnstile, stride quickly over the dirt road and up a couple of steps over the bank to the next field on the other side of the road. We are on the banana route now. The group is forced to run in almost single file by wooden fences on our right and left, which keep the cattle at bay. The grass is thick and high, but we follow a single red dirt path that has been worn over time and we reach a wider road. I am running on the path behind Lornah. Her feet point out to the sides; it does not seem the perfect foot-strike to the naked eye; but her world record over ten miles is proof that her "Ngugiesque" style is pure efficiency. Ever since the 1960s when Kip Keino, despite gallbladder problems, and absurd numbers of qualifying rounds, contested three Olympic finals, Kenyans have known that they can run like the wind. They simply know it. The boy that runs with us today knows it. He runs free; he does not have any doubts.

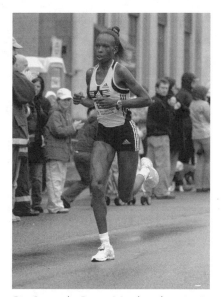

Rita Jeptoo, the Boston Marathon champion in 2006, here running to fourth place in 2007. (*Flanagan/PrettySporty*)

One day, not eager to walk the two kilometers to the Iten stage to catch the communal taxi to Eldoret, I asked a police officer if there was any way he could stop a car for me. I offered to buy him a soda. His thirst slaked, he walked into the middle of the road, stopped the first "nice" car that came along, and instructed the driver to take me to Eldoret.

I climbed into the comfortable car of a professor at the Moi University in Eldoret. His name eludes me today. I asked him why Kenyans are such good runners. "It is because we start life under attack, we fight for everything," he said. Nothing comes in Kenya unless you fight for it. We are born survivors; otherwise, we would not be here. When *you* run, then you do so for health, or as a serious hobby. When Kenyans run they are hunters, they are fighting, as they did from the first day that they realized life is a fight. That is the Kenyan secret."

We are now running well above a thin blue line of lucent mist that hovers over the rift valley. I am with a group of Kenyan hunters as we silently glide across valley and vale, on a quest to hunt for survival. The pace slowly starts to increase; I notice a faster leg turnover as we hit a larger road and turn right on Rita's Route.

You would take this road if you wanted to go to Rita Jeptoo's old place. The week before I had been running with Rita on this road, and somehow when she goes in this direction she always starts to fly.

The surface changes; this dirt road has many small loose stones on its surface. One stone immediately becomes lodged in the clef of my Mizuno shoe. I lurch forward like a giraffe with rigor mortis, whilst trying to kick the stone out on the run. Half the group at once says, "Sorry" for my fumble.

Their shadows are thin and long to the left; again, I notice the posture, how little core movement there is with the Kenyan runners. Inside Brother Colm's bungalow, on the left hand-wall when you walk in, he used to have a large collage of pictures—hundreds of running photographs stuck to the stone wall. There was one shot that always caught my eye. It was a black-and-white picture of four runners in a line; it was dark and the athletes were blacked-out silhouettes. Three gazelles, and one buffalo; one runner sat low in the hips and you could see he had a shortened stumpy stride with wooden-clog feet. "So you can spot the mzungo, eh?" joked Brother Colm. I think about this photo as I go galumphing along the road.

Now the shadows that run alongside the Kenyans ahead of me are dancing through the cornfields. The deeply rutted mud path, hardened and rougher than the usual paths in Iten, has been tortured by the tread of large agricultural tractors. I ponder Iten resident Michael Kapkiai. He invested in a couple of tractors after running well in the early 1990s. Michael was a brother to all, helping the up–and-comers. When injuries struck and the money slowed, the friends trickled away. Against all the odds Kapkiai, broke, was forced to attempt a comeback. As a 35-year-old, sporting numerous leg injuries, he won a few thousand dollars placing third at the Arizona Rock 'n' Roll Marathon in 2004. If ever there was a story about the power of the mind. . . anyway, seemingly everyone in Iten borrows Kapkiai's tractors now that they are working again.

We glide past a small *shamba*. There are three round mud huts, with a wooden-pole structure covered in a clay mud that becomes hardened in the sun. With a thatched roof that is surprisingly waterproof, as I found out when sleeping dry during a thunderstorm in Bomet town, the hut becomes habitable. The outer walls can be constructed in a day; the roof takes a bit longer. Although the inside room is small Kenyans like the feeling of togetherness. When I was renting a three-bedroom apartment in Lidingo, Sweden, Wilson Musto and Jacob Losian of Kapenguria came to stay for a series of races. I offered them a room each; they preferred to share one room. When another African arrived, I gave him the third room, and he instead moved into Musto's room. When I questioned Musto, he replied, "When you are alone there can be too much thinking. This is not good. When you are together worries cannot hurt you." Being a Kenyan runner seems to be a life-encompassing agenda.

Just a few circular huts with fencing around the ambit to contain a small amount of wandering livestock—I count three large black-and-white cows. Kalenjins love their milk. There is a hectare of cultivated maize. It looks oddly uniform in the pastoral setting. When you drive up to the Nandi Hills district and see the tea plantations, you see field upon field that are perfectly aligned; Iten is somewhat different. Our feet crunch over dry bamboo stalks. They have been laid over the path to make the muddy route, that has now dried, less treacherous. A cluster of jacaranda trees with indigo flowers vibrantly color and shade one of the huts. No voices come from within; we pass unnoticed except for a scruffy dog that comes jogging toward us. In Kenya dogs are not house pets; they are kept for security. As we run away from the *shamba* the dog, assured that there is no trouble, turns back.

There is a forgotten beauty that cradles rural Kenya, the purity of the calm and of the hush in a secure setting. People living without constant communications, in an environment free of the clutter of electronic noise and the twenty-four-hour availability that we have begun to crave in the Western world. A month earlier, I had been running with the governor of New York State, Eliot Spitzer, one of the busiest, hardest working men in America. As we ran around a reservoir with no company but the cherry trees, Eliot remarked, "I love running, because it is the one time of the day when I get away from the ringing phones." Eliot would love Kenya. When I was staying in Kapket with Joseph Chepkwony, we would have to run the telephone training loop if we ever wanted to make a phone call: 46 minutes in one direction to reach the nearest phone.

Lornah, or "the Simba," as we call her, is running free with her lengthened stride at the front of the group. Her ivory teeth flash as her head leans back slightly, reckoning with the body's acceleration. The whippet legs are majestic in their control, propelling her muscular 47 kilograms over the ground at speeds unmatched by any other woman in the world. It is an executive decision; the session has been changed and it is Simba time. Her quadriceps muscles ripple through her thin Lycra tights, processing the crisp Iten air and powering her size-40 Adidas shoes along the tractor route. I move to the far side of the path; I do not want to smear the shadow of these gazelles running in unison. I check on the form and note that, although the road is full of undulations, the pace and the stride of the Kenyan runners are ever consistent over these furrows. The runners are unaffected by nature's challenges. Then, as if in contradiction, one runner drops off the back of the pack, to waken me from my moment of daydreaming. I can just see a shadow pulling back; I do not turn my head to see who it is. You can be sure that the runner would never, ever call out to the group to slow, or to wait; that is not the Kenyan way.

We are climbing again, and as the sun is squinting over the horizon it is hard to see how long the hill will last. Deep breathing, rhythmic like African drumbeats, is now heard. The arm carriage of the runners now looks like a pack of boxers synchronized in ring practice. My mind shifts to Benson Masya, or rather to the spirit of Benson. The man who added a segment of "pushing the pace" to every training run. Masya was a former boxer; his father had whipped him when he started to run, telling him to concentrate instead on a "real" career. Masya had "the" running career. Even the day before a race, as when he won the City-Pier-City half-marathon in Holland in a few seconds over the hour, he would add some speed to the training run. The day before the race, thirty minutes of his prescribed jogging had turned into more than an hour, with the last twenty minutes run slightly slower than his perceived half-marathon race pace. So much for Bowerman's easy day, hard day theory. Who but a Kenyan would do a twenty-minute tempo run twenty-fours before an important race; then win it? Zablon Miano tagged along on that day, and ended up with a personal record of 1:00:50. Try to fully comprehend the Kenyan concept of running, and logic will betray you. Run with the Kenyan spirits, and you will succeed. When a Kenyan dies, people place the word "late" in front of the surname. Late Masya would have liked the run on this day.

We swing left now onto the Eldoret road. A dirt path runs parallel to the tarmac all the way from Iten to Eldoret. From post office to post office (as the distance between Kenyan towns is measured) is twenty miles. As legend has it, one day Brother Colm answered the door to José Manuel Abascal, who had ran from Eldoret to visit Colm. Later that year, Abascal won a bronze medal in the 1984 Olympics 1500m. I immediately decided that this would be a good challenge; the road winds from 2000m to 2440m— uphill all the way. The next day, early in the morning to avoid the hot sun and heat, Brother Colm and I set off for Eldoret in his car. The only problem was that Colm knows everyone and their dog in Kenya. We stopped seemingly each ten minutes to talk to people on the way. We finally arrived in Eldoret at nearly eleven a.m. The sun was perched on my shoulder, larger than life, when I set off. Purposely I had taken no money, so as not to be tempted to quit and take a taxi. As I set off I was already thirsty. Let me assure you, white people begging in Kenya are not taken seriously. I arrived in Iten just under two and a half hours later with a throat of sand and a skin that was scorched red and raw.

A quick crossing road and we are onto a route called the Jeruto Throughway. A large pond—collected from the rains—blocks the way. In perfect harmony, we all leave the path and stride up to run along the rim of a field avoiding the pond. A cactuslike plant called sisal, very common to the area, softly scratches my ankle as I brush past. The plant, like most, has its purpose in Kenya; it is used for making rope.

This twisting road, linking to the all-weather road, has one very flat stretch where runners like to do interval repeats, affectionately known as "flat stretch road." Iten was originally, called Hill Ten by the British settlers, referring to the topography. The Kenyans could not pronounce the "H" and the new name stuck. Another H, aka Hilda "Jepchumba Airlines" Kibet, is striking for home and has taken over from the Simba to push the pace. Hilda will get a world best soon for a road race, I just know it. At the camp a couple of nights earlier, all proudly watched a video of her beating world-champion Gete Wami and one of the Dibaba sisters.

This is not a race; the athletes are just taking turns pushing at the front of the pack. Mukche looks indifferent, he clears an enormous puddle with a single flick of ankle power; no wonder Kenyans are great steeplechase runners. Coincidentally we pass the home of Jeruto Kiptum, one of Kenya's best female steeplechasers. Jeruto is not at home; at least, her dark-blue car is missing. She is one of many athletes who train so hard some mornings that she returns to her home unable to eat breakfast for fatigue. When Anthony Edwards, the TV star who played Dr. Mark Greene on *ER*, came to visit Iten, I took him to Jeruto's home. I wanted to show Anthony the humility of one of the world's best athletes: how she lives in complete simplicity in a small two-roomed converted wooden hut, no larger than an average European kitchen. We flash by Nancy Kiprop's home on our left. I look at Lornah and remember a story that can still bring a tear to my eye.

Nancy was an excellent athlete, a World Juniors silver medalist. When I lived in St. Patrick's she was part of the women's training group coached by Colm. She, Edna

Kiplagat, and Jebiwott Keitany, "the three sisters" as we called them, were a boost to every afternoon's post-run stretch; they were always laughing and full of fun. Nancy, after a stunning junior career, drifted out of the picture, yet her fellow alumnae went on to conquer the world. In time, Nancy's mother fell gravely ill. An operation was urgently needed and Nancy had no money. She vainly sought funds to help her mother. It was not a tremendous amount of money, but nobody would help. That is, until she knocked on the door of Lornah and Pieter's house. Neither woman knew the other, yet as Nancy opened her heart, Lornah opened her purse.

We saw Nancy stretching in her front yard; with her foot pulled up to her butt she grinned and waved as we passed. Victor, her young son, ran crying to Nancy, probably thinking her mother would leave him for another training run. We passed quickly and the child's cries dwindled. Today Nancy has resumed racing and had just returned from a successful trip to Europe.

Swing right. A short downhill stretch—I'm glad the end of run will soon be in sight. We soar past four wooden cabins to our right—they are general-store kiosks during the day, selling everything from hardware, to sodas to farm produce. The huts are simple, with a small serving hatch, half covered in wire mesh. It was huts like these that athletes like Robert Cheruiyot and Martin Lel used to work. Money is not a necessity in the heart of the Rift Valley; many of the poorer families trade maize or milk, for the non-locally-grown commodities like tea and sugar. Rose Cheruiyot, no relation to Robert, tells of how when she was a child, her family would go weeks without a shilling being seen in their hut.

A left turn and we are on the All-Weather road. This was christened because, when the heavy rains fall, it remains the most usable non-tarmac road in Iten.

The All-Weather road is wide; another group of runners comes toward us, their legs zipping up and down like the needles of sewing machines: seven men, six of whose faces are writhing in agony. The stupefying Stephen Cherono is putting a chariot of his teammates, like a Roman centurion on a battlefield, at a killing pace. Cherono's idiosyncratic gait, has given him ten of the eighteen fastest times ever run for the steeplechase. He was born and bred in the Iten district. A week earlier, sitting in Freddie's Café, leaning on the formica tables and drinking an orange Fanta soda, Stephen had talked about running: "There's no place better than here, it is no one thing, or two. You have to run here to understand it." I knew exactly what he meant.

The runners sweep past us; no word is spoken. I look across at the face of a runner; I think he is called Kenneth Kandir—a tall, strong-muscled man with a chestnut face. I see real pain and suffering in his eyelids, the wrinkles at his temples. This morning he is burning, and I think of the words that double world champion Benjamin Limo had said as I sat in the back of a pickup truck with him and Olympic champion Ezekiel Kemboi last year. We were following a race in Paul Tergat's hometown. "Don't bother going to your race unless you have dragged your body to the last inch of survival in the training runs." Kandir looked as if he was there, running on the very lip of Satan's grave.

We pass the turnoff to the famous Kamariny track. It is the equivalent of New York's Yankee Stadium, or London's Wembley Arena. Kamariny cannot be condensed into a phrase like "a field of dreams," or "a venue of champions"; it is a sacrosanct patch of ground that would probably not catch the eye of any passer-by. All the Kenyan success stories of this region have paid their dues at this field. It's a rough chewed-up oval of 440 yards (slightly over 400 meters) surrounded, for the most part, by wooden stadium seats that are more likely to give you splinters than comfort. This is the Mecca, the Holy Grail, the Holy Kingdom of the distance runner's performance; the stadium of all stadiums. If you can make it here, you can challenge the very gods. Name a famous local athlete, and there is a story about his, or her, deeds at Kamariny. Only yesterday, we had been talking of the day when a then-unknown, Raymond Yator, came from the bush to defeat Stephen Cherono here.

Luke Kipkosgei overtakes our group and powers ahead. He looks as though he is finishing up a tempo run. Kipkosgei once ran the Stockholm Games 5000m in the 1990s, and after the race I had asked him how he developed the speed that enabled him to accelerate mid-race and pull away dramatically from the rest of the field. He told me that the secret of running, for him, was to be in shape to compete at the distance below your main event. Thus, in this instance, when we raced the 5000m, he was training with 1500m runners back in Kenya. His long stride is eating up the ground, thin knees leading the way to power his feet, which bounce off the road, and there is hardly an ounce of fat on his entire frame.

Another hill approaches and we to stride up; again the flamingo-like legs gobble up the meline. The Simba has re-taken control. Mukche is running just behind Lornah on her shoulder, with Sleepy Sylvia Kibet by his side. Sylvia's, undisturbed smooth steps remind me of a leopard padding through the bush. We call her Sleepy because once, during an interval session, it was her turn to lead the group up a steep 15-second uphill sprint. Hilda yelled "Go," and Sylvia set off as though she was running a marathon, forgetting the length of the interval. The group could not stop laughing, and the nickname stuck. Sylvia has one of those typical unbelievable Kenyan stories, the kind of story that even if you lived through it, still leaves you shaking your head. A runner does not start a comeback after nearly a year's layoff with goals of making the *Kenyan national team* and medaling in a major championship. Meet Sleepy Sylvia, 2006–07 African Games and Championship medalist and 2008 Olympian, finishing one place from a medal.

Doris, as is her custom, runs just behind Lornah, still seeming not to breathe. Her hip swing looks like those momentum balls that used to be popular on people's desks in the 1980s. No discernible effort can be seen. It is the exact same laissez-faire motion I saw when running in Albuquerque with Josiah Thugwane of South Africa who won the 1996 Olympic gold marathon. The only other person I can think of with this style is the legendary Khalid Khannouchi. Doris has the same liquid style as these two men. I begin wondering, how fast Doris could run a marathon. Pieter thinks she has more potential than Lornah, and watching her sashay over the dirt road, I can believe it. I hope the Simba is not reading my thoughts.

To the left is the house of Judith Kiplimo and Christopher Kandie, two typical Iten residents, she a 2:28 marathon runner and he a 2:08 marathoner but perhaps best known

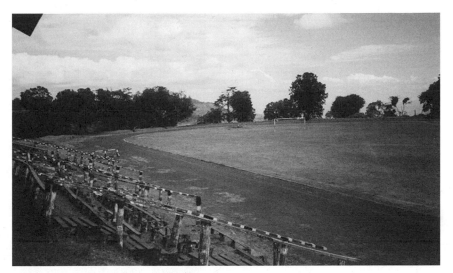

The famous Kamariny running track. (*Author*)

for pacing Paula Radcliffe to her out-of-this-world marathon record of 2:15:25. A year after that record, I spoke with Christopher about the day. From his birds-eye view, he rated Radcliffe's record-breaking run as more than astonishing: "She was fighting from many miles out. I was really wondering if she could sustain the effort, but she did. She is a fine lady."

Into the last 100 meters, everyone slows to a walk. There is no bravado of trying to win workouts in Kenya. Training is a true group effort: individuality pales because unity shines. We come to a complete stop and I am surprised to see that the group is about thirteen runners. Lornah invites all for a cup of tea at her camp; she and Pieter feed and support nearly everyone with fast-moving feet in the Kamariny district.

"Starbucks" is sitting in the Land Rover's front seat, the *Daily Nation* newspaper with an Elias Makori story open on the dashboard. He is holding a clipboard and a steaming cup of his favorite coffee, writing the schedules for the ensuing days. A whisker away from the 1984 Dutch Olympic team, several times an Ironman finisher, and fit enough to run a marathon on any given day of the week, he is the unofficial Mayor of Iten. He modestly dismisses his coaching talents (and any compliment you pay him), yet his athletes disagree. "Pieter is why I am here [running well] today," says Helena. "He is somehow making me run like a. . ." she pauses, looking for a word, then grins like a clown and shouts out laughing, "A Lion!" Lowering the coffee cup, Starbucks adds, "Well, that and the magic of Iten." It is another training run finished. One more paving stone is laid in the never-ending journey. In a sport of few or no guarantees, there is no time for standing still; the chances are out there, and they must be taken on the run.

Most of the runners now walk toward the camp. Doris, however, has turned and is adding some strides to the morning's program. She looks down the road with big russet eyes; her fingers are twitching. She drops her shoulders and I notice she is finally breathing. Then as I look in her direction, magically she is gone, like a dart to a target. One more time down the road, working toward becoming the person she wishes to be. The last glance I saw her take was over her shoulder at Lornah. The Simba does not notice; instead she lifts her arms and stretches like a newly woken wildcat. She removes her shades and uses her T-shirt to clean the sweat off the lenses. She is training for the World Cross Country Championships, which will be held in her home country for the first time in history. "It will be the cross country of all cross countrys. I am asking God, if I can win just once, then let it be in Mombasa. For this I am sweating today." Nothing comes easy in life, though somehow, the running in Kenya is its own reward.

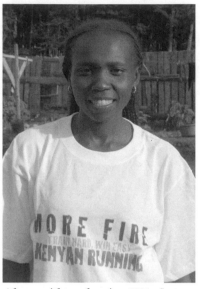

After qualifying for the 2008 Summer Olympics, Sylvia Kibet said, "I ran with More Fire! I was thinking, More Fire! (*Author*)

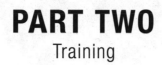

PART TWO
Training

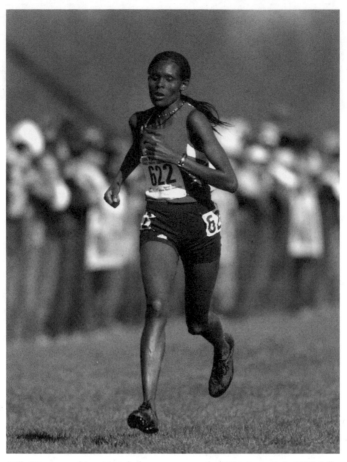

Sally Kipyego, at this writing, the hottest name on the NCAA circuit. In 2006, Sally Kipyego, of Texas Tech, won the NCAA Cross Country Championships, becoming the first Kenyan woman to win an individual NCAA title. Has she opened the floodgates? Only time will tell. In 2007, at the NCAA Indoor Championships, she took both the 5000m and the 3000m crowns. At the outdoor championships, she won the 10,000m. In her outdoor track opener, she ran a collegiate 10,000m record of 31:56.72 at Stanford University. Kipyego's roommate at Texas Tech is Chepleting Boit, daughter of Mike Boit. By the summer of 2008, she had won seven NCAA Division 1 titles, a year in which she set a personal record of 31:25:45 for the 10,000m. (*Parker Morse*)

Training Scenes

Believe. If you believe you can do it, you can.

The Moi Air Base residential training camp came to life for the second time that day. A shrill whistle pierced the hot late-morning air, calling the runners, who had been relaxing for about 2-1/2 hours since their early-morning run, to assemble before Coach Danny Kibet.

Runners dressed in an assortment of sun-bleached athletic attire drag their fatigued limbs toward Kibet, the resident camp coach, who stands stoically on the exit road. "Is anybody suffering from injuries today?" he barks. There is stony silence from the gathering of some athletes. Apparently everyone is in fighting trim despite the protestations of aches and pains that had been bandied about by the breakfasting runners—or at least no one wished to own up to any weakness or fallibility. "Okay, then, I want an hour run. Start off easy, especially on the tarmac. You can speed up a bit when you reach the dirt road. Off you go. Remember, easy at the start!" Kibet's words trail off as the large pack stumbles stiffly along the road at a pace barely above walking speed.

After the first corner is passed, the runners feel the soft red dirt road underfoot and the group steps up to a steady but not uncomfortable pace. One runner bursts from the pack and opens up an instant gap of more than 50 meters. No one comments. No one follows.

The route drops headlong into the basin of the Rift Valley, the heat intensifying as the runners descend. By the roadside, children interrupt their games to watch the large contingent of runners, who are continuing to accelerate. The breakaway leader boomerangs back to the assembly, which includes several world-class runners.
Stride length increases due to the continuing descent and the tight formation of the pack begins to rupture. A giraffe cranes his neck around to check out the approaching multitude, then idly returns to the tree he is lunching on. A small boy clothed in black rags and dust sprints to try to join the pack—he manages about ten dancing strides before abandoning his moment of glory.

After forty-five minutes, one of the leaders shouts out a command, causing the runners to skid to a halt and turn about. As they double back, the slower runners are rewarded with the opportunity to rejoin the pack. It doesn't take long for the pace to be restored to an intense level. Nearly everyone is breathing with the effort, beads of sweat spraying like raindrops.

The hellish climb back up the seemingly vertical Rift Valley wall approaches. There is no respite in pace, no allowance for the gradient. About half a dozen runners now govern the group, which is now well strung out.

Simon Chemoiywo, fresh from a sizzling performance in Brazil, is constantly pushing the boundaries of speed endurance. His expression is blank, his focus undivided. On his shoulder, stride for stride, are others quite willing to take on the leadership role should the pace diminish an iota. The scarcity of oxygen at this altitude is now becoming severely apparent, as the runners battle against the incline and the heat.

Round each bend another steep grade appears, the summit still hidden from view. Paul Tergat's actually looks like he's enjoying himself. Perhaps he is the only one not laboring in breath and muscle fatigue.

Finally the road planes out and the military compound can be seen. The tempo gently decreases as the runners float one by one into the encampment and past Coach Kibet.

Afterward, some athletes do some stretching, others chat. No one has much interest in more energy-sapping exercises. Tea is made, hot and sweet, and all seek refreshment. For most of the runners, today's principal session was run at competition-level intensity—the prize being the chance to do it all again the following day!

Perhaps the hardships of life take away the comforts of dreams. The Kenyans I observed do not sit around waiting for a lucky break or a miraculous transformation of athletic form. They believe in the input-equal-output ratio.

"Hard training is our secret." Ismael Kirui says, echoing the feeling of most Kenyan athletes. "Kenyans rely on training long hours and running over the hills," says Brother Colm.

"I was so happy to see my cousin [Susan Sirma] doing well and earning good money. I said to myself, 'One day I must be like her,'" says Sally Barsosio, explaining why she had begun hard training.

These runners simply believe that through hard work they will succeed at the highest of levels. William Kiprono, who has yet to travel outside Kenya, has been training and racing for many years. He won the Army steeplechase and finished second in the 10,000m on consecutive days in 1996 (against such notable runners as William Mutwol and Ondoro Osoro), and eleven years later he remains optimistic, hoping that one day he'll get a passport and a plane ticket to Europe. "I know I will win if I race in Europe," William says with an almost religious conviction. Year after year, teams are selected and he has remained behind. When asked why, against the odds, he continues to train, William answers, "I know I will make it with hard training."

Brother Colm points this out as a major factor. "They run hard because they love to run hard; they enjoy the practice and have great levels of perseverance. Life itself is hard in Kenya." The possibilities of financial reward and a ticket to Europe are definitely on their minds, but without the enjoyment and ability to endure long, hard training, there wouldn't be anything close to the legions of runners Kenya has supplied to the highest levels of world distance running.

Training in the Schools

Four of the most successful secondary schools—athletics-wise—are St. Patrick's, Singore, Kipsoen and Kapkenda. Each of the four is a boarding school. (These students, therefore, do not run a dozen miles to school and back, contrary to what Westerners have been led to believe.)

Physical exercise in Kenyan secondary schools is seen as an important factor in a child's upbringing. Thirty kilometers from Eldoret, there is a small girls' high school. Sing'ore Girls' is home to some 400 boarding students. Each afternoon, one hour is set aside for sport and conditioning. Hockey, running, and basketball are three sports commonly practiced. On Sunday, the girls are free to do as they like, but most of them choose to spend an hour at their favorite sport. When I visited, a group of girls who had planned a basketball game began by warming up with twenty minutes of vigorous running at various tempos before taking to the court—a sure sign of good teaching and a natural love for exercise!

Shortly after 6:00 each morning, a group of girls leaves the school's gates for a morning training run, many barefoot or wearing "everyday" shoes. They return before 7:00 to wash and eat breakfast before the day's regular schedule begins.

This "system" has produced astonishing results. In 1991, four girls from this school placed first, second, sixth, and ninth at the World Cross Country Championships for junior women, capturing the team title. Sally Barsosio who won the World Junior Cross Country title in 1994, is another Sing'ore prodigy. As you can seen in the statistical chapter, Kenyan junior women have won the world team title seven out of the eight years since this Championships division was introduced, so it's not just Sing'ore Girls' School that is turning out outstanding runners.

The schools in Kenya are well aware of the potential rewards and prestige involved with running, and training is encouraged. At Kipsoen Secondary School, the girls who are training have their own dormitory. Nancy Kiprop, fourth at the 1996 World Cross Country Championships (and third in 1995), points out the advantages. "We are not disturbed here, and we don't disturb others when we rise early for our training each day before school hours." Roommate and fellow World Cross Country medalist Jebiwott Keitany is quick to add that they receive no special privileges, with no leniency for time away from studies: "If we are late to classes, we will be punished like any other student." The young athletes motivate one another and are all present at each morning's run. Advised by Brother Colm, the girls train twice a day, before and after school hours. Tempo runs and hill repeats are on the menu nearly every day.

The runners at St. Patrick's High School have it a little easier, according to Martin Pepela, a student in Form Three. "Kwambai [one of the school's top runners] doesn't come to a lot of our lectures. He is usually relaxing, staying in bed." (Charles Kwambai eventually left school without graduating, in part because of his unwillingness to comply with the common school rules.)

The headmaster of St. Patrick's, Elijah Komen, is very proud of his runners: "The name of St. Patrick's is known throughout the world as the finest running school." In the 1995 African Junior Championships, two St. Patrick's students, Kwambai and Japheth Kimutai, captured gold medals at all distances from 800m to 10,000m, and their schoolmates took most of the silvers as well! The school record book is more like that of a large nation, not of a school in a small village. Take, for instance, 1:44 for the 800m! "At one time we had four sub-four-minute milers at the school at the same time," proudly smiles

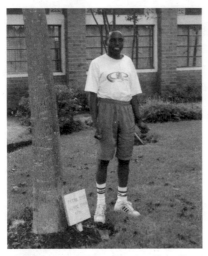

1988 Olympic 1500m champion Peter Rono standing by a Nandi flame tree planted in his honor at St. Patrick's School. (*Author*)

Brother Colm. This is not just dominance—it's another planet!

Growing in the central square of the St. Patrick's High School grounds is a thriving Nandi flame tree, planted in honor of Peter Rono's Olympic victory in the 1988 Olympic 1500m. A couple of meters away is the "Birir bush," another Olympic gold-medal commemoration (Matthew Birir, 1992 Olympic steeplechase). All students regularly pass this small garden of intentional inspiration. "So many great runners have been to this school—when you train with the runners here, you know that with hard work, you too can become a champion. Being at this school, you know it is possible," says one of the school's current middle-distance stars.

It's not just the secondary schools that are infused with a running ethic. As part of the induction course into the Tambach Teachers Training College, all students must be involved in a period of running training. "One of the days we had to run up and down a steep hill. It was very hard, as I hadn't run for many, many years," recalled one student. Running is indeed a part of growing up in Kenya.

The Ups and Downs of Hard Training

The typical running training in Kenya does not suit everyone. There are many runners who find the workload too hard to handle. Coach Elijah Langat of the Air Force says, "You have to be invited to join the military training camps. Sometimes runners come and after a few days of our training, they sneak out and go home in the night, finding it too tough." There is no idle chatter or fooling around during the training sessions. All the effort and concentration is geared toward running. Even at modest speeds, silence and seriousness are the norm.

Some Westerners believe that the Kenyans train too hard. The proof, they think, can be seen in the fact that Kenyans only last a season or two on the elite world circuit, with new runners quickly replacing the old. I don't believe it's quite this simple, however. There are so many good runners in Kenya that it is definitely a problem to remain at the top. It's rare that one athlete will win a series of races in Kenya; it is much more common to have fluctuating results, because of the incredibly high quality of the competition. That's one reason that elite runners sometimes do not perform well at a national trials competition and are left off the team (Daniel Komen in 1996 is a case in point).

Take also the case of John Ngugi. Although a five-time World Cross Country champion and a 1988 Olympic gold medalist, Ngugi never won a major Kenyan competition after 1987. One year he was 76th in the national cross country championships prior to winning the world championship. He wouldn't have made it out of Kenya that year if it hadn't been for his legendary status. Ismael Kirui could not make the podium at the Armed Forces Championships in the 5000m in 1995, and he just scraped onto the national team for that year's World Championships, which he won.

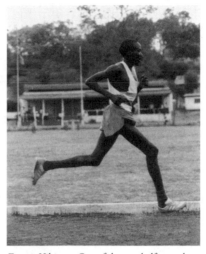

Francis Kibiwott. One of the new half marathon stars of Kenya running 59:26 In Berlin 2007 yet to be selected for a major championship. (*Martijn Venhuizen*)

To succeed in Kenyan athletics is incredibly tough. To remain at the top takes superhuman efforts. "They complained that we were training too hard. Kenyans would never complain." So spoke the great Moses Kiptanui about a group from the British national squad who came to train in Kenya. Kiptanui, the world's first sub-eight-minute steeplechaser, leads a training group in Nyahururu. Among his athletes was Daniel Komen, who broke the world 2-mile and 3000m records in 1996.

Kiptanui trained three times a day—an early-morning run of about 40 minutes at 6:00 a.m.; a quality session, often intervals, at 10:00 a.m., and a long easy run in the late afternoon. The Britons, however, should have visited a couple of years earlier when the amazing Kiptanui was logging four sessions a day. "I got up early and ran 10 kilometers, then before lunch I ran intervals on the track. In the afternoon there was hill training and in the evening a distance run." It's not much of an exaggeration to say that the effort many Kenyan athletes put in daily is similar to a week's worth of effort expenditure for the average American or European club runner.

Throughout the year, various competitions are organized around the country. It is not uncommon to see a world champion trailing the field. Kenyan athletes at home use competitions differently than do Westerners.

Prizes for competitions are usually of little value, so races are seen more as means to test fitness and progress. Ismael Kirui, after finishing third in a small 10K race in 29:46, explains, "Today was just speed work, that's all." Kirui echoes the thoughts of his brother, Richard Chelimo, that in the training period, you train. Placement in races is unimportant.

The Kenyans' race-completion percentage must be among the lowest in the world. Many Kenyans test themselves by starting at full speed, regardless of distance, and drop out as they reach exhaustion.

The Varieties of Training

In-Season Training

Once the period of hard base training is over, the great migration begins; the Kenyans hit the racing scene all over the world. Often the workload is reduced. Richard Chelimo, after arriving Europe, would run intervals reduced in both quantity and quality. "Once you have the form, it is very easy to ruin the shape with too much training," said Chelimo. Benson Koech is very careful to monitor his form. "If you train too hard, the season can be ruined; you must rest and begin the buildup again." Wilson Musto trains in Kenya for a few months, then flies over to Germany when he feels in form. When in Europe he races most weekends and runs just one session per week. An example of Musto's in-season routine from the 1996 campaign is shown below:

April	18	67 mins easy jogging
	19	57 mins easy jogging
	20	Travel to Holland
	21	40 mins easy
	22	60 mins easy
	23	51 mins easy with some sprints
	24	Same as the 23rd
	25	52 mins easy, 6x100m sprints
	26	44 mins easy
	27	Rest day
	28	Rotterdam Marathon. Pacemaker till 30K, with splits of 10K—30:27, 15K—45:28, 21.1K—65:27 & 30K—1:32:57
	29	Rest
	30	60 mins easy
May	1	45 mins easy
	2	56 mins easy
	3	Travel to Sweden, 46 mins easy
	4	47 mins easy
	5	Cross country race, 2nd. "Still tired from Rotterdam!"
	6	43 mins easy/46 mins normal
	7	45 mins normal/45 mins normal

Interval Training

Despite running fewer sessions, intervals or otherwise, on a conventional running track than do most international elite runners, the Kenyan men are world leaders on the track from 1500m to 10,000m. The percentage of Kenyans in the world's top ten performer list for 2006 demonstrates the fact: 1500m: 40%; 3000m: 60%; steeplechase: 50%; 5000m: 50%; 10,000m: 60%.

Formatted interval sessions are usually embarked upon after the cross country season is over, in April. Many of the rural runners do not run intervals at all. However, most of the runners in organized training groups, or in areas densely populated with runners, do run intervals. For the middle-distance runner, the distances are usually between 400m and 2000m. The number of repetitions is rarely decided until the day of training; even then the runner often will add more repeats if he feels the body has not been sufficiently exhausted.

A typical session for the Armed Forces team would be 20 x 400m at goal pace of 60–61 seconds with 200m jog rests. The marathon runners would increase the number of repeats, aiming for a 12K total of intervals, and slow the tempo by a second or two. A typical session will see a lot of runners burning themselves out in the first few intervals and barely running the last few. Some appear to attack the session with no forethought as to self-preservation, especially the runners who have not made it onto the international circuit.

Mark Wendot Yatich has a typical approach. "I ran three times a day every day except on Sundays. I never ran intervals, just fast runs and steady runs. After winning a road race, I came to the Air Force training camp. It was only then that I began with other kinds of training." This simple holistic attitude is perhaps one of the Kenyans' greatest assets, along with the ability to push their bodies past pain barriers and close to exhaustion. "Interval training is not always necessary in Kenya, as the runners reach the same intensity of work when out on a tempo distance run," noted Navy coach Danny Kibet. "You could go to the track at 10 o'clock in the morning and [Peter] Koech would be there running intervals; three hours later he would still be doing them. When he got too tired, he'd temporarily rest at the side of the track before resuming."

Intervals often are run on the red dirt roads of the Kenyan countryside. There are not many athletic tracks in the land, but this does not stop the Kenyans from being the world's best middle/long distance track runners! The tracks that are available are usually comparable to cow fields in smoothness and surfaced with cinders. "Intervals on the dirt roads help build up immense strength," notes Coach Mike Kosgei. "After running intervals on the tracks of Kenya I know I can fly round the tracks in Europe," Richard Chelimo pointed out.

The 1970s style of interval running seems to be the most popular form in Kenya, the runners recording huge amounts of intervals, working the rest period with a short jog. Moses Kiptanui, and Yobes Ondieki are famed in Kenya for their tough interval sessions. "Yobes could go out in the morning and run a hard track session, then run another hard track session in the afternoon!" remembers Patrick Sang. "Moses trains similarly; I had to take a week's rest after training with him!"

Spending an hour or more continually running intervals was not uncommon for these runners. Kirwa Tanui, an 8:20+ steeplechaser at altitude, explains: "Sometimes when we are training in a group no one wants to say this is the last interval, so we all wait for each other. Consequently the session goes on and on!"

Often if an athlete feels that he has hit good form on Kenyan soil, he will reduce the intervals and concentrate on steady runs of around 60 minutes in the forest instead.

"Peaking is an art; that is where we can help," says Coach Albert Masai of the Navy team. "The intervals must be planned, reducing in quantity as the main race period arrives." Here is a typical middle-distance schedule the week before the Armed Forces Track Championships, the major event for the Armed Forces men:

Saturday	6 AM	Easy 40 min. jog
	10 AM	Long intervals, 8 x 800m.
		Full recovery, run at 5000m race pace
Sunday	Rest day	
Monday	6 AM	Easy 40 min. jog
	10 AM	40 min. steady run in the forest
Tueday	6 AM	Easy 40-60 min.
	10 AM	5 x 400m, sub-60 sec., with 1 min. jog rest
		[a light session for the Kenyans!]
Wednesday	6 AM	Easy 40 min.
	10 AM	Cross country run over one hour, steady tempo
Thursday	6 AM	Easy 40 min.
	10 AM	Light 200m intervals, "stretching the legs!"
Friday	6 AM	40 min. "easy, easy!"
		Travel to competition
Saturday	Race day	

Note just two sessions per day at the most! Kenyans do taper! Of course, extra stretching and relaxing figure highly in the final days.

Tempo Training

Tempo training—runs of between 45 and 70 minutes at speeds close to racing efforts is by far the most popular form of training in Kenya. Before many tempo runs, the coaches will ask the runners to run at a predetermined pace: steady, moderately fast, or flat-out. However after twenty minutes someone usually starts to push the pace, and then another wants to lead. Inevitably, 90 percent of group training turns out to be a mini-competition at top speed. Even when a hard competition is within the next couple of days, the runners seem unable to contain their natural competitiveness. As the runners fly back to the camp at speeds blatantly contradicting the coaches' wishes, there are never reprimands; quite the opposite! The reasoning is explained by sub-28:00 10,000m runner Julius Ondieki. "Tempo running is practicing the pain we will face in competition; who wants to run slow in competition?"

As many as five sessions of this type of training can be undertaken during a week. A common form of tempo running has the runners start off fairly slowly, picking up the pace until the halfway mark, when the run becomes full-speed-ahead. As the runners typically are in a good-sized group, the pace never drops; each runner serves a spell at the front of the pack and pushes a little before the next takes over, not unlike cycling races. Simeon Rono, a member of the national cross country squad, points out that runners rarely win race after race because when a runner wins a race in Kenya he is usually training in one of the aforementioned groups. Thus, the other runners know they can stay with his pace. Back to the "belief" theme again.

The tempo runs tend to be over hilly routes, often with a speed injection at the start of the hill, underlining the competitiveness of the session. The red dirt roads provide a forgiving surface that allows the legs to cope with the endless miles. The tempo session is also undertaken by injured athletes. Whereas a runner may rest from an interval session, or a hill run, most of the runners participate in the tempo run. "You can begin slowly and in a little pain and as the pace heats up the hurting disappears as you concentrate on keeping up," says Haron Kerio of the Air Force team.

Interestingly enough, the runners who are often in the front of the pack on such training runs often become the "new" Kenyans to break through. This was true of Chelimo, Kirui, and Tergat. This form of training brings out the best in the strong individual runner but can be a nightmare to untrained or out-of-form athletes, though it will soon bring them back to form. "Runners in Europe were surprised how quickly I came back into form after a long injury time. This kind of training [tempo] really pulls you back into shape. There are no races in Europe as hard as the tempo runs here!" half-jokes Olympic champion Julius Korir.

Fartlek is also a very popular system of training in Kenya. The reflection of the philosophy to push hard when feeling strong brings out the strengths of fartlek. A fartlek run can be turned into a tempo run if the runner is so inclined—this kind of improvisation suits the Kenyans. Structured fartlek, such as a session of two minutes hard with one minute steady for 10K, are likewise used. William Sigei employs this method. In the training camps fartlek is utilized as a transition from cross country to track training.

The Long Run

Most runners from the middle distances upward do a long run once a week. The distance covered varies greatly. Benson Koech, a middle-distance man, may cover 20K, and Michael Kapkiai, a marathoner, up to four hours. The speeds also vary. Some believe in fast-paced distance, others in slow. Moses Tanui likes to run his distance at a steady pace with a fast five kilometers to finish off the run. Patrick Sang likes to run at an honest tempo from start to finish. The Armed Forces long runs often begin ,a pleasant rambling pace only to end up like a cavalry charge—all-out to the finish.

It is very rare to see Kenyans drinking on their long runs. They generally wait until the conclusion of the run before hydrating with Kenyan *chai* (tea). Due to the relatively low humidity, the runner does not lose as much fluid as, say, in New York at similar temperature.

Distances are irrelevant. The Kenyans run chiefly for time. The rural terrain typical of the Rift Valley is quite suited to prolonging or curtailing training sessions. During one training run in his hometown, Kirwa Tanui was asked how much more distance had to be covered before the training run was completed. "Oh, about two kilometers," smiled the steeplechaser. After fifteen more minutes of strongly-paced running, Kirwa was again asked. "About two kilometers!" was the sincere reply.

Hill Work

The Kenyans place great faith in hill work. To this Westerner's eyes, they appear to float, rather than labor, uphill with the greatest of ease and grace.

Much of Kenya's highlands is, of course, very hilly. More likely than not, one will encounter a few hills on any training run. These hills can ascend for miles and miles. Mix in the thin air and the heat and one gets a demanding session! In the organized training groups, there is usually a hill session once a week or more often. These tend to vary between the short-interval type, in which the runners will run up and down the same hill a number of times, and the long drag—a hill which can be up to 25K long.

Mike Kosgei, the former national coach, favors a very steep 200m hill, with a dirt surface to allow the runner to drive hard up the hill. "I like the seniors to run at least twenty-five repeats, the juniors twenty times, the women twenty, and the girls fifteen. When they reach the top there is no rest; turn and stride back down for the next repeat. This is a very tough session and the athlete should be rested before attempting it."

The Armed Forces camp uses a mountainside, the route taking twenty-seven minutes to climb when run at a good clip. The cross country runners ascend once, the marathoners return for a second effort. Moses Tanui drives twice a week to a gravel road where he starts his hill session at 1300m of altitude. The road relentlessly winds upward to 2700m in 20 kilometers. Tanui runs solo up this hill with his Toyota Land cruiser driven behind him. "It takes around one hour, thirty minutes," he says.

Up in the Nandi Hills near Kapsabet is a long, winding tarmac road over a similar distance. Here Patrick Sang returns each year a few times to fine-tune his winter buildup. "All the greats have run this hill. Ibrahim Hussein often ran up this hill; his house is at the top. Kip Keino used to run here, and Henry Rono ran his long run up this hill," remembers Sang's driver, a former national class runner himself.

Rest and Recovery

A major topic among running coaches is how to successfully balance recovery and hard training. Some athletes, like Rob de Castella of Australia, for instance, trained year-round; others, such as Great Britain's Steve Ovett, took a yearly break from training.

The Kenyan system works around the cycle of resting the body, building up, racing, and resting again. It is not uncommon for athletes to take breaks of three months or longer each year. Nearly every Kenyan athlete rests starting the month of October, with most not resuming training until December or January. Moses Kiptanui, who trained at superhuman intensities, always took a two-month break after the season to recharge his batteries. 800m runner Nixon Kiprotich took this opportunity to relax, put on a few pounds, and catch up on the family life he had missed spending the summer on the European circuit. Patrick Sang took the time for a family holiday before burying himself in the business he had been forced to neglect while abroad.

Be it for just relaxing, business, or family, this break is important to the athletes. Chelimo explained, "Training is time-consuming to us; when we train it takes all our time, a very intense period. Then we go over to Europe, traveling from race to race. When we return to Kenya we need to get back the energy." Cosmas Ndeti was another athlete who believed in taking long breaks. "The marathon recovery cannot be hurried; I like to eat well and spend time with my children, and then begin a hard buildup," said the three-time Boston champion.

Resuming full training, the athletes seem to return to form with incredible ease and speed, proving that non-active rest does pay dividends.

Rest During the Hard Training Period

Frequently a session of jogging is called for, perhaps after an extra-harrowing morning interval session or long run. When the runners have decided upon a jog, then the speed is quite slow—eight or nine minutes per mile is typical. Although at this pace the athletes could easily converse without raising the pulse, they jog in stony silence. "Training is training; talking is for after the training," explained Christopher Kosgei. Another example of the intense Kenyan focus.

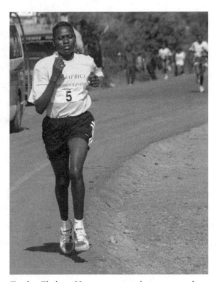

Emily Chebet, Kenyan national team member, here competing in Nyamira, Western Kenya. (*Pieter Langerhorst*)

Rest during the week is usually scheduled for Sunday. Many of the Kenyan athletes are deeply religious and attend church services on this day. Life at the Armed Forces camp on such a day is very tranquil. Many runners take the opportunity to stay in bed late; those who don't walk down to the local church often stay in camp reading the newspaper, writing home, or taking a stroll. Some athletes do train and omit a weekly rest day; these are in the minority, and they usually take an easy session on this day.

Before competitions, runners often jog easily the morning of the day preceding the race. A light session of 40 minutes is typical. If the race is an important competition, then the day after the race is also taken as a rest day to ensure full recovery. Paul Tergat takes a rest day after a competition, then two days of easy running before resuming his normal training schedule. Often the more established the athlete the more rest taken.

A team of the Second Army Brigade were to compete in the Iten cross country relays, which were scheduled to start at 10:00 a.m. At 6:00 a.m. two members of the four-man team who are still trying to make an international breakthrough, Kiprono and Kosgei, were out running 40 minutes of intense hill work. Kiprono was later to record the day's fastest leg!

An interesting concept used by a large majority of the Kenyan athletes is the employment of two training runs, both in the morning. By beginning the day's running schedule at six a.m. and finishing at roughly 11 a.m., the athletes are giving their bodies a much longer time to recover than the full-time athlete who conventionally trains once in the morning and once in the afternoon. Whether the two-a-morning regimen is superior or not, one thing is for sure: it works for the Kenyans!

Strength Training

At Nyayo Stadium in Nairobi there is in actual fact a weight room. Some runners lift weights—sprinters mainly, but a few distance runners do lift on an irregular basis. Gyms are as rare as hen's teeth in Kenya, however. Instead, the runners use forms of light exercise to gain strength, along with their actual running training, which many argue is the best form of strength training. The Armed Forces have some homemade strength equipment, as has Brother Colm O'Connell in Iten. Dumbbells made out of cement-filled paint cans joined by iron bars can be found. Looking at the arm musculature of most of the runners, however, one suspects that these are not frequently used. When a session of ten push-ups was called for before one training run, loud groans were heard. About eight in ten failed to complete the set. The strength of the Kenyans is certainly not in their arms. Not one of ten subjects managed more than two pull-ups!

Farm chores, such as hauling sacks of seed or plowing are undertaken by most athletes a couple of times a year. This work, which is performed generally without motorized machinery, is extremely rigorous and can take a week or more. It helps to maintain overall body strength.

Before training, and after a warm-up jog, the runners often perform in light calisthenics. This is repeated after the hard running session and the cool-down jog. One member of the group acts as supervisor and calls out a stretch or an exercise, then another runner comes up with a different one. The group follows along, and the coaches prowl around looking for anyone stretching incorrectly or not putting in a good effort. After a few of the exercises, the body begins to feel as though an interval session has been run!

William Tanui ran through a few of his favorites exercises with the ease and grace of an aerobics-dance teacher. "It is very important to have a flexible and strong body; this we get from these exercises. The stride becomes much more efficient with these movements."

There is often laughter among the athletes during these sessions. The Kenyans seem to derive from community and simple exercise. After about twenty different exercises and stretches, the group will either stand up and begin the running session or walk off and be glad to complete another day's training. Sometimes an exercise session will replace running altogether. This was the case if the runner had trained twice before mid-day; if the athlete was not feeling up for another run in the afternoon; a session of exercises was substituted. "Doing something is better than nothing!" says Kip Cheruiyot.

Below is a selection of the exercises and stretches commonly used. The stretch is usually held for between ten and twenty seconds.

Hurdles, 10 each leg.
Pulling air, 10 sec. each position.
Trunk bend, 45 sec., moving continuously side-front-side-back, etc.
Bent-knee bends, 20.

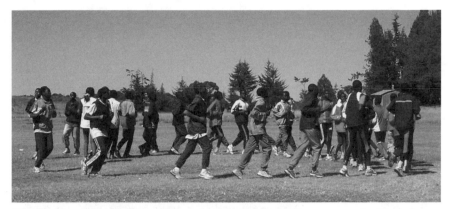

On the Iten location field, Brother Colm's runners go through a series of boot camp exercises. (*Author*)

Leg hold-up, 20 sec. each leg.

Slow trunk bend, hold 20 sec. each foot.

The stance, hold 20 sec., then increase distance between the feet. Repeat 3 times.

Sit-ups, 10-15.

Push-ups, 10.

Quad stretch, hold 20. sec and move head to the knee.

Rotating hips, 10 times clockwise and 10 times counter-clockwise.

Turnbacks, fast movements.

Sitting toe touch, hold 30 sec. 20-30 times.

One-knee sit-ups.

Leg hovers, 10 secs in each position.

Knee lifts, 1 minute rigorous.

Standing start, 30 times as fast as possible, movement arms + legs, with the legs coming as far forward as possible.

Personal Themes

Here are some quotes from people I met in Kenya who should be considered good sources of advice for the aspiring athlete:

Florence Barsosio: "Acclimatize slowly when training in hot conditions."

Robert Cheruiyot: "I thought I was training hard until I joined a group of runners who were racing faster than me, then I realized."

Ibrahim Hussein: "When hill running, use your arms and hips to work into a rhythm on the hill."

Jackson Kabiga: "Don't expect to live in your house when you are building it." [Don't race hoping for a personal best while training hard.]

Moses Kiptanui: "If you are not sweating, you are not training."

Daniel Komen: "Have patience; it takes years of hard training to get good results."

Christopher Kosgei: "Believe you can do it."

William Mutwol: "If you run and train as a team, you can defeat anyone."

Brother Colm O'Connell: "Remember, even 13-year-old girls are training three times per day."

Peter Rono: "Aim high, and then higher. Training hard—that is all."

Simeon Rono: "When you find the weight your body races best at, try to keep it."

William Sigei: "Learn to run when feeling the pain; then push harder."

William Tanui: "Train in an environment that is the best you can find."

Paul Tergat: "Ask yourself, 'Can I give more?' The answer is usually 'Yes.'"

Jack Daniels: "Passionate dedication."

Kip Cheruiyot: "Under race conditions, think about your stride length, especially if you want to catch a runner up ahead on the track; just gently increase your stride length, instead of your stride rate. If you feel good after 400 meters in a race, do not wait; push on. Regardless of what the other runners' advantages are, when you feel right, then go for it. If you want a long career, then race sensibly and not too often to avoid the all–too-common burnout syndrome."

John Litei: "Training is sacred; just a little training does not win the race. Training is a repetition and very hard, not like a race where you just go out once. You must put it in your mind that training is everything; you can even go four times per day if one session involves gym work. Training gives me proof, I can't go to the competition without proof; it gives me the knowledge and the belief. I know in my heart I will succeed, and through training, everything is possible."

Wilson Kipketer: "If you get any problems, or anyone hurts you, just touch your heart and continue. Never lose hope. If you work hard in the future you will be somebody."

William Tanui: "You need good flexibility for your stride to be effective."

Sammy Cheruiyot Kipketer: "Do not give up. You can make it as long as you are healthy and well focused."

Benjamin Limo: "My philosophy in training is to stick with the schedule that has been given to me by the coach without making an alteration to it. That is what all running is about—following instructions, as it will not lead to (my) destruction. I never calculate mileage, it does not matter. If I have a weakness, it is speed work, and that is what I have to work on. I would also like to get some good training partners for when I run the marathon training. Train hard focusing on [one key] good performance."

Richard Chelimo: "Never run more than one hard session a day, otherwise you will 'kill' yourself. Don't over train once you have hit good form; just keep the body ticking with some light intervals. You must not think about what training lies in front—just get it done. Never train alone with speed work or you will not make it to your best ability."

Christopher Kangogo Cheboiboch: You must ask yourself, 'When is it time for training, am I ready to do that hard training?' Because when I train hard then I win easy! I like to train in a group. My theory about the marathon is when the race is far, I must take it easy in the early stage, keep the gasoline in the tank. Thus when you get to the middle of the race you will find you are very strong.

John "King of the Country" Ngugi: "If I feel good then I run fast no matter what the session. Don't waste good time—if you feel good then run hard!"

Economics of Training

To the Westerner, renting an apartment in Kenya is inexpensive—exceedingly so, if one wishes to live somewhere other than Nairobi or Mombasa. Patrick Rono, a Nandi runner, rents a one-room house in Iten where he lives, often with a fellow runner from his home district. The rent per month, including electricity, is $7. Paul Kanda and Paul Kimutai share a small room and there is another room for their kitchen use, though there is no electricity. They pay a total of $5 per month.

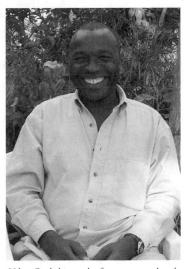

Yobes Ondieki was the first runner to break 27 minutes in the 10,000m. (*Author*)

A lot of athletes pay nothing, staying with family members or friends. William Koila, an 800m runner who had some international success, says, "In the last six months I've had two runners living at my house. The first just turned up, saying he was having difficulties at home, and asked if he could stay for a week. I didn't know him, though we'd met briefly at Brother Colm's training camp. That man stayed three months; he never paid for food or rent, nor did he help with any of the jobs."

Not only is the rent cheap but food is, too. As noted in the diet chapter, most of what the runners eat is home-grown. When athletes arrive in an area to train, they usually bring a sack of produce from their family *shamba*. Lydia Cheromei brought a huge sack of potatoes when she arrived at Brother Colm's.

Even if food has to be paid for, the price is right. In 1996, the cost, in Kenyan shillings, for a two-kilo bag of maize meal was 27 shillings, or about $.50 cents. In Europe, a one-kilo bag of maize meal would cost the equivalent of 180 Kenyan shillings!

The Kenyan is able, without finance or backing, to give athletics a real shot. The rewards are such that the gamble is well worth it—a season in Europe could result in earnings in excess of ten years' ordinary wages.

More and more assistance is being put forward in Kenya by the athletes who have been successful and earned a good income in the Western world. Three-time Boston Marathon winner Ibrahim Hussein started the Ibrahim Hussein Track Club, which provided assistance with training and living expenses to a group of local runners in Nandi District. Frequently the runners would turn up to "borrow" a little money to travel home from the training center. The food was free. Hussein would not reap any financial gain from this venture. "It is our duty to put something back into the sport," he said.

The late 10,000m world champion Paul Kipkoech had a similar group. Joseph Chepkwony remembers, "We got transport to any races, or if we needed a ride to a certain hill to do hill training, Paul would always provide a vehicle. This was very important because we could not afford to pay for transport. Without Paul we would have never got to any of the races. Moses Tanui is another Kenyan distance hero heavily involved in helping the young athletes of the Eldoret area.

Brother Colm O'Connell has virtual "saint" status in Keiyo District. While working half-time at the Teachers Training College in Tambach, Colm spends more than 50 percent of his wages on his beloved hobby of coaching the junior runners. Driving his car to pick up athletes from group training, following the group in case anyone has to drop out during a training run, transporting runners to races, paying for their food—these and many more services are provided by Brother Colm without a grumble, and it has been going on for twenty years. There is hardly an athlete in the region who has not been helped by the hand of Brother Colm in some way or another.

The Training Camp

There can be few more inspiring training sessions in a runner's life than charging along the red dirt roads of the Kenyan highlands in glorious sunshine with fifty world-class runners at your side.

Kenyans generally do not like to live alone. Large families are commonplace in Kenyan rural society. The family base is usually permanent, with the family members building their own houses in close proximity. Because there is an absence of the infrastructure found in many countries in the Western world, Kenyans have learned to rely heavily on family members. Therefore, their kindred communal way of life is quite impervious to change.

A Kenyan who is attempting to become an international-standard runner will often move to another to live and train with other runners. Frequently one will travel with another like-minded runner from their village and engage a lodging jointly. Living alone is seen as something incongruous. "I don't like it. All my life I've had lots of people around," says Patrick Rono, who welcomes Nandi runners to share his single room in Iten. Residential training camps sprout in the highlands like mushrooms in the dew. "You cannot make it to international standard if you are training alone, you need the company of others to push you when you are tired. If you are always training alone your body will take the sessions easier than you should," advised Richard Chelimo, who used to train with a large group of Army runners.

All over the Rift Valley Province there are small groups of runners training together. Often an established runner, such as Moses Kiptanui in Nyahururu, bases himself in the area with a couple of training partners. Then others, on hearing that Moses trains there, move to the area. Kenyans still have the hospitable touch, so even the poorest of runners usually manages to find a space to sleep and some *ugali* to eat. "When you run with champions in training, then you know you too can be a champion," says Ondoro Osoro.

The training camp is thus born. One main advantage of life in a training camp is that the runner is excused from everyday chores. "I moved away from my village to Iten because I could not train with all the jobs at home," says David Kemei, an international 1500m runner.

Brother Colm adds, "This especially affects women runners in Kenya. Often they run well in school and then on returning to the family farm they are faced with all the household work; there is no time or energy left to train." A woman is not often seen setting off from the family farm for a training run. "Living in Iten with the Iten running club makes training much easier," notes Lydia Cheromei.

Japheth Kimutai, a former world-class 800m runner, explains, "My parents can not read or understand English; they can not comprehend the chances I have through athletics." Living at home would have involved him in work that would preclude effective training; a training camp helped elevate him to world standard.

Kenyans have an amazing ability to relax most of the day; they do not need to be occupied, as so many Westerners do. Wilson Musto, who had some success on the European road race circuit, had a day schedule while training in Sweden that included going back to bed after breakfast and the morning run, rising for lunch before retreating to bed once again, taking an afternoon run, eating dinner, then returning to bed!! Often in the Kenyan countryside, children can be seen just sitting by the roadside for great lengths of time doing nothing but watching the world roll by. Therefore, at a training camp all energy can be directly channeled into training. Whereas mini-golf or a drive out to some nearby landmark might fill the afternoon of some European athlete away at a training camp, the Kenyan is content to rest up for the next session.

An important role for the camp is for the runners to bond, thus forming a strong team. Before the Armed Forces Championships, the coaches sit with the athletes and discuss the tactics that will be used during the competition. They draw them up with military precision. Perhaps no other country in the world has athletes who are prepared to give all for their team members in an individual sport such as running. World Championships team medalist Simeon Rono tells this story:

In Durham [1995] I was in great form; I think I could have got a top-five individual placing, but the orders were that on the third lap I should sprint to the front of the group and push the pace as fast as I could. The end result was that after I had done my effort I faded to 30th place; but anyway we won the team title.

A staggering sacrifice was made by Simon Chemoiywo in the World Cross Country Championships of 1994. "My job was to keep up the pace early on, then when Sigei broke from the group, not to go after him and take the Ethiopians with me, so I hung back till I was sure Sigei would get to the line before the Ethiopians." Only then did Chemoiywo let loose his lethal kick, which left Haile Gebrselassie a well-beaten third. "The important thing for us is that a Kenyan should win; that we must be sure of!" noted Chemoiywo. "When we live, struggle, and work together, a victory by one of us is for all of us."

The theory is that the coaches who have many high-level runners on the team, should be able to see which runners best fit their team aspirations at an international championship. Mike Kosgei, who was behind so much of Kenya's success from the mid-1980s to the early 1990s, had such a close rapport with his athletes that there was almost a family feel to the squad. This was a perfect scenario for getting runners to help each other toward a common goal—team and individual honors. "Kosgei is a master of cross country coaching. He knows it too well that I doubt any other coach can beat him," says John Ngugi, a man who has a lot to thank Kosgei for.

The Armed Forces Training Camp

"The Armed Forces camp was our ace. When we had the camp at N'gong, nobody could beat us. We need to train together, then Kenya is unbeatable." —Ismael Kirui, soldier, two-time world 5000m champion

Thirty kilometers from Nairobi are the N'gong Hills. Sitting at high altitude in an environment of lush vegetation is the Armed Forces training camp. It is here that many large weather-beaten green canvas army tents are erected from October through July. The camp is divided into three sections—Army, Navy, and Air Force. Each has its own central office and organization. The three sections train separately and the competition among them is fierce for national Armed Forces track and field and cross country honors. Living full-time at the camp are medical personnel, coaches, athletes, and cooks. The cross country and track runners arrive in October; the field athletes in March.

The large tents are basic shelter. There are no ground sheets to keep out the wind, and it's not uncommon for the tents to leak. They typically hold twelve to sixteen runners. Inside the tents are rows of steel-framed beds. Next to each bed are the athlete's personal belongings locked up in a tin chest. Running apparel is slung over every available space. The conditions are Spartan, or, in the words of Paul Tergat, "Here we live like animals."

In the center of each area is the outdoor cooking facility—a large open fire around which the food is prepared each day. The coaches, who are usually superior in military rank to the athletes, live together in one tent. "We are able to understand the athlete much better when we live in constant contact. How else can the coach really get to know his athletes?" asks Navy coach Albert Masai.

The daily routine, Monday through Saturday, for the camp's best runners is show below. Others who do not show as much talent or are not producing the best results often have camp chores to take care of, as well as training, such as fetching firewood or sweeping the dirt from the camp.

5:00-6:00 a.m.	Rise and run "how you feel"
7:00-7:30 a.m.	Stretch and change clothes
7:45-8:00 a.m.	Breakfast
8:00-9:45 a.m.	Relax, usually in bed
9:45-10:00 a.m.	Assemble for training
10:00-11:15 a.m.	Main training session
11:15-11:30 a.m.	Stretch/exercises
11:30-11:50 a.m.	Drinking tea, talking/social
11:50 a.m.-1:00 p.m.	Relaxing
1:00-1:30 p.m.	Lunchtime
1:30-3:30p.m.	Relax/sleep, laundry, etc.
3:45-4:45 p.m.	Strolling, jogging or exercise
4:45-5:15 p.m.	Showering, cold water basins

5:15-6:00 p.m.	Personal time
6:00-7:00 p.m.	Dinner
7:00-8:30 p.m.	Social. Drink tea or cocoa
8:30 p.m.	Bedtime
9:00 p.m.	Lights out

Examples of the Main Session

Winter

One hour of fartlek, varying efforts from 30 seconds to three minutes

Tempo runs of 50-70 mins at race pace for large portions of the run

Hill work, intervals or continuous

Steady runs of 60-80 minutes, though invariably finishing fast

Long run: distance covered would be individual, 1–3 hours.

Summer

20 x 400m track work at 60-62 sec. pace, 45 seconds rest

3 x 4000m, run at 3-min-per-km speed with a 1-2 min. rest

20 x 800m at 10K race pace, 1 minute or less rest • A session of 200m intervals, often neither timed or counted

A tempo run of 45 minutes in the forest

This camp lifestyle has been experienced by the best runners in Kenya. Most of the successful runners, like John Ngugi and Richard Chelimo, spent time at these camps. Some, such as Paul Tergat, live in close proximity and join the runners just for speed sessions. Others, like Simon Chemoiywo, live and train hundreds of kilometers, but come into the camp a month before a major competition or simply for sharpening up.

"When you are winning and doing well, the Forces put no demands on you as long as you represent them in the major competitions. There are no military duties for Army men such as Ismael Kirui," explains Simeon Rono, one of the team's star cross country runners.

Imagine: on any given day, at least 30 world-class training partners, food prepared for you daily, live-in coaches and medical staff, high altitude, and a perfect running climate—for an eight-to-nine-month span each year. Is it any wonder that Kenya is producing excellent results in the athletics world?

Control over the camp is left to the coaches who often have ranks of senior sergeant or higher. "I don't like loose morals in the camp. Taking one beer or two is okay as long as it doesn't become a habit, but if there is a lazy runner not committed to hard training, then there is no place for him here," says Navy coach Masai.

Certainly, a positive atmosphere permeates the camp. Encouragement is showered upon all athletes who are working hard, regardless of talent or results, and the harder you train the more respect you gain. The social talk rarely centers on personal achievements but more about life in general, family matters, and plans for the future. Although they have every right to crow a little, Kenyan athletes are very seldom boastful about their running successes.

The National Training Camp for the World Cross Country Championships

From 1985 to the spring of 1995, Mike Kosgei was the Kenyan national trainer. Kosgei had been a successful athlete himself, and his team thoroughly dominated the World Cross Country Championships. After a second-place finish in 1985, the senior men never lost another team title under his leadership. Many Kenyans agree that Kosgei's magic was sown, mentally and physically, in the last four weeks before each championship when the training camp was held. All runners selected had to attend. Ismael Kirui, who in 1994 was leading the IAAF World Cross Challenge series, chose to compete instead in Europe and was left off the team despite his status. The camp was run with military discipline by an ex-military man.

High altitude, hills and most important, according to Kosgei, suitable dirt roads were the requirements for the proper location in 1994. Embu, on the slopes of Mount Kenya in the Eastern Province, suited these requirements, and it was here, at St. Mark's Teacher Training College, that Kosgei would hold his camp. Talking and living daily with his runners Kosgei was able to develop a bond few other national coaches could comprehend. The runners would give everything and more for this man. "The coach must know and feel his runners. He must understand their emotions," explains Kosgei.

The food was similar to the Armed Forces diet—wholesome, plentiful, and nourishing. Cooks would be provided to prepare the food, but that is where the creature comforts came to an end. The living accommodation was basic school dormitory, metal-framed bed with foam mattress, and a few centrally located taps for water. Washing clothes was also the responsibility of the athlete; this job would usually be done weekly by the male runners, and slightly more often by the females. Attendance at the camp was by invitation only and the costs were covered by the Kenyan Amateur Athletic Association.

"The mentality is so much different when working with Kenyans. A Kenyan is happy if he or his teammate wins. This makes team tactics much easier than if you are working with a bunch of individuals."—Coach Kosgei.

The hard part of the camp life of course, was the training. Three sessions per day, six days a week. Sunday was a "rest" day with just one session. The senior men would often log in excess of 240K (140+ miles!) of running in the week. More amazing is the fact that over 30 percent of that distance would probably be run at a speed comparable to competition pace. Here is the shape of a typical day:

6:00 a.m. Morning run. For the men, around 10K, for the women 8K, and for a few of the elite, up to 22K. The run would begin at a stumbling pace, though the end of the run was inevitably swift. Kosgei would require the runners to wear short-sleeved T-shirts as preparation for conditions they might have to face at the championships.

7:00 a.m. Stretching and exercises, 15-20 min. A section of the day that Kosgei deemed very important. Flexible bodies lead to more efficient runners, he reasoned. Breakfast, then rest in bed.

10:00 a.m Typically the main session. Some examples:

10K fartlek—2 min. fast + 2 min. slow over hilly ground

Road intervals, 100–1000m, no predetermined number. The runners would run until they were "dead"

Dirt track intervals, 20 x 400m in 56-64 secs/10 x 800m in 1:58-2:08 Recover by jogging the same distance

Threshold work, 2 x 5000m at 15 min with 2-3 min recovery jog

Short intervals, 15K of 3:30 per K warm-up

Hill work, 25 x 200m, for senior men, 20 for the women, on a 40-degree hill. Stride back down, no rest!

Tempo run, around 20K with an ever-increasing pace. Usually after the first ten minutes it has become a full-blown race situation.

800m repeats. Usually 8-10 repeats, for the senior men, in about 2 minutes, with an equivalent rest

The long run. Typically between 20-25K. Starting slowly, and the usual creeping up in pace. A hill will often be the starting point for a strong upsurge in pace.

12:00 Lunch, followed by resting. "It is good to lie down; you need rest in hard training," emphasized camp regular Simon Chemoiywo

4:00 p.m. Usually 12-16K of steady running, though often speeding up toward the end. Could also be the main session switched from 10:00 a.m.

6:00 p.m. Dinner

8:30 p.m. Bed

After the interval session, the runners would include a 5K or so cool-down run. If any of the athletes was not completely exhausted by the earlier session, this too would often be run at a high speed.

The camp does have a competitive side. The team would be selected from this group of runners, thus they are of course eager to catch the eye of the coach by "performing" in training. Kenyans can often be quite competitive, and it's not uncommon to see a training session turn into a race at any given moment, with or without an audience. "The first time I went to the camp I trained too hard and injured myself; the next time I made sure I did enough to make the team, not more," said Tergat, who admitted to training so hard he thought he was about to faint!

Despite the severe training, recovery seems to be the theme of the camp. The day ends with exhausted bodies strewn about the school, yet mysteriously the next day the legs are again fresh and fit for battle. "This training makes any race seem easy because soon after one session is finished another begins—there is no rest," said Chelimo, perhaps explaining how he managed to "recover" while cruising at 62-second laps in 10,000m races!

The month prior to the 1994 World Cross Country Championships is looked at below in day-by-day detail. The morning run, at 6:00 a.m., is excluded due to its individuality. The distances are for the senior men; however, some male juniors train just as hard as the seniors.

March 1–26. Location: St. Mark's College, Mt. Kenya. 6,200-foot altitude. Hilly rough terrain. The exercises are done before and after the run. Stretching, in some form, is usually done at least twice a day. Each training day is from 10:00 a.m. to 4:00 p.m.

Date	*First Session*	*Second Session*
1	20K @ 80% effort.	Exercises, before and after the run
	20 min. rigorous 9K fast distance.	15 x 200m hill work hard!
2	15K "B" speed (75%), finishing fast.	Fartlek 15K, speed "A" (90 %+) stretching, 20 min.
3	22K steady + 20 min. exercises	10K easy + exercises
4	15K high speed, 20 x 100m	15K light fartlek + exercises concentrating on style.
5	15K high speed + 20 strength exercises	8K easy
6	Competition, cross country 13K	Rest
7	12K 75% effort, finishing fast	Strolling. + 20 min exercises
8	12K easy + circuit training	20K 6 min./mile + 20 min. exercises
9	12K high-speed fartlek + 20 min. 12K warm-up stretch. 30 x 150m hill work+ exercise.	
10	25K hilly distance run, supposed	Strolling, washing to be relatively easy. clothes, etc.
11	18K high speed, 90% effort, racing	12K fartlek, 75% tempo effort.
12	15K 80% effort + 20 min. exercises.	12K competition speed, flat-out.
13	20K high speed	Strolling/jogging.
14	15K run in around 50 min, hilly + hard, as above	
15	10K easy	10K easy
16	15K fast + 15 x 100m, 85% effort	10K fartlek, 80% effort + exercises
17	10K steady + 20 min. strength exercises	8K jog + 20 min. exercises
18	18K long run, 8K easy jog. run at a "conversational" pace	
19	10K, 80% effort	10K easy + exercises
20	10K fartlek + exercises	8K easy + exercises
21	15K @ 80-85% effort + exercises	10K @ 80% + exercises
22	15K high speed, tough and hard	10K @ 80% effort
23	Travel	
24	Travel 8K easy jog	
25	10K jog on the course "looking, strolling, learning." Running together.	
26	Morning jog as a team. World Championship domination.	

The Kenyans are well aware of their reputation and the respect that is accorded them, and a canny pre-race tactic is the group jog. Like a pride of lions they prowl the course reminding the opposition of their united force. A similar tactic is employed prior to the national championships. As the senior men await the start, the Armed Forces runners jog to the line with a flag bearer leading them as they chant in unison to remind their opposition—"Together we shall win." True to their word, win they do!

Running-Shoe Camps

All over the Kenyan countryside, shoe companies are opening training camps to recruit and nurture athletes who will represent their brands. Typically between four and thirty runners live together under the representation of one manager, funded by the affiliated companies. These camps follow the daily programs of the Armed Forces and national-team training groups.

Would the Kenyans dominate without training camps? Due to the Kenyan mentality of training and living together, the runners would succeed in any case, as lots of small "camps" would be formed. Certainly, however, larger camps do help create strength in numbers. "When you are tired there is always another man pushing and not letting you rest. Even if you think you are at full speed, you can always be pushed a little faster," said Daniel Komen.

The Kenyan Diet

Sunshine bathes the Kenyan fields, and purifying rainfall nourishes the land. The chemicals that saturate fields in the so-called developed quarters of the world are less common here. Farmers have financial difficulty enough trying to hire a tractor for plowing, let alone invest in quantities of expensive chemicals. The climate is advantageous for growing hearty crops. Maize grown in Kenya is larger than corn grown, say, in England, and looks far more edible, flushed by the sun rather than by alkali.

The price of land in Kenya is much more affordable than, for instance, a car. Most rural Kenyans own a plot of land called a *shamba*. This enables the family to produce their own food. William Kiprono, the 1996 Army Brigades steeplechase champion, explains, "We grow enough maize to eat the year round; it is sufficient just for home use. Like our neighbors, we don't grow to sell." When Rose Cheruiyot began to make money from running one of the first things she did was buy twenty-five acres for a family *shamba*. Kenyans often prefer to invest in the land rather than in the bank. "Inflation and economics are not so stable in Kenya," explains Paul Tergat.

The diet common to the average family from the rural towns and villages, where virtually all Kenyan runners grow up and live, is quite nutritious. But this is often because of economics, not necessarily preference. "I love French fries, I don't like *ugali* at all," admits Lydia Cheromei. "Hamburgers are great; I like to eat at the fast-food places when I'm living in London," says Benson Koech with a smile. "My favorite? A big steak with a plate of chips [French fries]," says Kip Cheruiyot. Kimutai Koskei, a 28:49 10,000m runner, gained over six pounds when posted to Bosnia for six months. "We had fried food every day and I grew to love it!"

The depth of the pocket is usually the dictator in Kenya. There are well-documented cases of Kenyan athletes becoming alcoholics after earning vast sums of money, and in some cases it is the same with food. Often the richer the athlete, the more varied his plate. With the current generation of runners nearly all coming from poor origins, this ensures at least twenty years of good food into their bodies.

Body Weight

Lornah Kiplagat maintains 11 percent body fat when at her skinniest. "My coach is not happy when he sees anything below 13 percent, it is just before a race I get low, but it is not too healthy." Following a marathon, Kiplagat does what she calls "Express eating" when she eats as much as possible, especially adding fats to help restore the body's strength. "I like to start my training at least three kilograms overweight. When you are back in training the weight will fall off before the race day, I never worry," said Lornah after boasting that she could out-eat any athlete. "Nutrition plays a very important role in my program." She goes on. We designed a diet with the right mix of carbohydrates, proteins, and fats. I eat a lot of fresh vegetables, and of course fruits." On race day, Lornah curbs her voracious habits. "I'll get up on race day at six (for a ten o'clock start) and take some breakfast. Probably one bagel with some black tea, or maybe porridge with a banana."

Phillip Chirchir, who has four 2:08-marathons under his belt, adds, "Don't be underweight, that will not work to run your best marathon. You'll find the best marathoners are also very big eaters, this is how the body recovers and accepts the hard training."

Twice a New York City Marathon winner, John Kagwe notes, "I like to race at 50 kilograms. However, following a marathon I rest and I load up to 54 kg easily with healthy eating. After the training has reached 50 kilograms I am back in form, but I use the training to reduce the weight, not any special dieting."

Moses Kiptanui advises, "You have to eat. You should be eating double what a normal person does when you are training. If you do not, then the body just will break down. I had a long career, much longer than most elite runners did. Why? Because I looked after myself. You should also be drinking three liters of water per day."

Elijah Lagat, today a politician, eschews the last French fries on the plate on Christmas Eve. "Now that I am not running, I have to be careful." The Nandi is remembering back in 1992 when his doctor told him that his cholesterol was through the roof, and he had too much fat around his heart. "I was near 160 pounds! So then I started jogging, and then running. The more I ran the better I felt, so I kept on adding, and adding." By the mid-1990s Lagat was competing, and well. In 1997 he won the Prague Marathon, and in the autumn the Berlin Marathon, setting his PR of 2:07:41. Following that event, at the post-race party in a Holiday Inn, he related how he had lost well over 30 pounds through by the love of running. "No pills, no avoiding foods, just running." Three years later, at the 2000 Boston Marathon, Lagat outkicked Gezahegne "Geza" Abera of Ethiopia who would go on to win the summer's Olympic Games. From an overweight non-athlete who could not walk without wheezing, Lagat proved that dreams do come true through hard work.

Key Diet Ingredients of a Typical Rift Valley Resident

Maize is the main crop of the Kenyan farmer. It requires little attention and thrives in the Kenyan climate. Once harvested, the maize is removed from the cob, dried for a number of months, then ground to form a flour called maize meal, which is cooked to produce the staple food of Kenya—*ugali*. From the *shamba* the maize meal is unsifted and rough in texture, but when bought commercially it is usually sifted and of a fine consistency. Some cobs are saved for roasting over an open fire to be eaten as a lunch, and some maize is boiled with kidney beans to be eaten as *githeri*, a lunch dish.

Some staples:

Ugali. A stiff porridge made from water and ground maize. Eaten at least once a day. Used as a Westerner would use rice or pasta.

Sukuma. Wiki Dark green cabbage plant. Eaten with *ugali*. Often mixed with wild dark green plants that grow on the *shamba*.

Uji. Porridge made from ground maize or millet, often fermented.

Maziwa. Lala fermented fresh milk.

Viasi Potatoes, often sweet potatoes eaten at lunchtime.

Maharagwe kidney beans, frequently eaten for lunch.

Githeri. Maize and kidney beans mixed and boiled together.

Muthokoi Similar to *githeri* but with pumpkin leaves and potatoes added.

Machungwa Oranges, regularly eaten when green in color.

Chai Tea, the leaves boiled with milk and sugar.

The nutritional value of the above foods provides an adequate diet, excellent for the runner. The *ugali* is pure carbohydrate. *Mboga* (green vegetables such as *sukuma wiki*) provide a plentiful source of iron and minerals. Proteins are found in abundance in the *maziwa lala* and *maharagwe*. Vitamins come from the vegetables and the *machungwa*. The fat content is extremely low. When boiling the *maziwa* (milk), the fat is skimmed from the surface and used for cooking.

Recipe for "African Cake" Ugali

Serves 5

4 cups of cold water

2 cups maize meal (unsifted is preferred)

Bring the water to a boil in a large pot.

Add the maize meal stirring with a large wooden spoon slowly.

Reduce the heat and continue to 'stroke' the thick porridge-like mixture. Reduce the heat, continue to stir. After a while there is a unique smell that comes from the maize meal burning on the bottom of the pot.

Turn the pot upside down onto a plate, and the *ugali* should plop out. Take another plate and squash the *ugali* down a touch by placing the second plate on top of the *ugali*.

Cut into chunks and serve immediately.

Moving with the times Lornah Kiplagat uses a microwave after stirring the powder into the water.

What's the Magic Ingredient of Ugali and Milk?

One of the world's leading authorities on the Kenyan diet is the Dirk Lund Christensen of Denmark, an exercise physiologist, with an MA in African Studies. More Fire asked Dirk if there were any secrets to the Ugali and the milk diet.

"Kenyans often mention their intake of ugali and milk as one of the reasons for their success in running. *Ugali* is without a doubt a main contributor to their high-carbohydrate intake, but the food in itself does not contain anything extraordinary aside from the carbohydrate. It is simply what they are used to eating. And as far as milk is concerned, it does provide the runners with some essential amino acids which their diet seems to otherwise lack in sufficient amounts, as their consumption of meat is rather low. However, the milk intake is not as dominant a part of their diet as they would make us, or maybe make themselves, believe. I think it has a lot to do with identity stemming from their Nilotic heritage (now we obviously speak of the Kalenjin). In Denmark we probably consume more milk and milk products than the Kenyans—including the runners—do, and yet we have no world-class runners."

Pills and Supplements

Increasingly, athletes from all corners of the globe are taking substances to enhance performance. Athletic journals often advertise some new potion that is certain to improve performance. Not so in Africa! Firstly, the information is very sparse in Kenya. There are no running magazines available, and the information on the most fundamental of matters is hard to come by. Apart from basic glucose powder, which Sally Barsosio admits was an inspiration to keep on competing (as the sweet powder was often served at the end of a race), substances, such as creatine or CO Q10, are simply not sold.

Vitamins and/or minerals are taken by a few of the runners who have lived abroad for a length of time, but even these are rare. Over in Europe, where a manager may pressure one of his runners to take supplements, a Kenyan's easy going nature would probably make him acquiesce. But in Kenya, the tablets would undoubtedly be left untaken. Most Kenyans know that the real secret to success is hard training. "There is no substitute to hard training, and more hard training," says Moses Kiptanui. Asked whether he used any sports drink while running and winning the 1996 Boston Marathon, Moses Tanui replied, "Just plain water!"

The Kenyans have a drug far more powerful—that of belief. It is not ignorance; far from it. They feel that with their training and way of life they can be unbeatable. A talk was held at a Kenyan running camp, on the subject of nutrition. A visiting Westerner, convinced that his sales would go rise like buns in the oven, intended to recruit some Kenyans to endorse his products. The windy speech lasted thirty minutes whilst the salesman cogently explained all the advantages to taking various special tablets, examples of which he produced from a black suitcase.

The Kenyans listened silently to his every word, not questioning or showing a flicker of disinterest. Graphs, charts, and diagrams of many colors were produced to illustrate the benefits. At the end of the pitch, the salesman looked to his audience and asked, "So, are there any questions about the presentation?" An old man, who had been sitting at the back of the room, stood up. In a clear voice, he asked, "So, you mean you want my boys to start eating these tablets so they can start running like the runners in your country?" Laughter erupted throughout the room; obviously, it had been the thought of many. No sales, or sponsorships, were locked up that night.

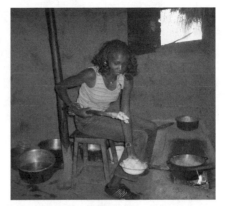

Hilda Kibet finishes off stirring the ugali for the day's lunch. (*Author*)

In Kenya's athletic history, there have been, just a couple of drug-infringement incidents. These cases in Kenya have usually been for a drug found in Kenyan common cold solutions available at most apothecaries around the country. "It is one thing we stress very carefully at our training camps; there isn't the information available when you go to the chemist [pharmacist] on what substances are banned and what aren't," says Brother Colm. Even the hospital in Iten, in one of Kenya's major running centers, was unable to come up with a list of banned substances. Therefore it is highly conceivable that a Kenyan can be a happenstance victim, since strict testing is enforced by the IAAF in Kenya the year round. Japheth Kimutai, a 17-year old schoolboy, barely managed to find a race in Europe in the 1996 season, but he was hunted down in the Kenyan highlands during the spring of 1996 by the drug testers. A member of the testing group, who wishes to remain anonymous, says, "Because of their incredible achievements we are pressured by other countries' athletic bodies to test, and retest, the Kenyan athletes to 'find' some excuse for their achievements. They are tested more often than most other athletes and 99.9 percent come up 100 percent clean!"

Typical Daily Diets

While the Western world moves away from the idea of eating excesses of red meat, cooking oil, fats, and salt, the Kenyans have no such notions. The Armed Forces training camps chefs are heavy-handed with the fats, salts, and oils. The beef stew is dripping in oil, red meat is served twice a day and well salted, and the morning sandwiches are slathered with of margarine. Western nutritionists would be diving for their stomach pumps after a day at the camp! This, however is not the typical diet of Kenyans *before* they arrive at the Athletic Camps.

If a family has money to spare, bread will be eaten for breakfast, though this is a luxury, and one most families go without. "We sometimes had bread at Christmas and on New Year's Day," says marathoner Mark Yatich. Most families buy just tea and sugar from the shop and grow their other supplies. There is a myth that most Kenyans eat a lot of meat. Nearly all the runners come from a background where meat was a scarce luxury. The majorities of Kenyans cannot afford high-protein diets. Although Benjamin Limo and Solomon Busendich now eat a large amount of meat, neither did in their formative years, "We could not afford it. Having meat on the plate, it was a rarity that was not counted upon," recalled Limo.

Most families are lucky if they get to eat meat once or twice a month. The usual meat is *kondoo* (sheep), though at ceremonies *ngombe* (cow), is eaten. Julius Korir recalls, "It used to be that if a visitor came, an animal from the farm was slaughtered; however, poverty does not allow that. We had only five cows and a couple of chickens, so we ate meat only a couple of times per year, though because we were typical of the neighborhood we did not miss it." A big advantage to the Kenyan diet, and that can easily be duplicated, is that most Kenyans eat fresh foods. They are plucking sweet potatoes from the garden, (or buying from a vendor who has), not from a supermarket's old stock. I can guarantee that none of today's successful Kenyan runners ever had a frozen meal when growing up. "You go to your fridge for pasteurized milk, we go to the field," says Rose Cheruiyot.

With more and more studies pointing toward the pluses of a meatless diet, this may be a blessing in disguise. There is something non-organic about the thought of powering the run with pieces of an animal's carcass in the stomach!

Three examples of daily diets are given below. Diet #1 is that of Paul Kanda. He has no income, has a small piece of shared land on which to grow maize, and relies on friends and family for any extra money needed. Kanda is typical of many Kenyan athletes who are trying to reach international standard. Diet #2 is taken from a day in the life of Moses Tanui, who at the time was a well-to-do successful runner. Diet #3 is a day's menu for the Armed Forces training camp. Since many of Kenya's best runners have developed at the camp, it must be a recipe for attainment!

Diet #1
Breakfast, 8:00 a.m. Two cups of black sugared tea
Mid-morning,* 11:00 a.m. One cup of *uji*
Lunch, 1:00 p.m. *Ugali* and *sukuma wiki*
Dinner, 7:00 p.m. *Ugali* and *sukuma wiki*
*This would only be taken if Kanda was training three times a day, as was his usual practice. Occasionally a neighbor or friend would donate a piece of meat or a jug of milk. However, these occurrences were neither regular nor plentiful.

Diet #2
Breakfast, 7:00 a.m. Bread, jam, and margarine sandwiches. Kenyan tea
Mid-morning, 11:00 a.m. Kenyan tea
Lunch, 1:00 a.m. Rice, bananas, and a beef, and vegetable stew, followed by more Kenyan tea
Dinner, 7:00 p.m. *Ugali* with meat and vegetables

Diet #3

Breakfast, 7:00 a.m. White bread and margarine, lots of Kenyan tea

Mid-morning, 11:00 a.m. At least a couple of mugs of Kenyan tea

Lunch, 1:00 p.m. a blend of rice, potatoes, and spaghetti with kidney beans and chunks of beef in an oily sauce; Kenyan tea

Dinner, 7:00 p.m. a large slab of *ugali*, potatoes, and a beef stew. Kenyan tea or cocoa.

The amounts eaten are frequently substantial. Kenyans do not typically worry about weight control; they believe hard training will take care of that. The regular-sized plate at the camp is usually heaped with food. The Kenyan women are a little more concerned about overeating than the men. Lydia Cheromei believes that during the cross country season her weight is not really a concern, though for the track season she makes an effort to reduce weight: "You need more strength to get up the hills and through the mud, but on the track it is important to be light." A week before finishing second in the World Cross Country Championships, Rose Cheruiyot was attempting to lose a couple of kilograms, one day substituting a lemon for lunch.

Diet on the Road

World Cross Country Championships silver medalist Simon Chemoiywo spends a large part of the summer months in Europe. Based in the London suburb of Teddington, Simon has adapted, along with a houseful of Kenyans, to British life. When asked about the differences in diet, Chemoiywo pointed out that the basic structure, and most of the food types, were similar to what he would eat at home on his farm near Kipkabus. "We shop at the local supermarket. The big difference is all the selections of brands for each article. We usually buy bags of rice, potatoes, and cornmeal flour to make *ugali*, vegetables, bread and meat." Sometimes if the runners are out for a stroll or away from home, then they eat out for lunch, though most of them try to make it back to the base for the important evening meal. "We can go to one of the fast-food restaurants and take a hamburger and chips. They taste very good and it is a light meal," says Lydia Cheromei, one of the many Kenyans who very much enjoy Western fast food. A sample of a typical Teddington day for Chemoiywo would be:

Breakfast A couple of slices of toast with margarine; tea

Mid-morning tea

Lunch Vegetable soup

Dinner Vegetables and meat, with either *ugali*, rice or potatoes

Simeon Rono, another London-based Kenyan from the national cross country squad, explains,

When we are racing on the track we usually do not eat as much as when we are in heavy training. I have to watch that I don't go up in weight with the reduced training. But when we are a big group it helps as we are all watching each other. If I am 65 kilograms then I know I will not run good, but if I am 62, aah! We all know at what weight we perform our best at and we try to keep that weight constant. There have been many cases of our countrymen coming over and eating their way out of form. They arrive at a hotel where for breakfast you can eat as much as you want. Maybe all their lives food has been scarce; the temptation can be big.

Some of the runners are a little superstitious about the power of *ugali*. Some even go as far as believing that Kenyan *ugali* is more powerful than European versions. The night before an important race, a bag of maize-meal flour brought over from Kenya is often opened on Back Road in Teddington as the runners gather round the "magic" food. Jane Kimutai, a 400m runner who in 1995 was voted the Kenyan schools' most valuable athlete, is one such superstitious runner. Jane even goes so far as saying that if salt is taken with the *ugali* the runner will not be able to run. One can salt the accompanying vegetables, however, with impunity!

Blood Link

Ingrid Kristiansen, formerly the world records holder at 5000m, 10,000m and the marathon, was a fond eater of blood pudding. Nutritionists have often wondered about the benefits of eating foods with a high blood content. Then came the news that the Chinese world-record-breaking women drank turtle blood daily to strengthen their bodies against the hard training. The Kenyans are at it, too! The Maasai tribe, who are spread over the southern Rift Valley, have long been known to drink cow's blood mixed with milk. The fresh milk, from the cow, is blended with blood taken from the throat of a living beast with a thin pipe, then drunk. Blood is also drunk straight.

The Air Force camp was expecting some superior to visit their training center. It was decided to slaughter a goat in the superior's honor and cook up a stew. The goat was hung up on a nearby tree and manually gutted. As the fresh warm blood flowed from the animal, a soldier collected the liquid in a large cup. A group of runners (not just the Maasai) gathered round and each took a gulp of blood before passing the cup along.

Kenyans do not particularly like sweet foods. Chocolates are often accepted with great relish then surreptitiously spit out. Confectioneries are not common in the diet of young Kenyans as they are for so many Western children; thus many Kenyans never develop a palate for such foods. An Army 10,000m runner named Kosgei remembers his first, and last, encounter with chocolate. "I won a box of chocolates in a race in Finland, so in the evening when I was back at my hotel room I opened the box and ate them. The next day I was feeling very bad in the stomach. If I were to take this food to my children and friends and they were to experience such feelings they would think me a bad man for giving them such food, so I threw the rest of the box away."

Mombasa: The World Cross Country Comes Home

Sisi tuko tayari kwa kazi (We are ready for the job)

It was a tradition that a country that won the World Cross Country Championship would often be offered the rights to host the following year's event. Kenya won the World Cross men's team competition in 1986, and started an eighteen-year domination of the sport never equalled in a any other sport. Twenty-two years later, the championships were finally held in Kenya for the first time. Journalists the world over called it the homecoming of cross country. Fifteen years earlier John Ngugi had stood at the N'gong race track outside Nairobi explaining why the Kenyan nationals displayed such a fervor for high-class running, "This is the athletes' time to shine. You know, when we go abroad we never get the real cheers we get in Kenya. If ever the Worlds come to Kenya, then the world will see us really run!"

However, the solid foundation of Kenyan cross country had started to show cracks. In 2006, the mighty Ethiopians had swept all four senior titles, and with many of the team returning in 2007, the outlook worried many Kenyans. Suddenly Eritrea, Uganda, and even Qatar were promising to bump Kenya from the podium. Kenyan chances looked less convincing after a relatively weak rostrum of stars turned out for the February nationals in Mombasa, and in March many established names failed to impress at the country's trial race. Kenya was left with a virgin team to face the world.

The obligatory three-week national training camp was based in Embu, but the runners were transported to Siakago, near Masinga, to meet more muggy conditions on the advice of Tergat to help acclimatize to Mombasa-like conditions. The three coaches, John Mwithiga, who is based at N'gong and is credited for discovering John Ngugi, along with Julius Kirwa and David Letting, had been in charge of the national squad for the past couple of editions of the World Cross, thus there was no experience lacking in that department. They knew the country wanted two things, individual and team winners. "Anything less than complete success will be seen as not good," warned Kirwa, noting the thin line that separates finery and fiasco in athletics. Coach "Warm–ups" Mwithiga was more blunt; "We *have to* have the win. It is on us to do it, the world will be expecting to see Kenya winning, and we will not let them down. The team spirit is to win and we will hold it. I have been working on the mental strategy very much."

The Championships began with an athletics symposium held by Dr. Mike Boit. This attracted not only a number of the world's leading professors on sports research, but many of the Kenyan old guard, some of whom flew as far as from the States and Britain to see cross country come home and to meet old friends. At every hotel breakfast table, former Kenyan legends outnumbered non-runners.

The energy was simmering as face after face appeared. Lord Sebastian Coe, Richard Nerurkar, Sonia O'Sullivan, Hicham El Guerrouj...it was the golden gala of the running world.

The Tanzanians arrived somewhat miffed that the IAAF had been offering free full-board training camps in Kenya only for European squads. Suleiman Nyambui, the 1980 Olympic 5000m silver medalist, bemoaned, "We could not afford to hold a national training camp this year for our team. I am sure *that* was not a problem for any of the European teams!" The Qataris came looking for team gold. Richard Yatich quipped, "That's the team orders! They want a color, gold." The Ugandan chaperone, Rehema, said her team's sights were set on collecting at least one individual and one team medal. The most secretive were the Ethiopians. Coach Dr. Kostre Woldemskel, the International Association of Athletics Federation coach of the year for 2006, was asked of his team's plans. He only nodded his gray-haired head, saying, "We shall see. We shall see."

The day prior to the Worlds more legends continued to roll into town. Tegla Loroupe drove in with her sisters and manager Volker Wagner from Nairobi. She needed credentials for her vehicle parking. The CEO of the local organizing committee, Isaac Kalua, promised that they would be brought. Kip Keino, in a loose black-and-white shirt and with his hallmark smile, was explaining how he arrived on the athletic scene; "Nobody discovered me; I came, fast from the bush!" Sitting next to Kip, and looking exactly the same as he had a decade earlier when he had ruled the European tracks, was Daniel Komen. Sammy Koskei, the African record-holder in the 800m at 1:42:28, sat on the sofa. Billy Konchellah, together with a Maasai general, came to the hotel talking about how to bring athletics to Kilgoris and the Maasai lands: "Nobody helps the Maasai progress, they think we are a tourist attraction only. I believe people want us to remain behind, even in athletics!" Wilson Kipketer, slipping unnoticed through the lobby, stopped to talk about his new role with the IAAF as an anti-performance-enhancing drug educator, and how in the upcoming summer he had to drive his car from Monaco to Copenhagen. Back at the athletes' camp copious amounts of bottled water were being swallowed and the athletes, like resting lions, lazed under the shade of the trees dreaming the day away at the beautiful African Safari club hotel complex. Energy was definitely being conserved in the East African quarters.

Robert Cheruiyot and Paul Tergat had driven from Nairobi with their manager Federico Rosa, and Robert explained, "It's okay, we had a Lexus." Unlike Kipketer and the others, Tergat, whose presence transcends running, caused a stir in the lounge as fans immediately recognized the star and cameras came out.

At the afternoon's press conference, the whole stage centered around one man, the Ethiopian Kenenisa Bekele. Senegal's Lamine Diack, the IAAF president, spoke of Kenyan cross country: "They have dominated like no other. It seems their favorite pastime! Cross country has come home, to Africa." Isaac Kalua spoke eloquently and said that Kenya was fulfilling the dream that people had waited decades to witness. Moreover, when the inevitable deluge of questions fell to Bekele, he answered all with panache and grace. He respected the Kenyans, he had never raced in Kenya, but had enjoyed being in Kenya before, and he professed to be very happy to being in Kenya to race.

Moses Mosop, nicknamed "The Big Engine" and Pamela Chepchumba came to the IAAF press conference to represent the home team. Mosop admitted that he was not really prepared for the heat: "It was a bit of a shock to feel the heat in Mombasa. I was not expecting this." Pamela Chepchumba, sweating heavily, was dressed in a full tracksuit despite the weather being a reported 35 degrees celsius with 94 percent humidity. Sweat rolled from her brow. "God willing, I will perform." The women's team captain looked anything but confident.

A tree planting ceremony at the Mombasa Golf Course was next on the agenda, whilst down on the race course, the full Kenyan team took the opportunity to walk the 2K circuit. Coach "Warm-up" led the way, shouting out instructions as Coach Letting waived a hoisted flag. "Warm-up" halted the troops to voice his strategy for each section of the twisting course. IAAF veteran John Velzian had done a first-class job designing a challenging route. Barely a teenager, Chebet Cheptai from Kapsait, the younger sister of Pauline Korikwiang, walked along with the older athletes; she had qualified for the team by placing third at the trials, though at fourteen was not old enough to satisfy IAAF regulations. She said it was her dream to represent her country and could not wait until she was old enough to enter the junior division. Wearing a green Safaricom cap Matthew Kipkoech Kisorio strolled along at the back of the pack. Matthew had won the team trials in Nairobi, and he spoke about how he would like to win just a medal. I wondered, as he silently isolated himself lingering at the back, whether he was thinking of his late father Some Muge who, back in 1983, had become the first Kenyan to win an individual medal at the World Cross Country Championships.

As the group came to the finishing straight, where "Warm-up" was shouting, "Here you sprint till the power has left you," the world champion Ben Limo was waiting to greet and motivate the athletes. He had driven down from Nairobi that morning. "I am not running this year as they have got rid of my event, the short course, but I am here to lend my support," he said, shaking the hands of all the athletes, offering words of encouragement. Marathoner Chris Cheboiboch joined Ben. "Run hard tomorrow, run for Kenya!" He grinned, running on the spot.

An elderly couple stood at the finishing line. It was the first time they had left their home district up in the Rift Valley. They had sat in an old overheated bus for twenty hours driving over some of the worst roads in Kenya, which wrench the backbone and torture the knees, to come and watch the race. "Our daughter is running, how can we miss it! We have not seen her run before," the man said. And what an event Mr. and Mrs. Kosgei had chosen to see Mercy Jelimo run!

On the morning of March 24, 2007, African drums of heat hammered Mombasa as the thermometer crept up to its performance-crippling norm. Nairobi had been ruled out for the World Championships, apparently due not to its 6,000-foot altitude, as many had presumed, but to the city's inability to provide enough hotels for appropriate accommodations. Given the choice, the altitude, some 2,800 feet lower than Mexico City, where the Olympic had been held, would have been a far easier option. Even the acclimatized camel called Henry who gave tourists rides along the beach had collapsed under a palm tree. The three Kenyan coaches, usually bubbling with brio, were slumped in easy chairs in the lobby of the hotel, asking only for more boxes of water to be sent to the team's meeting room. A few Kenyan, Ugandan, and Tanzanian athletes sat together talking about how it would be possible, if all came together, to defeat Bekele. No one appeared confident. Boniface Kiprop, the Ugandan hope, summed up the general mood: "We are going to die out there!"

Two miles up the coast, at the Severin Hotel, one Kenyan was upbeat. "I have been training for this day for six months, and it has been in my head for much longer," she said, pouring over the country's largest newspaper, *The Daily Nation*, which had a large picture of her wearing a Shoe4Africa T-shirt in the day's edition. Lornah Kiplagat had meticulously prepared for this day. Up in Iten, she had spent hours sweating and suffering in a sauna to acclimatize whilst still training at altitude. She was booked into this hotel, and had brought cooking utensils, so she could prepare her usual food instead of staying with the athletes in the official hotels, fighting in the buffet lines for overcooked foods. She had made three trips to Mombasa to train on the course. Most important, she had not lost a cross country race in Kenya since 1996.

The security presence, due to some pre-event terrorist threats, was high. Boarding the athlete buses all persons were subject to airport-style checks. When loaded, the buses were not able to leave the gated compound until the drivers received police clearance. The athletes sat for an hour plus, sans air conditioning, with most of the Kenyan team in their full nylon rain jackets, on the stifling bus. The sweat poured off the face of Pauline Korikwiang, the defending world champion and the Kenyan junior 5000m record-holder at 14:45.98. Naser Jamal Naser, a Tanzanian, now representing Qatar, removed layer after layer of clothing. Still the bus refused to move. Never, in long memory, had an athlete bus been so deadly quiet.

The bus arrived one hour and forty minutes later at the oldest golf club in Kenya. The 1911 course, with its Indian Ocean side setting, was a spectacle to behold. Leaving the team bus, the Kenyan squad, with flags waving, walked down a tarmac road to the course entrance and on to the tented call-room area. Tens of thousands of Kenyans, in trees and packing the landscape, many unable to afford tickets, cheered at the very tops of their voices, "Ken-ya, Ken-ya, Ken-ya!" with such passion and empathy that tears were rolling down the cheeks of the emotional Kenyan team. It was truly a most moving experience. With every bit of breath in their lungs, the crowds were yelling out hope, dreams, and desire in one word, "Kenya!" The team members were visibly taken back at the profundity of passion.

It was the first time in history that a world-championship event of any sport had come to Kenya, and the fact that the event was one in which Kenyans were the world leaders was ideal for the public.

The cheers continued as the team made their way onto the grassy course. Pens of spectators, pushed together by makeshift barbed-wire fencing, screamed their hearts out for their compatriots. Vivian "Kadogo" Cheruiyot was having a halcyon season with victories on the IAAF circuit; she had won the IAAF World Junior Cross Country Championships in 2000 as a 17-year-old and was now looking for a senior title. She was handling the pressure of being a favorite in her home country with ease: "I may win, I may not, we shall see," she laughed as a well-wisher called to her from the crowd.

As they arrived at the call up area there was a surreal moment as one of the Kenyan reserves, former world champion Eliud Kipchoge, who had just ran the fastest time ever for a 10K on the roads, albeit with a net drop that cost him the official record, had been the Kenyan favorite for today's event. However, at the training camp he had not been able to impress the coaches and had been named as a reserve. He walked up to the start list and ran his finger down the names, perhaps looking for a loophole.

Moses Kiptanui, dressed in an Arabic shirt, walked around overwhelmed by the huge crowds. "What a day to be a Kenyan," he said, glancing at the sun, "But I am glad I am not running." Kipchoge did not seem to share that view.

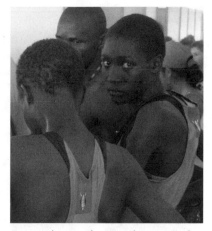

For once, the ice-cool reigning champion, Pauline Korikwiang, showed signs of nerves. (*Author*)

Junior Women's 6km

The first event, at 3:30 p.m, would be the most brutal, weatherwise. The Kenyan team, after warming up with some strides, all looked anxious for the day to begin. They were dressed in black uniforms and stood patiently in line as the race staff checked their names off the start list. Pauline Korikwiang, the favorite, was grabbed by Coach "Warm–up" and whisked away from the other girls. "Remember the race is yours," he said. "You know it. Now win it." Korikwiang did not answer, her wide eyes for the first time showing nerves.

The coaches voices were made to seem louder by the total silence of the team. In comparison, the Ethiopian women chatted wildly. The pressure was mounting. There was a slight hiccup as the officials at the check-in pointed out that all the Kenyan juniors' numbers had been incorrectly placed and harassed the young ladies to hurriedly change. Nimble fingers fumbled with the pins. The rush would be without cause as the officials then discovered they had no starter's gun. After a ten-minute holdup, the race was on. Coach "Warmup" said that the Kenyan strategy was to start cautiously, but to make sure they were positioned in the front group. "We'll let the Ethiopians lead."

That was exactly how the race played out—except for the defending champion, Pauline Chemning Korikwiang, who made a rash move because of miscounting the laps. Pauline's surge took two Ethiopians clear of the pack, but Mercy Kosgei later said she at once realized her teammate's folly, so did not attempt to follow the pace: "She was sprinting as if to finish the race, it was clear she had made a miscalculation, and the rest of us just relaxed." Arms raised Korikwiang thought she had won the race and came to a stop with the two other Ethiopians. The three following Kenyan women glided by to begin the last lap. Although Pauline tried to recover her position in the lead group, the effort proved two much; she staggered off the course, took a few steps forwards, then a few backwards, and collapsed from heat exhaustion a kilometer from the finish.. As she crumpled to the ground a dream was shattered. The crowd, transfixed, gasped in horror.

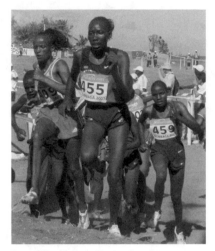

Linet Chepkwemoi Barasa. Linet's surname is now Masai, like her brother's. (*Author*)

However, even without Pauline, the team swept the podium, with Linet Chepkwemoi Barasa, from Mount Elgon, claiming not only the title, but her first-ever victory!

Linet, whose brother Moses Masai Ndiema, a 26:49 10,000m runner, is a former national cross country champion, deserved the win, she helped drive the pace from the gun to the tape. Linet worked for her gold, pulling her teammates along to team gold.

Junior Men's 8K

The crowd of a conservatively estimated 34,000 was joined by a loud chorus of tens of thousands who lined the perimeter of the golf course. Even the president of Kenya, Mwai Kibaki, was standing and cheering. The junior women's race had been a perfect start, and high expectations were on the junior men. The team was visibly bolstered by Coach "Warmup's" brief synopsis of the first race: "We won, I told you. Now you!" The men were surer of themselves than the ladies had been. It seemed that the clean sweep of the previous race had given them the assurance they were looking for; a conviction that the training camp's schedule had been a success.

It was little surprise that the men began at full tempo and immediately controlled the front of the pack despite the coach's advice to hold back. This is more remarkable considering that virtually the entire squad of these world-leading runners were newcomers to their national team. From the gun to the tape, it was Kenya all the way, and the men outdid their female counterparts by getting a perfect team score. Unbelievably, it was also the first ever win for Asbel Kiprop*, a 17-year-old son of policeman David Kebenei, a sub four-minute miler from Uasin Gishu. The late Some Muge's son took the bronze.
*Five months later the world youth silver that Asbel won in 2005 was upgraded to gold, as Taher Tareq Mubarak of Bahrain was disqualified after his age was questioned.

The Kenyan team with finishing positions: 1. Asbel Kiprop, 24:07; 2. Vincent Kiprop Chepkok, 24:12; 3. Matthew Kipkoech Kisorio, 24:23; 4. Leonard Patrick Komon, 24:25: a perfect sweep!

Senior Women's 8K

As the women's race got underway, there was a beautiful undulant sea of strides along the high coastline as a cascade of African legs controlled the front. In the lead, ahead of a quartet of the favored Ethiopians, was Lornah Jebiwott Kiplagat, now wearing the bright orange of Holland, had one tactic in mind: "I was afraid the Ethiopians would clip my

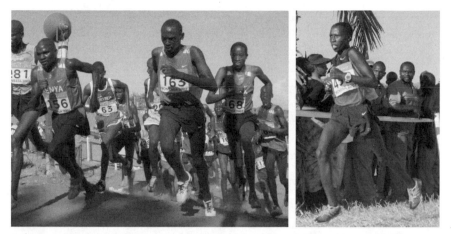

Left, Vincent Chepkok (bib 156) and Matthew Kisorio (bib 163) were the Kenyans in control for a large part of the 8K. They were rewarded with both individual and team medals. Right, Florence Kiplagat made the difficult transition from the junior to the senior ranks by leading the Kenyan team home. (*Author*)

heels, as has happened in road races, so I thought for the win, 'Let me make some space.'" Tirunesh Dibaba of Ethiopia had out-kicked Kiplagat in the last edition of the World Championships. The plan was to open a gap that would not allow Dibaba to repeat this trick.

With the first four Kenyans following Kiplagat, the three Ethiopians and the day's announcer, and the crowd, thought Kenya would win the team title, as the fourth Ethiopian was nowhere to be seen. However, on the last lap Ayalew Wude became the MVP for Ethiopia as she somehow chased down a score of runners in the final lap to place tenth and close out the gold-medal winning team for Ethiopia.

The season's new find for Kenya, Florence Kiplagat, who although not related to Lornah, was born a stone's throw from her birthplace, made an excellent transition from the junior to senior ranks and led the Kenyan team. Her coach and manager, Valentijn Trouw of Holland, was exceptionally pleased: "Anything in the top ten would have been fantastic for her!" Moments after finishing, Florence, looking as if every ounce of energy had been drained from her muscles, could only muster the words, "I tried to go with them, it was too hot, the speed, the weather. . ."

The fancied Kenyan who had performed so well in Europe prior to the championships, Vivian Cheruiyot, whose nickname, "Shorty" relates to her height, did not have the best of luck, as she kept slipping from the lead pack and had to run in no-woman's land. Valiant efforts, overextending herself to try and catch Lornah and the Ethiopians, drained her speed.

Lornah, in a devastating performance, had reduced the field to tatters, as only three runners managed to finish within a minute of her. "It may have looked easy, but it was not. I was very strong. Pieter was worried about my training because I have been going very,

very hard for this race. I reached 160 miles one week." She would recall later eating a steamed fish after the race and celebrating with a bitter lemon soda in a restaurant overlooking the Indian Ocean. "Kiplagat number two" was the second Kenyan home as the entire scoring team finished one after another all in the top ten.

Senior Men's 12K

It was Kenya against the five-time reigning champion, Kenenisa Bekele of Ethiopia. Half of Mombasa did not appear to know whether the race was a marathon or a cross country event, but everyone knew that Bekele was coming to town to race the Kenyans. It was a day to either immortalize the gracious Ethiopian, or destroy his invincible aura.

The cheers of "Ken-ya, Ken-ya!" rose even higher when the legend began his warm-up strides. Ethiopian Getaneh Tadesse, husband of former world cross country champion Gete Wami, and a former national-class athlete who had run in the World Cross back in 1992, was worried for his squad: "Dehydration will be a problem," he said, handing out chunks of ice for his athletes to cool themselves in the warm-up area. However, almost nobody doubted that Bekele would control the day's fortunes. Even Tergat, in his backyard, had picked the ten-time senior Ethiopian world individual cross country medalist for victory. Only John Ngugi, a five-time winner himself, seemed to believe that a Kenyan would win. On the course the day before the race, he had spoken not only of his historic runs, but also of the power of the Kenyan crowd: "They will pull Kenyans to win, you watch."

The opening quarter-mile was mind-boggling to watch as a fervent field of 170 bolted across the flat grass in front of the partisan masses, who now were crying for Kenya *and* water. The heat in the air continued to hang like thick hot steam. It was no surprise that Africans forced the pace, or that Bekele, and the reigning world road champion, Zersenay Tadesse of Eritrea, who had an individual World Cross silver, were at the front.

Bernard Kipyego and Gideon Ngatuny led the Kenyan chase. Kipyego, took a silver in the 2005 juniors, had wished to progress to the marathon distance, but had been persuaded by his former manager, Dutchman Michel Boeting, to wait a few years; it was turning out to be a sage decision for the 20-year-old. Ngatuny, a tall Maasai who is based in Japan, had planned to follow fellow Kenyan Moses Mosop after finishing second in the nationals and the trials. Yet it was Mosop who was following Ngatuny. Mosop, who had the most international experience, having medaled at the World IAAF Track and Field Championships 10,000m behind Bekele and placed seventh at the 2004 Athens Olympic 10,000m, had noted at the press conference the day before, "We're not really arranging anything special [to run as a team], but we really have to work as a team. But not to look at the others, and not for someone to work as a pacemaker."

The crowds whooped with delight as halfway through the race it was evident that Kenya, with its entire team in the top ten places, was going to win the team gold barring a complete disaster. Kenyan captain Mike Kipyego, a Marakwet like Mosop, was now towing six Kenyans, eight if one included the two Qatari Kenyans Richard Yatich and Albert Chepkurui. The crescendo rose when Bekele dropped out on the final lap. He was one of four Ethiopians who failed to cross the line. It would be the first time since 1980 that Ethiopia would fail to score as a team in the men's senior 12K. Tadesse sailed away unchallenged to a 23-second win in 35:50 ahead of Mosop, who had lost a shoe a lap earlier but gallantly charged on to receive the largest applause of the day. The six scoring Kenyans all finished in the top eight spots. Mosop expressed the thoughts of the crowd: "This was a huge victory for Kenya. We said we would win, and we did. We showed the world that on our home ground we would never be beaten."

Despite losing a shoe in the early stages of the race, Moses Mosop powered home to lead Kenya to the team gold. (*Author*)

Train Hard, Race Smart

The best racers in Kenya compete sparingly, especially at the longer distances. The trend began when Moses Tanui trained for months without a race, then won the Boston Marathon. "We started to change the workings of how to successfully race. Before it was common to race frequently, but then we noticed that the better runners did not compete so much before their best performances," said Mike Kosgei. Two notable practitioners of this methodology are Paul Tergat, who raced just twice in 2006 (a 59-minute Lisbon half marathon in April, and a third place finish at the ING New York City Marathon in November) and Felix Limo, who seldom runs any races apart from his biannual 2:06 marathons.

The top steeplechaser, Stephen Cherono likes to compete only half a dozen times per year. Isaac Songok, despite having run a world-leading 12:55 5000m in June, refused to expand his season past the three 5Ks he had planned. Top Kenyans have a trait of not over-racing and of making that big race count.

What people call the free-spirited Kenyan approach to athletics certainly does not apply to race day. The athletes, although still totally relaxed, approach the warm-up and the race in a detailed manner. Ninety percent of Kenyans always do a thorough warm-up, going through the phases of preparing the body before the race with meticulous care.

Warm-up

A significant difference in the Kenyan method of pre-race preparation is that many Kenyans rise very early (often 5 a.m. for a 9 a.m. start time) on the morning of the race for a pre-pre-race warm-up. They go out and run for twenty to forty minutes at a very easy pace before returning to shower, stretch, and eat breakfast. Forty minutes to an hour before the race, the second warm-up jog begins. Some of the leading non-Kenyan athletes have recently started adopting this method.

The Pre-Race Warm Up Routine

The whole process of the warm-up usually takes a good hour from the arrival at the warm-up point to the gun. After checking their bags in the elite-athletes tent, the runners typically take a short run. This stage, twenty to thirty-minutes of jogging, is usually painfully slow at the start, with the feet barely moving faster than a walk, but after a few minutes the pace increases a little, and in the last couple of minutes it reaches a brisk speed to raise the heart rate. Stephen Cherono, as noted in this book, never increases his pace past a jog until the final strides. Joseph Kimani, a prolific winner in the 1990s, would run the last 800m of his-twenty minute jog at about six–minute-mile, after an initial two and a half miles at at eight-minute pace.

Paul Tergat and Tegla Loroupe's pre-marathon warm-ups are a mere ramble. Most warm-up jogs last only twenty minutes, though Benson Masya would often extend his forty minutes. Catherine Ndereba likes to jog for ten to fifteen minutes at a very easy pace in her sweats prior to her race.

Ten minutes before the start is when the athletes usually start stripping off the layers, and Kenyans use plenty of layers regardless of the temperature. They strongly believe in keeping the muscles warm. Even on a hot day, when others are warming up shirtless, it is not uncommon for a Kenyan to wear a full tracksuit, with skintight suit below, and a shirt. This was clearly apparent in Mombasa. Then, after a change to lightweight racing shoes, some strides, typically four to five of 80m, are run before the athletes line up.

The Race and Its Structure

For many years, the Kenyan race tactic at most track and road events was to to fly from the starting line and play the catch-me-if-you-can game. In 1974, the year that John Kipkurgat won the Commonwealth Games 800m in 1:43.91, only a couple of tenths from the standing world record (1:43.7), he also ran the second-fastest 600m mark of all time, 1:13.2, en route in an 800m race at a small meet in Pointe-a-Pierre, Trinidad and Tobago. Tim Hutchings himself a former world-class 5000m runner, commentating during Daniel Komen's 3000m world-record, reported on the Kenyan spirit of racing: "This is fast, this is world record pace for a 2000-meter race, never mind a 3000-meter. It is aston-ishing." The brave do–or-die tactic makes for great spectating, but it was not always the best scheme for securing the first-prize pot.

Athletes like Paul Bitok, Paul Tergat, and Moses Tanui started to change this front-runner approach. After Charles Kamathi out-kicked Haile Gebrselassie (the man rumored to have the best kick in the business) to win the 2001 World Championships 10,000m in Edmonton, Canada, more and more athletes have started to believe that Kenyans can win coming from behind, and win with a fast sprint finish.

In the mid-1990s, it was common to hear that athletes were training for surges, and practicing holding a continuous hard pace to burn off the competition. A decade later, it is common to see groups of Kenyans training to develop a killer finishing kick.

During the race, Kenyans will often talk to each other and evaluate the situation. Ben Limo and Daniel Yego both talk in this book about mid-race dialogues that took place in major competitions. In many cases, the Kenyans will try to assist each other.

This is not always the case, in the 2006 Boston Marathon there was the incident when Ben Maiyo asked his countryman Robert Cheruiyot to help maintain the leading pace, reasoning that the third place man (Meb Keflezighi, of the USA), might catch up should the pace slacken. Cheruiyot, on that day, was not interested in making small talk or helping with pace duties. But in more cases than not, as Joseph Chelang'a expresses, there is a team theme: "There is a bond between fellow Kenyans at the front of the field, and we are always thinking of not just ourselves, even though it is a race."

This ethic probably stems from growing up in an extended-family situation where a community cares for each of its members. John Ngugi says, "To be born a Kenyan is an honor indeed, to help each other is God's request." When Rita Jeptoo won the 2006 Boston Marathon, the defending champion, Catherine Ndereba, who had not been invited back to defend her title, was at home sitting on the couch yelling for Rita. "I was so happy that a Kenyan won. When I heard that I could not go, I prayed to God and asked, 'Let it be a Kenyan that wins.'"

The Cool-Down

Following the race the Kenyan athletes—pending obligatory press responsibilities—are sure to cool down with an easy jog to remove the lactic acid from the legs. About twenty minutes is the usual. "This is a must; it takes the stiffness out of the legs. How else can we do training the next day?" asked Tom Nyariki. "We are told in the training camps in Kenya that it is compulsory, so we do it." Patrick Boiyo, who raced in Scandinavia frequently in the 1990s would wait until he came to a flat grassy field to do his cool-down, "You must have no pounding for the muscles, just gentle jogging on grass for forty minutes." Even if Patrick had to wait until after the travel home, he would do the cool-down this way, believing that a cool-down on the roads causes further unnecessary muscle damage.

Road Racing, Kenyan Style

Tiger Woods might have a private jet, and Carl Lewis would often turn up at track meets in stretch limousines, but for Kenyans the ride is often not so easy. There is story that one Kenyan, stuck at the U.S. immigration office, who had to pull out a copy of *Train Hard, Win Easy* to prove that he was an elite runner. Even championships winners get a rough ride; there is a certain airline that one Kenyan Olympic medal-winner will not use because of a bad experience. Often the Kenyan elite racers on the U.S. road circuit come to the starting line in anything but a smooth manner.

In the 1990s, Thomas Osano, an All-Africa Games 10,000m gold medalist, a 60:36 half-marathon runner, and the winner of nearly all the major U.S. road races; Delillah Asiago, who is a female equivalent of Osano (and also his wife) and I were traveling to Clarksburg for a road race. We flew from Albuquerque to Cincinnati. There was no direct connection to Clarksburg, so we had to travel to Pittsburgh to take another flight. There was no bus, but a gypsy–cab driver agreed to take us there. When we got there after a two-hour drive, the plane had taken off. So we sat in the airport for a while.

It was late, so a further ride had to be taken into the nearby city to get a hotel for the night. Neither of the Kenyans had any money for board or food. The next morning we took a bus back to airport, and then we took the flight to the closest airport to Clarksburg. When we arrived in the afternoon the day before the race, the organizers had not, understandably, scheduled a pick-up, so we sat at the airport for a few hours, not even sure of what host hotel we were headed for. Late, late in the afternoon, after a multitude of phone calls, a van came and picked us up. However, the driver had to wait for another couple of hours because another runner was arriving at the airport. Finally, at about 10 o'clock in the evening we checked into the hotel. The next morning, after 10K of running, and 18 beers (blame Delillah), we began the homeward trip—twelve hours after we'd arrived.

Another time, Olympians Salina Chirchir and Helen Kimaiyo were invited to a race in Kansas, but there was no budget for travel or accommodation. The prize money was decent, and these women made a career out of finishing in the money. A car was rented and off we popped, driving all day from Albuquerque through Colorado, *nearly* speeding the entire way with eagle-eyed Salina watching out the front window and Helen out the rear. We arrived in Kansas, ran the race, bought five liters of Mountain Dew, and drove back home. These are two of many road-trip stories—tales to think of the next time you see a Kenyan on a starting line.

Kenyan Pioneers

Major Michael Rotich, from Marakwet, was sixth in the Kenyan Olympic Trials back in 1972 behind such stars as Kip Keino, Cosmas Siele, Mike Boit, and Ben Jipcho. He talks about the training at this time in Kenya:

"You must remember in those days we had no information on training, any books or magazines or educated coaches. We slept and woke at 6 a.m. [at the military barracks in the 1960s] to find the athletes like Wilson Kiprugut in bed, so we would relax and take another hour's sleep. Little did we know Kiprugut had already trained and was now in bed resting. What we saw is what we did; slow learning. At ten o'clock, there would be group training where a sergeant would stand at the top of a hill and we would have to run up. That was how training was back in those days. When we ran competitions, we won blankets or cooking utensils. Very few of us took athletics seriously. We had no information on training, or running. If only we had had the help of a training manual. When I got a trip to Portsmouth, England, it was academics first, sports definitely second."

Kip Keino, the Legend of Legends

"If you want to win races, then you should learn to burn in training, else you will never win."

Although neither Kenya's first international athlete nor first Olympic medalist, Kipchoge Hezekiah Keino ranks as one of the most famous and most influential of Kenyan runners. Keino inspired a nation, indeed a whole continent, with his international success. And his post-athletics life has further enhanced his legend.

Keino was the first black African to run consistently and successfully in America and Europe. In the late 1960s, he became enormously popular with Western track crowds, as he ran with great personality and flair— not to mention great accomplishment.

First seen on the Olympic stage in 1964,

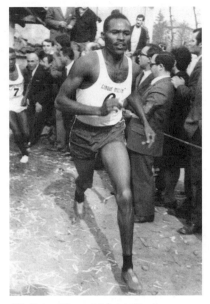

Kip Keino. (*Cinque Mulini Archives*)

Keino finished fifth in the 5000m in Tokyo. It was to be at the shorter 1500m event that Keino would gain true world recognition at the next Olympics. Jim Ryun, the world record-holder in the mile and the 1500m, was the favorite for the 1500m gold in Mexico. However, going into the 1968 Olympics, Ryun felt he was at a disadvantage. "Always in the back of my mind remained the phantom of Kip Keino, born and bred in the Kenyan highlands which gave him an edge in Mexico City's thin air." If Ryun wanted an equalizer, he had more than one to chose from: Keino went into the Games with a gallbladder infection, and in eight days he would attempt the 1500m, the 5000m, and the 10,000m events!

The Games began badly for Keino. With three laps to go in the 10,000m, he collapsed in the infield clutching his stomach in agony. As the doctors approached, he sprang to his feet and rejoined the race to finish last. On medical grounds, Keino was advised to withdraw from the remaining events. But Kip had other ideas. He could eat no solid food his stomach could tolerate only milk and soft drinks while he rested for the 5000m. In the 5000m final, he and Mohamed Gammoudi of Tunisia raced shoulder to shoulder to the finish line, with the Tunisian finally edging Kip by two-tenths of a second.

Still without solid sustenance, Keino prepared for the 1500m. "How could I go home failing?" he asked. Keino reached the 1500m final, running an unencumbered five seconds faster than he needed to in the heats! Ryun also qualified for the final as did the German Bodo Tummler, who had been all-conquering in the last twelve months.

When the gun sounded, Ben Jipcho, Keino's young teammate, shot into the lead. Keino slipped in behind him. Ryun, who was expecting a more tactical final considering the altitude, the distance Keino had already covered in previous events, and the African's infection, lolled in the back of the field. The first lap was a very swift 56 seconds—3:30 pace! As the world record was then 3:33, surely this was a suicidal pace at altitude. On lap two Keino passed Jipcho and the 800m split was 1:55.3. Tummler was hanging in four meters back with Ryun pursuing a further 15 meters behind.

Still at world-record pace, Keino strode round the third lap. *Track & Field News* reported, "He [Keino] was expected to fall flat on his face at any moment." Ryun was now in full flight, but despite a 54-second final lap the American could not catch Keino, who won by 2.9 seconds. It was Keino's first victory over Ryun. His 3:34.9 clocking was a new Olympic record. It was to be the fastest 1500m of Keino's career!

On returning to Kenya he was promoted by the police department, and in the midst of being paraded in the streets of Nairobi, he fainted from stomach pains. It took six months for Keino to be restored to health.

He returned to the Olympic forum at Munich. In the 1500m final he was passed in the last 100m by the Finn Pekka Vasala, who ran a 1:48 last 800m and, nipped Keino by a half-second. However, six days earlier, Kip had competed seriously for the first time in the steeplechase. The Kenyan's style was ragged, but the result was impeccable—gold in a new Olympic record!

Keino's Olympic at Mexico City is not only mind-boggling, it is likely never to be repeated. Kip ran considerably more than a half-marathon worth of track racing in eight days(!): 10/13/68, 10,000m; 10/15/68, 5000m heat, 21st place, 14:28.4. 10/17/68, 5000m final, 2nd place, 14:05.2; 10/18/68, 1500m heat, 1st place (by nearly five seconds), 3:46.9. 10/19/68 1500m semi-finals, 2nd place, 3:51.4. 10/20/68, 1500m final gold medal, 3:34.9, Olympic record.

Date of birth:	January 17, 1940
Birthplace:	Kapchemoiywo Village, Nandi District
Height/weight:	5'-9-1/4", (176 cm) 143 lbs (65 kg)
Personal bests:	1500m–3:34.9, Mile–3:53.1, 2000m–5:05.2, 3000m–7:39.6,
	3000m Steeplechase–8:23.6, 5000m–13:24.2, 10,000m–28:06.41
Honors won:	1966 Commonwealth Games champion, 1 mile and 3 miles
	1968 Olympic 1500m Champion (2nd, 1972)
	1968 Olympic 5000m, 2nd
	1970 Commonwealth Games champion, 1500m
	Order of the Burning Spear, 1970
	1972 Olympic Steeplechase champion
	World records, 3000m and 5000m

Comments

To be active in many sports was an important factor to Kip. In the off-season period Keino participated in such sports as volleyball, tennis, basketball, and swimming. According to Keino, in 1996 his weekly mileage was a mere 50K, and in some books he has been quoted as saying he ran as little as three times per week. Keino's philosophy was to put quality before quantity, not to tire the body with endless kilometers. In interval training he felt it imperative that the athlete "burned" while running. Keino reasoned that unless this feeling was experienced in training one could not expect to run through such pain in competition. "I had good speed. I could run 21-second 200s. By running lots of intervals I kept that speed fresh. A lot of runners lose their natural speed through too much mileage."

Training Week
Location: Kiganjo Police Training Center. Altitude: 2000m. Surface: dirt tracks. Training in spring for the track season.

Monday	AM 6K steady. PM 5K steady.
Tuesday	AM As above. PM 10 x 400m, run in 55-60 sec., 200m jog rest.
Wednesday	AM As above. PM 5K fast/steady.
Thursday	AM As above. PM 15 x 400m, run in 55-60 sec., 200m jog rest.
Friday	AM As above. PM Hill work.
Saturday	AM 5K fartlek or a session of 4 x 800m run in 2 min. with a similar rest.
Sunday	AM Long run, 10K good pace.

As the competition season approached, interval sessions would be adopted. "In the summer, I would run many 400m sessions, fast." Although Keino was not renowned for having a great sprint finish, he did have excellent speed endurance, which was usually enough to wear down his opponents. More often than not Keino ran his sessions solo. When questioned about Kenyan dominance in distance running, Keino had the following to offer: "The Kenyan runner is free of pressure. Whether he wins or loses over here [in Kenya] it does not matter. They develop naturally. In Europe the young runners are told "win, win" all the time. With no forcing, the athlete enjoys the sport much more. If you have no interest then how can you train hard?"

Jim Ryun on Kenyan Running

The man closest to Keino's astonishing Olympic record in Mexico was Jim Ryun, now a U.S. congressman. His 3:58.3 to win the mile at the 1965 Kansas High School state meet is still the record for the fastest time ever in a race contested only by high school competitors. Ryun gives his thoughts and reflections on 1968, himself, and Kenyan running.

More Fire: Do you remember first lining up against the Kenyans? And what was your impression of their racing?

Jim Ryun: I remember Keino, a very worthy competitor. I raced against him the year before Mexico, in 1967 [when Ryun was 20] at a Commonwealth meeting in Los Angeles, and then in London at the White City Stadium. My strength to beat Kip was to stay with him and out-kick him in the finish.

MF: And this tactic was not obviously possible at Mexico, right?

Jim Ryan: Right. I knew I would get into oxygen debt if I went out at too fast a pace. I knew it was going to be different, the altitude advantage. Ben Jipcho came up to me after the race and apologized; he said, "Jim, I was really pushed by the delegation to take advantage of the altitude." I would say that was very courageous of him.

MF: Can you remember the day?

Jim Ryun: After the first lap I was about four or five seconds back. It was a matter of whether I could catch them with 600 meters to go, as I knew I could kick from that far out. I did not. I have the silver; it is the same size as the gold medal.

MF: Do you think things would have ended differently at low altitude?

Jim Ryun: Undoubtedly, and it was not just I that thought so. I had run some times that year that confirmed that. I would have definitely gone out with Keino and Jipcho had the Olympics been at low altitude.

MF: Apart from Kip, are there other Kenyans you remember from that era?

Jim Ryun: Kip was a great athlete. The "door opener," a little like Dr. Roger Bannister. You always admire the first one.

MF: What is your theory on the Kenyan running success, and did it in any way link to your own ideas at the time?

Jim Ryun: Well, it is more than altitude! They have tremendous dedication to their training, and they make the big commitment. My whole approach was doing it (training) legally, train hard, give yourself the proper recovery and that gets the good results and my mom's cherry pie!

MF: Can you see any "Kenyan" attributes in your own lifestyle back in the 1960s?

Jim Ryun: As a student I always walked, I never rode the bus. I walked everywhere. For me it was a choice, something I liked to do. As far as diet, I had a typical Midwestern diet, not as regimented as many have today. I think it was the right thing, not a scientific answer. I mean, running one hundred miles per week, you are trying to get calories in.

MF: Is there anything you think we can learn from the Kenyans?

Jim Ryun: Well, I didn't know so much about what they were doing, but in running, it is a matter of finding what works for you and sticking with it. Sticking with the program. I was lucky that I had a very good coach, Coach Timmons, from high school onwards. He told me something, after only my fourth-ever mile [4:21 on a cinder track], on the bus on the way back from a competition: "You can run faster." And I was thinking 4:19, and he said to me, back then, "You can run the first high school sub-four-minute mile." I was very fortunate to have such a man to provide direction.

MF: So you could say, belief.

Jim Ryun: Definitely, most important in running.

Henry Rono

"I was an intense athlete; I wanted to see how far I could push my own limits."

Kipwambok "Henry" Rono was born in 1952, in Kiptaragon village a small Nandi settlement nestling at a 7,600-foot altitude. As a youth Henry played soccer and was a high jumper. At the age of 18 he turned his attention to running.

"I saw Kip Keino running well and I thought, why not me? I think I have done as well as Keino now." President Jomo Kenyatta awarded Henry the burning spear, an honor that had also been bestowed upon Keino.

Studying industrial psychology at Washington State University, Rono was a shy, silent, and hard-working student with average grades. John Chaplin, the school's coach, first heard of Rono through hurdler and fellow Kenyan Kip Ngeno in 1976.

Chaplin brought Rono to a favorite training site called the Canyon. Rono far out-distanced his teammates, zooming up the hill with ease. Rono had a burning desire to set foot where no man had before, and he began to train his body ferociously.

In 1978, he captured the 5,000M, 3000M steeplechase, the 10,000M, and the 3,000M world records between April 8 and Jun 27, a period of only 80 days. Back in his heyday he weighed 142 pounds standing at 5'8". He trained 120-140 miles per week. Rono's philosophy on running is "to be consistent in training. Train like a team of bees working together to make honey."

Henry has this advice about competition: "During racing, race as a person who is taking the message to the promised land."

He has never lost the dream to be his best. Early in the morning, far earlier than need be and just like in the old days, Henry can be seen running up Copper Hill to the Sandia mountains. He is much heavier now than he was 20-odd years ago, but the fire in his eyes remains, his arms pump with the same vigor, and he still believes totally in himself: "People look and they see a big man. They can not believe I can run so fast, but I can run much faster!"

Ibrahim Hussein

The first African to win the New York and Boston Marathons was a Kenyan named Ibrahim Kipkemboi Hussein. Hussein was an economics student at the University of New Mexico, and during his stay in America he earned thousands of dollars on the road-racing circuit. In addition to three wins at Boston, he also won the Honolulu Marathon three times.

Hussein trained hard! Neither quality nor quantity was neglected. Many long road sessions on tarmac were run in his marathon preparations. Long hill runs and intervals were also practiced, as was fartlek. Though he could be out of shape and too heavy for competition a few months before a major race, with extremely hard training—often three sessions per day—he would haul his body into form in a couple of months.

Hussein would regularly run a predominantly uphill route over a tarmac road to his hometown of Kapsabet, covering around 22K. "If you work the hills, then running on the flat is easy," he reasoned. He also employed tempo road runs of 1-1/2 hours. "Running fast and hard on the roads is the best way to prepare for racing on the roads." Long runs could be up to three hours. "I would often run fast, not much slower than my racing speed." Hussein won over 40 percent of the marathons he contested.

Other Pioneers

In addition to the four influential runners profiled above, mention must be made of other Kenyan pioneers who made significant impact on the international running scene.

Wilson Kiprugut was the first Kenyan to earn a medal at the Olympics, taking the 800m bronze in Tokyo in 1964; he did himself one better the following Olympics, with a silver in the 1968 800m. Kiprugut also earned a silver medal in the 800m at the 1966 Commonwealth Games.

The first Olympic gold medalist from Kenya was **Naftali Temu**. He won the altitude-affected 10,000 meters in Mexico City in 1968 and also won a bronze medal in the 5000m. He was the six-mile champion at the 1966 Commonwealth Games in Kingston. Temu earned two *Track & Field News* number one rankings, in 1966 and 1967. He retired after the 1972 Olympics when he could only manage to run 30:19.6 in the heats, a time he considered a disaster.

Amos Biwott started the string of Kenyan steeplechase triumphs with his eccentric victory in 1968. He was eccentric because, to the delight of the crowd, he never got wet at the water jump, preferring to launch himself off the barrier completely over the water on each lap. Biwott returned in 1972, to finish sixth. He worked for the Kenyan Prisons, then as a security watchman, after retiring from athletics in 1973. He married Cherono Maiyo, a pioneer of women's athletics in Kenya who traveled to the Munich 1972 Olympics and was eliminated in the first round of the 800m, running 2:04.9, and the 1500m, clocking 4:20.9. The couple had five children, one of whom, Beatrice, was a high school sensation winning three Kenyan Senior National sprint-hurdle titles (twice the 100m and once the 400m), whilst still at school, and taking gold in the 1995 African Junior Championships 400m hurdles.

Dr. Mike Kiprugut Boit: "When I first started running in the 1960s, you were not supposed to train. It was something embarrassing, especially if one met ladies out running. Kenyan people did not understand it. It was expected that you went to a race and did your best, no training was needed and any running talent was enough for the races. So I would train in the evenings when it was dark, and nobody was about. Well, one day I was flying down a hill and I crashed straight into somebody and knocked them over. I quickly ran away fearing it was a woman. You see, if I had been caught, I could not have explained, what I was doing. They would not have believed I was training for running races."

At school, it was not much better: "We trained in four seasons. One month before the athletics championships, we did track. Other times it was soccer and other sports, just PE classes." There was no information available on coaching or methodology, so that was how it was done.

"I very much improved in 1970 when I finally got two coaches, a huge improvement," recalls Boit talking about the influence of Englishman Bruce Tulloh and Scotsman Alex Stewart. Boit was ranked fifth in Kenya, but in his own words, "I was close to giving up, as I thought I was not good enough, and to take a position as a high school teacher. These men made me reconsider." The incentives in those days were only of international travel and no financial reward, yet that was enough for Mike to continue with the sport.

European 5000m Champion Bruce Tulloh takes up the story.

"Mike was doing orthodox interval training—interval 400s, 300s and 200s. I introduced a few new things—a long weekend run for endurance, and also "situation practice."

With an American runner, we made Mike practice tactical situations—leading and fending off a late strike, following and putting in a mid-race kick, following and putting in a fast last 200—all at close to race speed. As there was not much competition, I had time trials, and in January 1972, he ran two times 800 meters in 1:53 and 1:52 on a bumpy school track, at 6,000 feet, with only five minutes in between. I knew than that he could be a great middle-distance runner, and I think that I gave him self-belief, because I had competed for many years at world level. If he had one key session, it was the eight times 300-meters, which used to start at 42 seconds and work down to 36 or 37 seconds."

At the 1972 Olympics, Mike took the bronze in the 800 and placed fourth at the 1500m. He shined at the Commonwealth Games, taking an 800m silver in 1974, gold in 1978 at the same distance, and bronze in the 1500m in 1982.

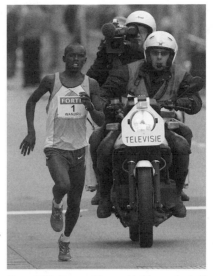

Samuel Wanjiru, world record-holder at the half marathon, here improves on his own record on the streets of Den Haag. His 5K splits: 13:40 - 27:27 - 41:30   55:31 for a time of 58:35. Wanjiru, Olympic champion at age 21, is fated to be a Kenyan legend. (*Robert Lejeune*)

Olympic Bronze, August 26–September 2, 1972

Aug. 26	a.m.	Munich opening ceremony
	p.m.	4 x 400m (52.8, 53.5, 53.5, 52.8) 3-min. recoveries
Aug. 27	a.m.	Light jogging
	p.m.	2 x 600m (81+82), 4-min. recovery
Aug. 28	a.m.	Light jogging
	p.m.	2 x 200m (23.9 + 23.9) Long full recovery.
Aug. 29	Easy jogging	
Aug. 30	Easy jogging	
Aug. 31	first round; first, 1:47.3	
Sept. 1	second round; first, 1:45.9	
Sept. 2	rest	

Sept. 3   finals; first, , 1:46.0 (winner's time 1:45.9). "I got boxed in with 200 meters to go and lost the opportunity to shoot for the gold medal."

Ben Wabura Jipcho of Mt. Elgon, who represented the police and was a teacher and school inspector by trade, was Kip Keino's 1500m pacemaker in 1968. He was responsible for taking the race out fast for the eventual winner. By the following Olympics, with a change of discipline, Jipcho, then 29, won the silver medal in the steeplechase. In 1973, at the All-Africa Games, Jipcho collected gold at both the Steeplechase, where he set the world record of 8:20.8, and the 5000m, beating the legendary Miruts Yifter. Later that summer, in Helsinki, Jipcho lowered his steeplechase record to 8:13.91 after skeptics had doubted the validity of the Lagos track and the height of the barriers at that event. In 1974, the ever-ambitious Jipcho tried for a trifecta at the Commonwealth Games. He won the steeplechase by an unheard of 16-second margin, just nipped Brendan Foster in the 5000m for his second gold, and then lost an entrancing duel in which both Filbert Bayi and John Walker had to beat the world record to leave Jipcho with the bronze in the 1500m.

Forty years later, Bayi recalled that race: "Jipcho was the *toughest* competitor. At whatever distance, he was there fighting."

Shortly after the Commonwealths, Jipcho followed the lead of Keino into the professional ranks, becoming a star of the circuit. Later he became a groundsman at the Moi International Sports Complex in Nairobi before retiring.

The Coaches

Few would doubt Kenya's dominance over the past dozen or so years in distance running, and no other country can match their achievements. Behind the "stones," there are always the architects.

"The coach advises in Kenya; he doesn't rule like a European coach," so spoke Moses Kiptanui. Middle and long distance running in Kenya can mean big money, comparable to winning the lottery. Even mediocre athletes can return home from a racing season with enough money to allow ten year's leisure. Coaching is taken very seriously. The job is not well paid in Kenya, and the coaches are often "forgotten" by their former athletes when they strike gold, but due to the lure of prestige, travel, and opportunity there are many people still wanting to become coaches.

The good coaches are involved mainly for the love the sport. Elliott Kiplimo, a successful Army coach, has been in the game for well over a decade, and many top runners have been nurtured under his wing, including the late world champion Paul Kipkoech. He has yet to receive more than a sports cap from any of his runners, however. Brother Colm O'Connell has to work a job in order to support his coaching.

Mike Kosgei, after being sacked by the national federation, coached in Finland for a few years and has now returned to Kenya, where he works with runners at Kaptagat. When employed by the Kenyan government, Kosgei received a meager salary and a government house to live in next to the national athletics stadium on the outskirts of Nairobi. Danny Kibet, of the Armed Forces, has perhaps one of the best squads of athletes any team could ever muster for distance events. "I have no car, and the way things are going, the likelihood is I'll never have one, either—it is something a coach does not dream of." "Sacrifice" is a word heard often in Kenya. The athletes believe that if you wish to succeed, you must put everything into your goal. The coaches follow this approach. Many live in sub-standard conditions away from their families for months to be with the athletes day and night. "If the runner sees you also are giving all, they will too," noted Albert Masai of the Navy coaching staff.

An important role of the Kenyan coach is as an organizer and a creator of structure. Kenyan athletes are often neither punctual nor organized. When left to their own devices they might reward themselves with a two-week holiday or simply miss training sessions due to other commitments. However when an athlete is plugged into an organized training plan and has someone checking his progress, he or she will give everything and more to training. Brother Colm O'Connell noted that the Kenyans simply enjoy training. "You have to give the European a motive to train. Maybe it is to win a race, or make a team, but with the Kenyans they will train just because they love to run."

In Kenya, the personal coach does not exist. Paul Tergat may be the star of the Moi Air Base squad, but he receives exactly the same program, advice, and help as all the other athletes in the squad. The training sessions are never set up designed to help a particular individual, and there is never the one-to-one relationship that can be found with elite athletes outside of Kenya.

The system does not work for every athlete. Perhaps the great number of athletes hides the failures in this scheme. Mark Wendot Yatich was a neighbor, in Kenyan terms, to the Olympic gold medalist Matthew Birir. Birir was the first to encourage Yatich as a runner. In the first important race Yatich ran, he defeated a highly talented field including such stalwarts as Simon Chemoiywo, Andrew Masai, and Ezekiel Bitok. The unknown runner was immediately recruited by the Moi Air Base team and brought to their training camp. Yatich's form plummeted. The training simply went against the grain for his body. Later he left the camp and reverted back to his old schedule; the results began to pick up.

Pieter Langerhorst: A Dutch Mind, But the Kenyan Way

Christopher Cheboiboch sits in his living room pointing to various medals. His eyes linger on the silver medal he won at the Boston marathon. "I owe that medal to Pieter—I was trained by him. Also the silver medal I won in New York the same year. I was using his training plan." Cheboiboch plans to use the schedule again, as it produced his 2:08 PR. He continues, "Rodgers Rop was training with me too, and he won both those races. I think it was a very good schedule!" Then there is the story of Kimutai Kosgei: Pieter coached him to a 2:07:26 win at Amsterdam in his debut run. Soon afterward Kimutai left to coach himself, and, like Cheboiboch, he never ran sub 2:10 again. Same with Linah Cheruiyot; with Pieter's methods, 68 minutes for the half-marathon, a change of coaches and she slowed to 73 minutes. and let us not forget the results of triple world champion Lornah Kiplagat, Pieter's wife! Pieter has one of Kenya's most successful coaching records. So how does his methodology work?

> My coaching? That is pretty easy. I base pretty much everything on endurance.
> Long runs at a pretty slow speed. Twice-a-week Fartlek sessions, and some-

times we go to the track. It all depends on the athlete you are coaching of course, and on the distance at which they will compete. For Mombasa, I have done mainly endurance and twice a week fartlek but then the "Kenyan" way. That means sometimes one minute fast, one minute easy, and sometimes one minute fast, 30 seconds easy or two minutes fast and one minute easy.

We have done only a few times track work, and then mainly 400-meter repeats, or a combination of 400 meters and 2000 meters with short rest in between. It is pretty much marathon training, but after seeing the course in Mombasa I knew that speed was not enough. You need also strength and endurance.

I further believe very strongly in exercises and the gym, we do that almost every day. The most important part, however, is the mind. I do not have to teach my athletes how to run; who am I to tell them? I do give them confidence and peace in their mind. I never put pressure on an athlete. If I have to tell my athletes to do their best or to push it, then it means the athlete does not have the right mentality and character. I only work with people I have to slow down in training-isn't that easy?

Walter Abmayr: German engineering on the Kenyan mind and body

Walter first arrived in Kenya in September of 1980. The German government, to the commissioned him for a Culture and Sports position with the Kenyan Ministry. The primary goal, apart from being appointed the National Coach by the Kenyan Athletics Federation, was to implement a coaches' training program. Over the ensuing years, Abmayr estimates he trained approximately 550 coaches in Kenya. "[Upon arrival] I saw great potential, but no guidance."

He noted that the schools had "little to virtually nothing" in to the way of physical educators in the schools, "But there were a lot of interested teachers." Walter cites the double Olympic boycott for being a possible lack of sports development in Kenya at this time.

"My aim at first was to provide more information and knowledge in terms of scientific as well as practical approaches in training," says Abmayr, who had six years prior experience coaching in Ghana and Nigeria. Walter, did however, come to Kenya with an open mind. "It would be arrogant and silly, coming to such a potentially rich place, and not evaluating and examining the current structure and approach of the training by the local people before applying a training program."

The German discovered that where there was formulated training, as in the Armed Forces (Army, Air Force, Navy, police, prisons) the athletes' intensity had to be modified "to keep the athletes alive longer." He noted that too many young athletes were being burned out by being pushed well past their athletic limits.

Although overburdened by coaching the coaches, Abmayr did have time to train a select number of Kenyans, notably Julius Korir, who won the Olympic Games steeplechase in 1984; Some Muge, who won Kenya's first individual World Cross Country medal, and the late, great first World Track and Field champion, Paul Kipkoech, who took the 10,00m gold in 1987. He was also the coach of Kipkemboi Kimeli, Kenya's first-ever World Cross Country champion in the 1985 junior men's race. "I found him as a stranded boy and helped him, and he later followed me to Germany and stayed with me." Walter instigated a framework training plan that was later used nationwide. Mike Kosgei followed the program with great results for the national team from 1986 up to about 2006. Abmayr is an emotional coach: "I coach by love and am a friend and a partner to my athletes. I hope this explains my feelings and approach to train sports people. [I use] quality, in terms of needs, before quantity."

Walter was integrally responsible for the birth of the Kenyan coaching in a country that he stresses is rich in athletic tradition and environment. "A wide heel bone, which enables a better force transfer in the stride, and an inborn running skill are examples of why Walter feels success has flooded Kenya. He adds also natural living and diet. "I can only say this in German: Bewegung ist awestruck der freude des körpers." (*Movement is the awestruck joy of the body*)

Boniface Tiren: Shoe4Africa Moses Kiptanui Training Camp

A coach in Kapcherop, Marakwet, who proved by learning that he was then able to teach; becoming one of the area's best coaches, Tiren has a junior camp that is a who's-who of junior steeplechase runners, yet he coaches on a thick, grassy, undulating playing field without a track! "I did not let that discourage me. And for the steeplechase practice, I constructed my own barriers and put them on the flat road."

Up in the Cherangany Hills, he has had unparallel results: the last three Olympic steeplechase champions have come from his camp. He explains:

My first athlete to coach was Richard Chelimo, and the second was Ismael Kirui. I started coaching as a schoolteacher at Chesubet School. I was not knowledgeable in training methods when I first started, and there as nobody to ask. I sought out the former 10,000m world record-holder Samson Kimobwa and listened to how he trained, and then I found a book on coaching, and was soon able to formulate some plans. I went to Brother Colm and we had a camp in Iten. I asked Moses Kiptanui [a neighbor] to assist and KIM came in to support the camp. My own thoughts are, 'do not pressure the athlete too much, you ask what is their aim, is it to train or to try to become the best athlete.' If they want the latter then you ask, "Are you prepared to be in the field a long time as it is not easy. Education comes first with my runners, they must not miss school. I also keep my young athletes fresh; we do not run over an hour. My training motto is 'Be fresh for speed,' else with no speed you will not succeed. Three sessions are run per day when the runners are in camp with an easy run at six a.m. each morning, and medium-paced runs and two quality sessions per week at 10 a.m. Jogging is done in the afternoon.

"This environment," Tiren's arm stretches out toward thousands of miles of green rolling hills and rusty red dirt trails, "is the unspoiled secret of Kenya. The girl that is doing well now in America, Sally Kipyego? She learned to run here, as did her brother Michael Kipyego, as did Solomon Busendich, Raymond Yator, Moses Mosop . . ." Tiren's tongue continues to reel off a never-ending spool of champions, as his new team of soon-to-be champions come racing up the grassy slopes. The runners follow his instructions to a T as they close another session. For the next hour, while Tiren and others continue to talk, they bask in the sun, stretching, talking, and relaxing. Tiren proudly looks over at the group and adds, "This is why this is the place to make the champions. That is the way to recover properly from hard training. No rushing off to check emails, going to town, stressing with problems, just enjoying the Kenya life!" Two months after this interview, the latest protégé from the camp, Willy Komen, won the All-Africa Championships 3000m steeplechase gold, beating Ezekiel Kemboi to the line in Algiers.

Renato Canova: The Leonardo of coaching

One of the most innovative coaches in Kenya is Renato Canova of Torino, Italy. Listening to Renato talk training is to hear methodical, proven, and stimulating ideas. He is quick to mention that he has also learned a great deal from coaching Kenyan athletes: "I always try to learn, and to explore something that I don't know. And, before coming to Kenya, I didn't know many things—not about scientific training, but about the interpretation of training. I have to thank my African athletes for this new knowledge."

After a lifetime of experience, his knowledge, methods, and execution have proven to be sublime. Renato was a steeplechaser who was a stride away from making his national team. He began coaching and was soon working for FIDAL [Italian Athletics Federation]. His roster of athletes throughout his forty-year career is stellar, and if you mention the words "technical coach" in Kenya, everyone knows that Renato is being talked about.

Canova, who has an apartment in Iten on the edge of the Kerio Valley, does a lot of philanthropic work, helping and supporting people outside the parameters of his professional life. He recently opened a camp to house athletes just off the Iten-Eldoret road.

Brother Colm O'Connell

This native of Ireland first came to Kenya in 1976 to teach at St. Patrick's High School. He knew next to nothing about athletics, but the day after his arrival he attended a track meet and his interest was stimulated. The British Olympian, Brendan Foster's brother Peter was in charge of the training at St. Patrick's, and during the first two years, Colm simply watched and learned: "I depended upon what I observed." This was invaluable, as it gave him a perception of the athlete instead of just athletics. A quarter-century later, his walls are full of photographs of runners who have succeeded at the highest level.

"I think it is very important to get to know the athlete, to understand the runner. Of course, I spend a lot of time with the runners because they board at the school [Colm's house is on the school grounds]... My first [top-class] athlete was a chap called Ibrahim Hussein; he won Boston three times and was the first African to win the New York Marathon."

Colm went from success to success. He coached Peter Rono and Matthew Birir, who went on to win Olympic gold medals. Wilson Kipketer left Colm's stable to become a world 800m champion. Today no doubt there are others in the wings. Modest as always, Colm places the credit on the Kenyan mentality. "Kenyans are very responsive to any sort of challenge; it is easy to motivate them. The funny thing is that I haven't the qualifications for the job; I would have never have been given the opportunity in England or Ireland."

"There are three things I don't like for my runners," says Colm "Steep hills, heavy weights, and tarmac." For hill work Colm prefers that the runners accomplish a greater number of hill repeats but over a lesser gradient, citing possible damage to the knees. Weights are not found much in his program. Colm argues that the strength of running comes from running; the exercises that the athletes do without weights, such as sit-ups and push-ups, are ample, he believes.

"Tarmac kills the young legs," he says. Certainly, avoiding tarmac in rural Kenya is not a problem, and experts, with the possible exception of Arthur Lydiard of New Zealand, have long believed that a soft, forgiving surface is much more beneficial for training.

Colm talks to each athlete a lot, and about a wide variety of things. At his training camp he showed the athletes a movie about racial disharmony instead of the usual athletics video. "I talk more about losing than winning," he says. This is not negative talk, far from it, but Colm tries to educate his runners to the realities of becoming an athlete, part of which is accepting defeat, something that Kenyans do with grace and humility in more cases than not. "They know it is only one race, another will follow." Analyzing a race is not a subject that appears on O'Connell's agenda. "It's not a positive thing to talk about problems or be analytical. When the race is over, it's over—until next time."

When asked why the Kenyans are dominating distance events worldwide, Colm offers the following comments.

In Kenya the resources are perfect for running. Long-distance running is perhaps the least technical of all sports. You can just go out and do it. In Europe the young adult has many sports to choose from. Not so here in Kenya! Westerners are not as tough as they used to be. Fifty years ago, around the times of the Great Wars, people had to struggle much more; it was a much hardier breed. Now life is easy, but for Kenyans the struggle continues. There are very few distractions here in the Rift Valley. It is easy to keep a focus on hard training.

Colm's thoughts do move with the times: "The new approach is more to "train lighter, win easy these days, as we do a lot less running than we did do, and more exercises." Not that Colm's earlier approach did not achieve remarkable success, as Peter Rono's, Matthew Birir's, and Reuben Kosgei's Olympic gold medals prove.

In the early season, his runners are doing bounding exercises and strengthening, working from the hips. "We spend a lot of time there, as that is where the power comes from." Colm has tried to cut back the excessive mileage, not just going out and running miles as was often the Kenyan way. Many of the runners, even the 800m and 1500m runners, do cross country in the early season. A mainstay of the program is lots of nice easy runs of 40 to 50-minutes.

"I think Kenyans tend to over-train, too much emphasis on mileage. There is little attention, or none, paid to running technique, or freshness of mind; they are not mentally sharp when they come to the competition," says Colm. He does, however, state that changing with the times does not mean allowing clutter and confusion into his plans, "Oh no, we still use the old-fashioned method of using the eyes! Do you need a machine to tell you you are running out of gas? Twenty years ago, a Swedish team gave me a heart rate monitor; it is still hanging unused in a box in my room. Everything seems analyzed and quantified, almost to the point of an obsession in the Western world of coaching. We still keep a quite simple approach to it all."

The training starts with 1000m repeats, and Colm watches the runners who are instructed not to run at top speed. "I look at their eyes; are they relaxed? If not, I stop the session." He notes that the Ethiopian girls have perfect form from the gun to the tape, whereas the reverse is often true of Kenyans. "They cannot hold the form through the competition. [So] four times per week, we work on exercises."

Colm watches alignment; are there problems of leaning, or over-striding? These are problems easily fixed if noticed. He does not work in a gym, but uses Pilates-type exercises in an open field, runners using their own weight as resistance. The Kenyans have long done exercises, but not with the scientific approach that Colm now uses. "Six years ago, the level I could take the runners to was reached by pure running, then you reach a plateau. So how do you take them higher? By exercises."

Controlled intervals are now a key element of the program, rather than all-out speed. Colm insists that this way the runners are fresher at each session. Brother Colm looks at the foot of each athlete to check if it is relaxed and there is no tension. If there is tension, he gets athletes to jump barefoot on a sports trampoline to develop a "relaxed action." He also uses a sloping board for the foot to strengthen all its muscles.

At the camp there is an acronym, F.A.S.T., that is often talked about. It stands for:

> F–Focus. In the morning the runners do a Sun Salute, a series of yoga stretches for concentration and meditation. "The Kalenjins used to worship the sun long ago," adds Colm. "It helps to get the freshness of the mind."
> A–Alignment. Is your posture correct? Is your back straight? Don't hunch, and if you lean do so without hunching the back. Do not reach out with your stride; the weight when you land must be vertical.
> S–Stability. Do exercises to strengthen your stability.
> T–Timing. This is time that the foot spends on the ground. Is the foot relaxed? When the foot hits the ground it has to come right off again quickly.

These facets are worked upon on daily. There is a strong emphasis on teaching the athletes how to train correctly. Colm believes that otherwise they will leave the camp and forget all that they have learned, and he would have to teach them again at the next camp. "To attend, you must be willing to learn," he stresses; "Don't be in the program unless you understand what you are doing. I'm not a technical coach, I'm learning a lot myself, but you have to be able to understand the principles!"

William Mutwol: Elite Olympic Medalist Coach

Mutwol won the Olympic bronze medal for the steeple chase in 1972. Now a coach, Mutwol reflects on the changes in Kenyan athletics since his heyday in the early nineties; "My aim as a coach is to bring back those days when we ran not caring who won as long as he was Kenyan, when we willingly helped each other in the middle of the race, when we ran together as lions." The Marakwet tribesman, whose name translates as "someone who is small" was inspired to run by his compatriots' success. "For sure we have great role models in Kenya, mine were world record-holders Henry Rono and Samson Kimobwa. You know if you sacrifice yourself

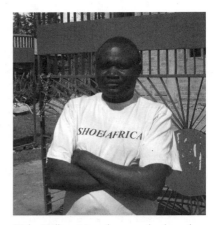

Today William Mutwol runs a school, coaches, and is an Ambassador for Shoe4Africa. (*Author*)

to training you can make it." And make it big the small man did. Mutwol trained with Richard Chelimo, Patrick Sang, Matthew Birir, and Ismael Kirui, to name a few. "We had such great groups in the old days; you don't see that so much anymore in Kenya. We have lost our unity. That is why the Ethiopians are unsettling us now, I think." The race William is most proud of is not his 5K world road record, which has only been broken by two men since 1992, nor is it his Olympic steeplechase bronze medal, it is his World Cross Country silver medal. Below is the training he used to win that medal. "It was the first time I had seen snow, it was −7 degrees Celsius. None of our team had run in such conditions, the Europeans were rejoicing, but it was an East African top three!"

The Mutwol Method

Set your mind on one thing, if it is rest then make sure you are resting. Do not disturb resting by doing jobs, or socializing. If it is training then focus one hundred per cent solely on training, die for that day. When training for the steeplechase use the barriers only once a week. Once a week at the track do a time trial of 1500m or 5000m, the former for if you want to improve speed, and the latter for improving endurance. My race tactic? Always go from the gun!

How do you know if you are in shape to run 13:12 for 5K on the roads? "I ran a session in Nairobi the week before Chelimo and I left; I did 10 x 800m [at altitude] in 1:55 with two-minute rest jogs.

Mutwol's best advice: "Before a team race for Kenya, the national coach said, 'You know why you are here today 30 million people back home await your result. Will you let your people down? Do you know how many Kenyans want to wear the colors of the national team? Go run—make not only yourself, but also your country, proud.' So in a word, run with your heart, and when you compete give it every thing, every. . . thing," he says drawing out the words from his soul.

Claudio Berardelli: Resident coach for Team Rosa

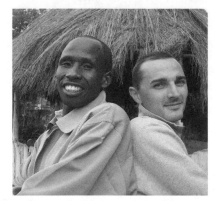

Claudio with perhaps his best known athlete, Martin Lel. (*Author*)

Claudio Berardelli is a very modest man. He praises the works of others rather than his own the successes. His athletes, who include Martin Lel, Joseph Ngeny, David Kipkorir, Benson Cherono, James Kwambai, and Patrick Ivuti, to list a small number of the squad of thirty or so (the slowest runner questioned was a 2:12 marathon man) speak with high admiration for the Italian.

"I have a hands-on approach, which is why I live in Kenya for most of the year being a coach for Dr. Rosa. Each day is different, and more so in Kenya, where a heavy rainfall can really alter the plan. Being here, every day I find something new to discover in the training. [Whenever you coach,] runners often say, 'I ran fast' when they ran slow, or vice versa, so that is why I believe it important for a coach to be with his athletes. I can make many changes. I am basically using the Dr. Rosa plan, with adjustments."

"The plan involves adding new stress to the body, breaking the balance. If you are not adding, you are not improving. In Europe often you have a program and the value of it is similar to the result you get, not so in Kenya. The value you get in Kenya is extra because of extreme conditions. Ask anyone who has run in the mud here; it is like glue to the foot. Then also, the dirt roads' surface, it is clay that is always unshaped. Every morning the foot has all these movements that are uncommon in Europe."

"Also in Kenya you have to categorize your runners. Inside a group, the training is very different. Look at two of my 2:07 men: Benson Cherono runs 250 kilometers per week, and Patrick Ivuti only 220 kilometers per week, but a very similar performance; why? Because you have a group with every one a single person that needs to be looked at, and that is the most important thing for me with training."

When planning Lel's for the London marathon, Claudio explains, "I do not believe the common conception that runners coming from a track background are always the fastest in the closing stages of the marathon if it comes down to a sprint finish; but I believe that if you are ready to run any pace you can save energy and to use it for the final sprint! Thus I will not have Martin working for a sprint finish. I will have him training to be comfortable operating at a high speed throughout the race." Thus it was little surprise to Claudio to see Lel run away from his competitors at the final stages of London.

Key Points to the Dr. Rosa Method

Long runs of two hours 30 minutes; a long run is 25–38K typically. 40K is the longest we do.

Fartlek. We do the typical two minutes hard, one minute easy, or the one-one routine. If a runner needs more speed, I will substitute this for 20 x 400.

Hill work. We do the Fluorspar run. (See Hilda Kibet's training, page 254.)

Speed work. This can be 10-14 x 1000 averaging 2:50, or 3-4 x 5K, or a 16–18K steady-state run.

We average 26-32 kilometers per day, usually split in two sessions. We live at altitude. Three weeks will not do it. We work with a three-month program of increasing intensity. Hilly, progressive runs are a mainstay of our program.

To see a weekly plan of Claudio's, see the section on Martin Lel (page 220).

Best Advice

"Most important, you must remember that adaptation to the marathon will take time, and fuel!"

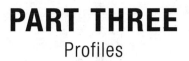

PART THREE
Profiles

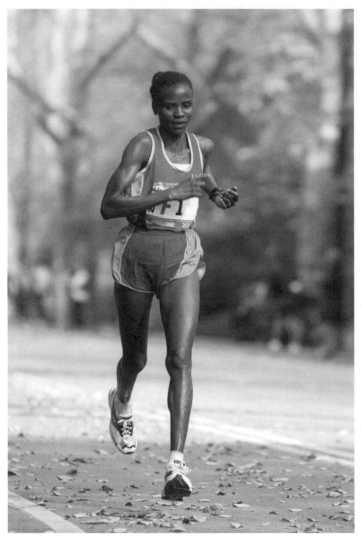

Joyce Chepchumba. (*New York Road Runners*)

800 Meters and 1500 Meters Events

National Records—800m

Sammy Koskei 1:42.28, 1984
Wilson Kipketer* 1:41.83, 1996
Japhet Kimutai 1:43.64, WJR, 1997
Pamela Jelimo 1:54:01 WJR, 2008
*Though Kipketer ran this race for Denmark, his country of residence, he was still a Kenyan citizen at the time.

National Records—1500m

Bernard Lagat 3:26:34, 2001
Cornelius Chirchir 3:30:24, WJR, 2002
Jackline Maranga 3:57.41, 1998

Olympic Medals 800m: Paul Ereng, 1988, William Tanui, 1992, Wilfred Bungei, Pamela Jelimo, 2008, gold; Wilson Kiprugut, 1968, Nixon Kiprotich, 1992, Janth Jepkosgei, 2008, silver; Wilson Kiprugut, 1964, Mike Boit, 1972, Fred Onyancha, 1996, Alfred Yego, 2008, bronze. *1500m*: Kip Keino, 1968, Peter Rono, 1988, Noah Ngeny, 2000, Nancy Jebet Lagat, 2008, gold; Keino, 1972, Lagat, 2004, Asbel Kiprop, 2008, silver; Stephen Kipkorir, 1996, Lagat, 2000, bronze.

World Championship Medals 800m: Billy Konchellah, 1987, 1991, Paul Ruto, 1993, Alfred Yego, Janeth Jepkosgei, 2007, gold; Wilfred Bungei, 2001, silver; Billy Konchellah, 1993, William Yiampoy, 2005, bronze. *1500m*: Wilfred Kirochi, 1991, Noah Ngeny, 1999, Bernard Lagat 2001, silver; Shadrack Korir, 2007, bronze.

Paul Ereng: The Story of Olympic Gold

Paul Ereng was not the favorite at the Olympic 800m final in Seoul 1988. "No, I was the new person on the block. There was [defending champion] Joaquim Cruz, [world 1500m record holder] Said Aouita, and the world championships silver and bronze medalists Peter Elliot and José Luis Barbosa. And Johnny Gray had just run a world-leading 1:42. Nevertheless, this field of champions did not intimidate Ereng; he thought he was fast enough to match the very best. "I wanted to see who had the best speed, I knew my speed was very good as I had run a 45.6 for 400 meters in Nairobi, done a 300 in 37.6 as a work-out, and had had some 200 meters repeats under 21 seconds, so I thought I was fast enough to run with anyone."

Ereng came from the Turkana tribe. He was the first runner to make a name for him-self from that region: "I looked outside for my role models. I admired Sebastian Coe very much, and also Cruz after I saw him win the Los Angeles Olympic 800m. And everyone wanted to be like Carl Lewis!" It was at Starehe Boys Center boarding school in Nairobi that Paul started to run. "I was not serious until near graduation. I would train by running ten times 100 meters with 45-seconds' rest, but that was good enough to give me 45 seconds for the 400m."

Moving to the States Ereng took his training more seriously whilst on a scholarship at the University of Virginia. In the spring of 1988, he moved up to the 800m from the 400m. "I used the coaches' method of training, because then I did not know about training," he says. "I thought I was doing a lot, but on reflection, 36 miles per week was not that much. No, I certainly did not over-train!"

Paul barely made it onto the Kenyan team, finishing third in the trials. The format in 1988 was four consecutive days of competition for the 800m. A week prior to the Games, he had run a 400–200m time trial with a scant thirty seconds rest clocking 47.0 and 21.6. A couple of days before the Olympics started, he ran 6 x 150m, averaging 15.6, so the tough schedule did not worry Ereng. "I knew I was strong, and that speed gave me confidence."

Lining up on Monday, September 26th, Ereng, only 22, was not befuddled by nerves. "I was thinking just to run with these people because they had run 1:42 and I had never been there, just run and stay relaxed. I thought I could run 1:40, as 25, 25, 25, and 25 did not seem too difficult to me."

The gun fired and Barbosa and Kiprotich took it out hard, Nixon's elegant stride gobbling up the tartan as Barbosa, the Brazilian, matched him stride for stride, shoulder to shoulder, racing to control the inside lane. Kiprotich recalls, "Yes, we were definitely going too fast, but it was a battle to see who would take the lead. In those days, that is how I thought you had to win the race." They passed 200m in a scorching 23.6, Ereng recalled, "I thought to myself, 'Stay relaxed and hit 25.' I hit 24.9. I remember thinking whilst I was in the final, 'It is possible to do 1:40.' I was thinking it would be a 47 first lap: I was running last." After 300m, Ereng moved to seventh place, and as he passed 400m he noticed 49.3 on the clock. "I thought, 'They are slowing down somewhat,' but still 1:39 is possible.' I looked about me and saw Said Aouita; [other runners had] told me that this man never loses a race, so I knew I am doing okay. At 600 meters I thought 'I am just wasting time here, I have so much energy,' so I pushed forward, but unfortunately I was boxed in on lane one. Aouita goes by on the outside. 'No wonder he never loses a race,' I remember thinking. Everyone was getting slower. I was thinking, 'Get out, get out.' Then between Nixon and Peter a gap opened and I dodged through. Cruz was leading, and with 50 meters to go I got in front and won in a PR of 1:43.4, my second PR in two days, as I had run 1:44.55 in the semis."

The following year, Ereng would win the World Indoor Championships 800m, setting a new indoor world record of 1:44.84 and besting the time of one of his heroes, Sebastian Coe. He would retain the title in 1991. In 1990, Ereng was awarded the highest honor bestowed on a Kenyan, the Order of the Grand Warrior.

Billy Konchellah

Konchellah's record of two golds (1987, 1991) came in the era when the championships were held four years apart, instead of two so that number could have easily been three under today's format. For good measure he also took a bronze six years after that first gold in 1993. It is a record unequaled in the event.

Billy went to Upper Hill School in Nairobi. "I was told because I was a Maasai that I should do the javelin! I also did the long and triple jump, and in the jumps I was the best in Nairobi." It was a fortunate day when, at a track meet, the school's 400m runner failed to show and Billy volunteered to run. "I tried to get some points for the secondary schools regional, and I ended up winning the heats in 53, and the finals in 52 seconds."

"The training in school for sprinters involved a lot of goal-post-to–goal-post sprints, 200m and 150m sprints, and very little endurance. We never ran farther than one kilometer," he remembers. "I was lucky we had a good sports teacher. She was called Muiru, and she encouraged us." Konchellah had planned to join the Air Force, but a talk with Ed Moses at a Nairobi Grand Prix track race, where Billy finished second at only 17 years of age, changed the mind of the Maasai man. "Then I wanted to go to the States for a scholarship. My father was very much against this, but finally he agreed. A lot of invitations had come, and we took potluck and chose Iowa. I really don't know why."

Konchellah would skip around schools, from Iowa (too cold) to California to Texas, but it was in the States that he learned to train correctly for track. "I also changed to the 800 because of picking up injuries in the 400. I ran my first-ever 800 with 57-second and 48.2-second splits and found the event easy. I ran 1:46.4 as a debut, finishing second to Mike Boit!"

Konchellah's Training Philosophy

"I would start the season by doing cross country; I really enjoyed the sport, and would run at the back, and just push the last bit to win. The training during this part was fartlek, 4K of 800 hard, 800 slow, 800 hard, 800m slow, and a fast 1K at full speed at the end. This was a key session. By the way, I never trained indoors. In track season, I would do lots of boot-camp drills for form. As far as running, in the morning I would run 4 to 5K easy jogging, in the afternoons on Monday, Wednesday, and Friday I would do stuff like 15 times 200 in 27 to 28 seconds with 30 seconds rest, split in two sets with 10 minutes of rest between the sets. Or 150-meter repeats in 16 seconds with a walk-back recovery. Other speed work would be 10 x 400, or 3 x 600, five mins rest, or 600-500-400 cut-downs. Tuesday and Thursday might be 10K runs. On Saturdays, one hour at medium speed or competition, and on Sundays always church."

"I ran about 70 miles per week—quite a lot for an 800 man. However, I am sure I could have been a great sprinter had I had the right training. I loved the form of Carl Lewis; I tried to develop a style equal to his for the 800. My handicap was asthma, which affected me throughout my career. I would train hard for one month, get a one-day setback; it would take me three days to get to feeling good again, then another attack. I was always playing the catch-up game. You know, the 800 is an anaerobic event!"

The Racing Philosophy

"I am a big man, 6' 2" and 70 kg. In 1991, coming into the World Championships, I was worried as I was two kilos overweight and out of shape. So I thought the best tactic to use was to stay behind so people cannot see me; this way firstly I know they will be worrying about me, and number two you never show someone your weapons. It worked: With 150 meters to go I was last, and I managed to win. Even if you are in shape don't show yourself to the others. Dictate from the back."

Konchellah asks you to watch the Olympic final of 1984 to see what he rates as his best performance.

"I finished fourth in 1:44.03. I had not trained for a month, as I had a hip-flexor problem, so I was constantly resting, just wishing it would go away. Look at the video and you will see the man who limps the whole race, that was me! With the belief, I managed to get fourth, and I really believe that on that day if I had had not been injured it would have been the world record, for sure."

Peter Kipchumba Rono of Kapsabet: Olympic 1500m gold

"I can still remember walking into the stadium in Seoul, people were yelling and screaming, "go Peter, go Peter!" I could hardly believe it, as no one was giving me much of a chance, but here were thousands and thousands of people. I thought they were cheering for me, I did not realize there were three Peter's in the race! That gave me great confidence, but down in my heart I knew I could win. I had not lost a race all year and had run 3:35 in Nairobi to win the trials. Yes, I had a shot and I believed in myself. When you walk out, as I did, with twelve people for that Olympic final you must go with faith, as all the athletes are fit and well trained. The tactic was for [Joseph] Chesire to take the pace, but he did not, so I thought, "I have to do something," as I knew many of the other guys had a good sprint, better than mine if I left it late. I kept looking back; 21-times, I counted later, as I did not want anybody to pass me. I ran 39 seconds for the final 300 meters but no one was getting close to me."

"To win an Olympic final does not really sink in until you are standing on the podium at the medal ceremony, with the anthem playing and every one in the stadium giving just you a standing ovation. That is a moment when you, as a man, can cry. Two people believed in me: Brother Colm, my high school coach who told me after I won the trials in Nairobi, 'You are as good as anyone.' And James Deegan, who was my coach in America at Mount St. Mary's. He told me after my warm-up for the finals, 'There are three people who can win this race, and you are one of them. If you run smart you can win.' He was a mentor, coach, and like a father to me. If I ask myself why I won the Olympic gold, it is because I truly believed in myself that I would win."

A true case of not hoping to win, but acting to win.

Training for the 800m and 1500m

"Hey, I have no magic formula but hard work!"—Fred Onyancha, Olympic 800m bronze, 1:42:79

One notable attribute that all Kenyan 800m runners have is a certain grace to their stride;

this may be due to the long time, and the willingness, dedicated to drills. However, watching Meretei Gregory Konchellah (new Bahraini name: Saad Kamel) run as an untrained athlete in 2002, it was clear that even untrained he was fated to follow in his father's footsteps and run a world-class 800m. Whether he'll win two World Championship golds as his father did remains to be seen.) Even with no style drills, his form was pure grace. Benson Koech, Japheth Kimutai, David Rudisha, Wilson Kipketer. . . these athletes, albeit with great natural form, style work(ed) for hours each week on style drills. Nixon Kiprotich talked about how, even when on an easy jog, he was analyzing every inch of his body, looking for tension, searching for a more relaxed form. Olympic Champion William Tanui mentioned how when he was running he would watch his feet constantly, checking for perfect placement. Another similarity is that the majority of Kenyan middle-distance runners are great cross country competitors, even those never seen on the international circuit.

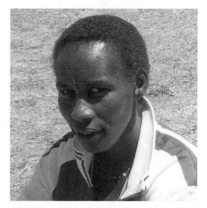

Janeth Jepkoskei relaxes watching a local race in Kenya after a hard season on the track—setting a new Kenyan 800m record. (*Author*)

Janeth Jepkosgei Busienei
"The Eldoret Express"

Date of Birth: December 13, 1983
Birthplace: Kabirirsang, near Kapsabet
Home: Eldoret
Height/Weight: 170 cm, 47 kg
Personal bests: 800m–1:56:07,
                   1000m–2:37.98,
                   1500m–4:11.91
Honors won: 2002 World Junior 800m
                     Champion
                   2006 African
                     Championships 800m gold
                   2006 Commonwealth
                   Games 800m gold
                   2007 World Champion 800m.
                   2008 Olympic 800m silver
Longest run: 70 min.
Tough session: 3 x 800 in 2:12 with 6 min.
                   recovery at altitude

Janeth was a major star for the Kenyan Commonwealth team in 2006. Nobody expected her to win the gold, yet she proved invincible even when lined up against arguably the world's finest 800m star, Maria Mutola. As Janeth lined up for her first major senior championship, Maria, with twelve world titles, was, as the two-time defending Commonwealth Games champion, expected to dominate the event without challenge. Jepkosgei, known for her front-running, this time sat behind and outkicked Mutola and the Australian Kenia Sinclair to take the gold in the final 50 meters of the race. Mutola at once cited fatigue from the World Indoors Championships, run just ten days earlier as the reason of her loss.

However, proving it was no fluke, Janeth also beat Mutola at the African Championships later in that year, and ended her season with the world's fastest time of the year. It was the springboard to far greater things at the 2007 World Championships. Jepkosgei began running at the Sing'ore Girl's High School just outside the village of Iten, famous for producing a slue of good runners. However, it was after hooking up with Claudio that the big breakthrough happened.

Monday	AM 45-55 progressive run; when feeling fine, a high intensity.	PM Diagonal sprints, technical work and a 30-minute jog
Tuesday	AM 2 x(3x400) in 56 sec.,	PM Easy jog, 40 min. with 6 min. recovery and 10 min. recoveries between sets
Wednesday	Repeat Monday's session	
Thursday	AM 12 x 200m in 26-7 sec. with a 3-min. recovery jog	PM Easy jog 40 min.
Friday	AM 12 x 450m up a slight incline jog down for the recovery	
Saturday	Easy day, two runs of 40 min.	
Sunday	AM Long run of 70 min., fairly easy pace	

Comments: Janeth does have good natural speed, being able to pull off a 52-second 400m. The plan is for Janeth to run the 1500m in the future. She also practices passing runners on the curves of the track. For instance in a session of 6 x 300m to be run in 44 seconds with a pacemaker, the goal of the workout was to sprint by the pacer on each repeat. The training is based to try to make her reactive in the competition, not to increase muscle weight.

Janeth's In-Season Training

AM	45 min. easy	PM	12 x 100m in 13 sec. walk back recovery
AM	50 min.	PM	2 x (6 x 20 sec.) up hill sprints, 5 min. between sets
AM	55 min.	PM	35-min. and 15 x diagonals
AM	2 x 500 (1:13, 1:15)	PM	45 min. very easy jog

5 min. recovery between,
then 6 min. recovery, 2 x 300 (42 sec.),
3 min. between, then another 6 min.,
and 2 x 200m in 26 sec. with 3 min. rest.

AM	45 min. easy	PM	6 x 100m to open up the stride
AM	Flight	PM	jogging with some diagonals
AM	Rest	PM	Competition, 1:57 800m

David Lekuta Rudisha

Date of birth: December 17, 1988
Birthplace: Oloibor-Soito, Maasai
Height/Weight: 6'2", 70kgs
Personal best: 800m–1:43:72; 400m–48:20
Honors won: 2005 silver East African Youth Championships 400m
                   2006 Champion World Junior Championships 800m.
                   2008 African Champion 800m

On David's nineteenth birthday he drew his padded jacket closer to his body. It was cold, much colder than he was used to, "Kenya is getting somewhat different in the climate. Back home we never have this weather!" he retorted with a hand wrapped around a chipped mug of thick Kenyan tea. Sitting in Brother Colm's garden, he is attending the famed winter month-long training camp, now in its last week. His arrival on the world's athletics stage has been anything but cold, a meteoric move from a local-standard decathlete to a world-champion 800m runner in barely a year. It was Brother Colm that suggested that the lanky Maasai try the 800m, and he did so at the Kamariny dirt track as a fresh-faced 18-year-old striding over the ruts and clods of dirt to clock a winning 1:49m; outstanding, taking into account the 2440m altitude. "Brother Colm told me, 'You have a long stride that is swift, this is good for the 800' so I thought, Why not!"

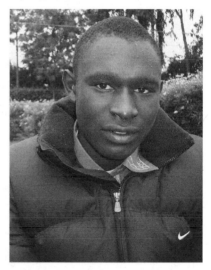

World junior 800m champion David Rudisha hopes to follow in his father's footsteps and medal at the Olympics. (*Author*)

Rudisha had started in athletics only a few years earlier. "I started running in primary school standard seven. I did not struggle; I realized I had talent and enjoyed the sport very much. My father was very encouraging for me to get into athletics." That father, Daniel, had won a silver medal in the 4 x 400 relays at the 1968 Olympics.

There was no need for David to push his body; like a well-oiled wheel, it ran by itself. With a little Irish intervention, he found the distance that suited him.

Training to Win the Junior World Championships

Monday	6AM	6K easy jogging
	10AM	40 min. at medium speed
	4:30 PM	Plyometrics and field exercises, some strides and foot pattern running
Tuesday	6AM	8K easy jogging
	10AM	10x120m up hill sprints
	4 PM	30 min. easy jog
Wednesday	6AM	8K easy jogging
	10AM	Working on a field technique, at running technique, lots of stride type drills pushing very low and plyometrics
	PM	Pilates class working mainly on core strength, 40 min.
Thursday	6AM	7.7K easy run.
	10AM	Diagonals, fast strides across a field
	4 PM	Exercises
Friday	6AM	6K easy.
	10 AM	4 x 600m in 1 min. 30 sec. with 90 sec. rest, 5 x 400m in 56-58 sec. with 90 sec. rest, 4 x 300m in 39-40 sec. with 60 sec. rest, and 2-4 x 200m in 25-26? with 60 sec. rest. Run to and from the track, 3K
	PM	Rest
Saturday	6 AM	8K slow in 40 min.
	10 AM	Long run, 1hr 20min followed by stretching
Sunday		Total rest.

Comments:

The emphasis is on quality, and not too much quality. Brother Colm's plan for David is focused on the 2012 Olympics. The program is centered on perfecting David's form and developing the talent slowly. "Watch out for this one!" winks Colm, and the last time the Irish coach said that about an up-and-coming athlete, the runner, Japheth Kimutai, developed into one of the world's best 800m runners.

Best Advice: "My Father told me that discipline is a must, and that respect and obedience are important for life. This advice I have always remembered and lived by."

Noah Ngeny

Date of birth:	November 2, 1978
Birthplace:	Ziwa Village, Uasin Gishu District. Nandi.
Height/weight:	5' 9" (176 cm), 121 lbs. (55 kg)
Sessions per day:	Two, the first at 10 a.m.

Length of long run: 1:30:00

Hardest session: 300m repeats

Personal bests: 1000m–2:11.96 WR
1500m–3:28.12

Honors: 1999 World Championships 1500m, 2nd
1999 world record 1000m, 2:11.96
1997 world junior record 1500m, 3:32.91
1997 world junior record one mile, 3:50.41
2000 Olympics 1500m, first

The back of Noah Ngeny's head is well known to Kenyans. Ngeny was a popular pace-maker on the Kenyan circuit before he surfaced with a World Junior Record in the 1500m at Zurich in 1997. Abel Nzimbi, an 800m runner of national caliber, remembers, "Even if he lost the first position he would fight and fight to try and regain the lead." When Vincent Malakwen ran a Nyayo (translation: "footsteps") Stadium record in the 800m, it was Ngeny who set out at a bold pace.

Living in the tough inner lane left Ngeny with an ingrained hard racing ethic. When he ran the 1000m world record, it was his twenty-fourth race of the season!

At Sydney, world-record-holder Hicham El Guerrouj was a strong favorite in the men's 1500m. He had a 12-0 record against Ngeny. One man, however, saw a different ending. Ngeny had promised gold in December 1999. Claiming his speed to be superior, Ngeny was certain that he would be crowned the Olympic champion.

The start was quick—a 54–second first lap. Then the pace slowed to 60 seconds before the great El Guerrouj took over. Ngeny patiently hung on the Moroccan's heels before unleashing a fierce kick down the homestretch to take Kenya's first Olympic 1500m title in twelve years. To sweeten the moment teammate Bernard Lagat took the bronze. (Four years later, Lagat would upgrade that to a silver.)

Typical training week in the off-peak season

Monday	AM	1 hr 30 min.	PM	40 min. Easy.
Tuesday	AM	Fartlek, 3 min hard, 1 min	PM	1 hr. easy run in the easy, for 40 min. evening
Wednesday	AM	40 min. at high speed	PM	55-60 min. easy run.
Thursday	AM	1 hr. steady run	PM	sprinting diagonals for 45 min. across a grassy field.
Friday	AM	30 min. at high speed	PM	20 min. easy run.
Saturday	AM	Long run on a hilly route.		

Comments:

"I like to train hard intervals with a group." Ngeny professed to "getting bored" with running distance, though his concentration is total when on the track. Ngeny blamed the physical nature of the 1500 in the 1999 World Championships for his lack of gold and vowed to run more aggressively in future races: "In the 1500, there can be a lot of shoving and pushing, and I lost my stride. Next time I will be ready for those tactics," he said then. It was an accurate prediction.

The Steeplechase

National Records

Bernard Barmasai 7:55.72, 1997, former WR

Eunice Jepkorir 9:07.41 (2008)

Stephen Cherono 7:58.66, 2001, WJR

Ruth Bisibori Nyangau 9:25:25 2007, WJR

Olympic Champions: Amos Biwott, 1968; Kip Keino, 1972; Julius Korir, 1984; Julius Kariuki, 1988 (8:05.51 Olympic record); Matthew Birir, 1992; Joseph Keter, 1996, Reuben Kosgei, 2000, Ezekiel Kemboi, 2004; Brimin Kiprop Kipruto, 2008.

World Champions: Moses Kiptanui, 1991, 1993 and 1995; Wilson Boit Kipketer, 1997; Christopher Koskei, 1999, Rueben Kosgei, 2001; Stephen Cherono, 2003*; Cherono, 2005; Brimin Kiprop Kipruto, 2007.

*Cherono, Kenyan-born, won this race for his adopted homeland of Qatar, running under his Qatari name, Saif Saaeed Shaheen.

Mark Rowland, world-class British steeplechaser, on the Kenyan Olympic team:

> You always knew that every time you stepped onto the track amongst the Kenyans, especially in the steeplechase, it would be a momentous challenge, both physically and mentally. A body-battering of the legs and a soul-wrenching, grinding torture of the psyche. The Kenyans had, and have, an abundance of talent would display elements of crazy unpredictability on the track.
>
> The aim was always to focus on my own tactics and ignore the others. That may be easy to say, but once you encountered the charging Peter Koech, hurdling the water jump on the final lap, with fatigue grabbing your b—s, it is as challenging a moment you may ever wish ever to imagine! Sheer surprise and beauty for me, and to be witnessing it first-hand inside a stadium of 80,000 screaming, yelling, and passionate fans under a vortex of that chance to win an Olympic medal. I was close to utter euphoria. It was also the first time for me in an Olympic final! All I could do was watch in withered desperation as I Koech's back disappear into the distance and fight with Kariuki for the Olympic record, and the gold! However, the most overwhelming feeling from competing with my Kenyan friends is how magnanimous and humble they were in either victory or defeat.

Matthew Kiprotich Birir—Olympic Gold Medalist, 1992

Birir ran in the Kenyan trials for the Worlds in 1991 and failed to make the team, but he gave the runners a clear warning that he would be a threat in 1992. "I knew all the top guys would be ready, so I had to be ready, too." In January, he was training to be in top shape for cross country. Then in March he was already doing track workouts. The first week, one session; the second, two sessions; until he had three solid sessions of speed per week. He was focusing on running races without interrupting the training plan at all; thus he would do a 1500m or a 5000m just concentrating on improving his times, nothing more.

The main sessions Matthew ran were 3 x 1000m in 2:30 to 2:33 with 90 seconds rest, and also 12 x 400m in 58 seconds with one minute rest. His best piece of advice? "When you know where you want to go, you will definitely know the way and the means to the place."

In the Olympic final, Birir never thought about one specific athlete, but he felt under pressure from everyone. Even his shoe sponsor was putting pressure on him to produce a winning result. Knowing that he was in excellent shape, and winning races, including the Olympic trials in Kenya, Birir also put pressure on himself. Even in the resting hours his mind would wander to Barcelona. "When I dreamt, I dreamt about being in the final and winning the Olympics," he recalls.

After he reached the final, the day came.

"When I was warming up for the final I was totally weak, I guess from being extremely nervous. After one lap, passing the point where I had hit the barrier in an earlier steeplechase race, I was fine. Then the Algerian runner Azzedine Brahmi stepped on my leg as I was lifting it, spiking me and half-tearing the shoe from my foot. Somewhere there I thought, "I have lost everything." However, by the fifth lap I had gained control and was running comfortably at the front. The last two laps I started pumping up the speed, so with only 100 meters to go, when I looked around, I had just Kenyans with me. With 50 meters to go, I knew I was going to win and I started celebrating. After the race I could not even walk to pick up some food, I needed assistance because of the wound. I had a tetanus injection."

The secret to his success? "What I know is, hard work pays, so I always tell runners, 'work hard if you want success. I ran with more fire!'"

The Kenyan record of success is obvious in all running events, from 800m through the marathon, but it is in the steeplechase that Kenyans have been truly dominant. Kenyans competed for nine Olympic steeplechase titles from 1968 on and won all nine. They have won six straight World Championships steeplechases, including three in a row by Moses Kiptanui. The Kenyan run was stopped by Kenyan born Stephen Cherono who won Qatar's first-ever track and field golds in 2003 Paris. Kenyans have won all the Commonwealth Games steeplechase gold since 1974, except for Edinburgh (1986), when the Kenyan team joined a boycott against the Games. This is truly "the Kenyan event."

Why are Kenyans so exceptional in this event? Purists frequently cringe as many of the Kenyans "hurdle" the steeplechase barriers. Kip Keino joked that he jumped the hurdles like an old horse. Patrick Rono, a national-standard runner, thinks he has the answer. "A group of us were sitting watching a local competition one day. . . A British runner was over here in Kenya running against us. We noticed first the big difference in leg structure; his legs were like oak-tree trunks whereas ours were like willows. When we jumped we floated over; when he jumped it was a major upheaval." Though willow-like legs are not the exclusive property of Kenyans, perhaps Rono does have a point. The Kenyans do seem to skip over the hurdles with ease, regardless of form, and this conservation of effort could be a key to Kenyan steeplechase success. Many have criticized the Kenyans for their seemingly ungainly style of clearing obstacles, but style marks are not needed to win this event.

Kirwa Tanui, a steeplechaser, speaks of the Kenyan belief in themselves: "A lot of Kenyans choose to run the steeplechase event because we know we are unbeatable; maybe we have some doubts in the 5000 or the 1500—we know that Kenyans are often beaten in those races. But when we run the steeplechase, we know that we shall win—no problems!"

Some Kenyan Steeplechase Wisdom

Olympic bronze medalist William Mutwol: "I don't train so much over the barriers. I train with 1500-meter to 10,000-meter runners—we all do the same training. Running in the country builds strength for the steeplechase.".

Bernard Barmasai, an 8:08.56 steepler: "There is no secret to our success in the steeplechase. To be competitive in the steeple today you have to be able to run a 5000 in around 13:15, but in most countries if you run 13:15 you are a 5000-meter runner—not in Kenya!".

Christopher Kosgei, 1995 World Championships silver medalist: "I train often with Ismael Kirui. We do the same training but compete in different events. . . I do no specific steeple training.".

Julius Korir, 1984 Olympic champion: "Cross country training and running over the hills is the best preparation for running the steeplechase event. Good strength is very important. Run hills often."

The Marakwets—Sui Generis

The Cherangany Hills, an Elysium for runners, in the Marakwet district of the Great Rift Valley has a startling ability to produce the world's finest steeplechase runners. This area of Kenya virtually owns the steeplechase event. Since Moses Kiptanui's stunning international debut of 8:07 in 1991, this small sub-tribe of the Kalenjin has amassed an amazon hoard of championship gold—the 2000 and 2004 Olympic victories (for good measure the tribe also took a medal at both the 1992 and 1996 Olympics), the World Championships in 1991, 1993, 1995, and 2001, and nearly every world junior championship. Reuben Kosgei, Ezekiel Kemboi, and Michael Kipyego all from a radius of a few miles, ran the Paris World Championships Steeplechase for Kenya. Kipyego, the only man of the trio not to have an Olympic gold was *just* a junior world champion—that's how good the Marakwets are!

The deluge was started by Joseph Chemaringo, the first known Marakwet steepler, who competed at the 1970 Commonwealth Games. Chemaringo, who today is a tea farmer, has long since retired from sports, but his legacy is the strongest dynasty in steeplechase history.

Marakwet District Records

Junior Record 8:03:72 (currently second-fastest all time, Raymond Yator 2000)
Senior Record 7:56:16 (currently fourth-fastest all time, Moses Kiptanui 1997)

Moses Kiptanui

Date of Birth:	January 10, 1970
Birthplace:	Kaptalamwa, near Kapcherop
Height/Weight:	5' 9", 56-57 kg.
Personal Records:	1500m–3:34.44 (3:34.0 hand timed, in Nairobi–the second-
	fastest ever recorded at altitude), Mile–3:52.06
	2000m–4:52.53
	3000m–7:27.18
	2000m–8:13.40
	5000m–12:54.85
	3000m steeplechase–7:56:16
Honors Won:	1990 African Junior Championships 1500m, gold medal
	1990 World Junior Champion 1500m
	1991, 1993, 1995 IAAF World Champion steeplechase
	1991 All Africa Games, world record steeplechase (2), 3000m, and
	5000m
	1994 Goodwill Games 5000m, gold medal.
	1996 Olympic steeplechase, silver medal

Although long retired, Kiptanui is still in shape today to run a sub- 30- minute 10K. "I run to only maintain the 60 kilograms," he laughs, patting his stomach after running with a group of Junior National team members up at the Shoe4Africa Moses Kiptanui Training Camp in the Cherangany Hills. We come to a manmade barrier and Kiptanui clears it just as if he were back in an athletics stadium competing before a crowd of 60,000. A lone goat, who is disturbed from his morning grass-munching, and perhaps ten runners are there to notice that perfect stride. Kiptanui flashes a smile, realizing he has impressed. "I've still got it, huh? I can still run!"

Kiptanui has always been able to run, ever since he was a young boy tending to his father's cattle in the fields. In school, he excelled at soccer as Shadrack Kosgei, a school-mate, remembers: "He was very good, talked about at school for his talents on the field. He could play any position." Following high school, Kiptanui looked for a job to pursue. Although he was good at sports, it did not seem that soccer in Kenya could generate enough wealth for a career. Moses happened to be training and running well at this time. "I knew my cousin Chelimo and thought, 'What's so special about him? He is shorter than I am, and if he can do it, why not me?'" and I became interested in training. Not as a pastime, but as a way to make money." Kiptanui had no TV set or sports newspapers lying around the house when he was growing up. "We heard about one or two men from our region running well, but it was hard to relate to that. Of course, every school child in Kenya knew about Kip Keino, too."

In 1988, Kiptanui joined the Army and met the likes of John Ngugi, William Mutwol, and Paul Kipkoech. "It changed my entire life. I got serious, and I started search-ing out training manuals and books to learn more." Following a hill session one day, Kiptanui knew the training was not enough for him; he needed more speed. He decided

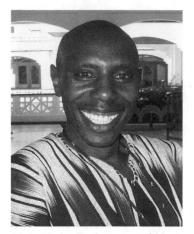

Moses Kiptanui, today a successful businessman, and still able to run as fast as a Kenyan! (*Author*)

to start training himself. He would question other athletes to gain knowledge and listen to the coaches talk, then concoct a formula that suited his needs. "I thought, 'if I am to beat the others, then I have to be training better than the other runners.' You know, Train Hard to Win Easy!"

In 1990, Kiptanui was sent to Bulgaria to run the World Juniors 1500m. Little did he know that his life was about to change dramatically: "I won the race and a journalist approached me. He told me a man called Kim McDonald wanted to talk to me and find me races, and could I come to England? I drove with that journalist for seven hours in a car across Bulgaria on bad roads. Our driver was falling asleep on the road; it was so bad that the journalist had to take over driving. I was sitting in the car thinking, 'What am I doing!'"

Kiptanui was taken to Newcastle, where he waited for two days in a hotel until Kim appeared. "He put me in a 1500m race. Imagine, my first race and I see Peter Elliot and Steve Cram, people like that on the starting line. Straight from the gun the pace went high, so fast that immediately it was single file. I could not even see what was going on at the front; I finished in 3:40, dejected. Kim consoled me and said, 'Hey, these are big guys, don't worry, it is your first race!' And he was right; in the next race I was third in a much better time. I went back to Kenya with money; I was elated." Although Kiptanui returned to Kenya and won the Armed Forces cross country (proving he could have been a legend over the country had he wished to perform at that discipline), McDonald advised the Marakwet runner to concentrate on the indoor season instead. "I flew back to England and competed quite well, but also I got five running kits and five pairs of training shoes, and thought, 'Now I am set, I have all the facilities—let me train.'" He also won $5,000, a veritable fortune back in Kenya.

When Kiptanui returned for the summer season, something happened that changed the face of steeplechasing: "I was sitting next to Kim on the plane and we were going to Stockholm. There was no place in the field for me to run the 1500, so I said to Kim, 'Why don't you enter me in the steeplechase?' I convinced him that I could run it, as I had done so earlier at an Armed Forces meet, winning in 8:46.6." Although the time may not have seemed worthy of a Grand Prix meet in Europe, McDonald knew that times on Kenyan soil meant nothing; it was the position that counted, and if Kiptanui could win the Armed Forces race, he would surely be a worthy competitor in an IAAF meet.

The meet director of the DN Galan, Rajne Soderberg, takes up the story:

Kim McDonald had for a couple of weeks tried to enter a "new talent from Kenya" into my 1500-meter race. That race was very full and I could not accept any more, so this athlete was told "no possibility." Not even when Kim told me that he was the World Junior Champion at 1500m did it make it possible to accept him. Regardless of this, Kim brought the athlete to Stockholm, hoping that I would be able to accept him once he was there. The day before the competition, the answer was still no. In the afternoon of the competition day, Kim approached me and said the guy can also run the steeple if I have an opening there. I did have a place there, so I said yes, entered his name, gave him a bib number, and went to the stadium. I forgot to tell the result service and media about this late entry. So, in the steeple, this guy from Kenya took off and was leading the race in world-record time. The media could not find his number in the start list. They called me and I understood it must be Kim's Kenyan, but I had not put his name on my mind and could not recall it. Anyway, he ran a tremendous race and barely missed the world record by a couple of seconds but was not identified until after the race. That is the story of how Moses Kiptanui became a steeplechaser, and he went on to be one of the great steeplechasers of all time!

Kiptanui, under a cool Scandinavian sky, simply flew from the gun; "I was on world record pace the whole way until the final 400. Kim was in the stands; he was stunned with my 8:07." Four days later, Kiptanui entered the steeple at the Oslo meet, again winning and improving his PR to 8:06. The following month, Moses was a world champion at the event, beginning a domination that would last for years.

In 1992, Moses started a camp for Kim McDonald at Nyahururu, and then Kim asked if Moses could also handle training the group. Moses agreed. "I had time during the day to write out the schedules." Like Moses Tanui, and today the likes of Lornah Kiplagat, it did not bother the man that he was coaching athletes whose sights were set on toppling the coach on the playing field.

"I was in the perfect position, I knew what training was needed, and I watched the form, like sitting in a class watching, analyzing, and coordinating the whole body. More than just the practical, I also did the theory for the group." It was the recipe for success. Kiptanui was responsible for starting one of the first running camps in Kenya, outside the governmental-run sites. Kim took this protocol worldwide and created a running-team dynasty that would dominate the track world right up to his premature death in November of 2001.

Before this, the Kenyans who went to America used to think of themselves as being superior. We changed the whole playing field. "You are leaving Kenya? Why? For facilities? We have the best running environment here in Kenya." Suddenly you found Kenyans training along the side of the roads, you would drive into the towns of Rift Valley, and everyone was out training trying to succeed. They saw it could be done by staying in Kenya. We created an explosion by offering possibilities. We are lacking only "training facilities" like running shoes and equipment.

A big disappointment in the year of 1992 was a knee injury that kept Kiptanui from a shot at the Olympic gold. "However, I was determined to show who was best in that year, so I came back strong. Ten days after the Olympics I set a world record over 3000 meters in Cologne, 7:28.96, and three days later I got the steeplechase world record, 8:02.08, in Zurich."

Kiptanui crests a hill, yet there are a hundred more hills to climb. The Cherangany Hills, near Kiptanui's birthplace, have probably bred more running champions than any other district in the world. There are a thousand reasons why a person would wish to run free in this paradise. Kiptanui thumps his heart. "Running comes from inside of our soul. Why are you doing this? It has to come from the heart if you want to succeed. We created the 'do it here in your homeland' [attitude], and you saw that from 1992, all the medals now came from Kenya-based Kenyans in the championships."

At this time email and cell phones did not exist, and landlines have never been brilliant in Kenya (more like dire); thus communications were improved when all the runners trained together under the coach's eye at a camp. "Suddenly we had two hundred world-class athletes in the camp!" says Kiptanui.

Moses' Training to Break 13 minutes in the 5000m and the 8-minute Steeplechase Barrier

Monday	6 AM	60 min. medium speed
	10AM	Hill work, between 200-300m, working on strength, not speed, so don't run slow down the hill.
	4:30 PM	30 min. easy and for warm up some aerobic exercises
Tuesday	6 AM	40 min. to warm the body
	10 AM	Track: 5 x 1 mile, 4:30-pace easy and talk with a 200m jog recovery
	4 PM	Run easy with friends, jog easy and talk.
Wednesday utes.	6 AM	60 min., but if you missed the track yesterday then 75-minutes.
	10 AM	Tempo work, 3 min. fast, 3' easy for rhythm
	4 PM	Easy run, 40 min. and aerobic exercises
Thursday	6 AM	40 min. warm-up.
	10 AM	Track: 2 x 600, (1:28), 200m recovery jog, 2 x 800 (2:01, or 1:56 at low altitude), again 200m jog, 2 x 1000 (2:31, 2:26 in Europe), 200m jog. 400m jog between sets.
	4 PM	Rest
Friday	6 AM	40 min. easy.
	10 AM	Fartlek, after 30 min. of jogging then 30 min. of 2-min. fast, 2-min. easy, or 2, 1. Warm down
	4:30 PM	Easy jogging
Saturday	10 AM	Track 16 x 200m (27-28) with a 30 sec. jog recovery, or 10-16 x 300m. "Near to a race I would have a time trial here."
	4:30 PM	Easy jog
Sunday	AM	One run of 1:15-1:20 min., medium speed.

Comments

"Long Hours, long preps. There are no shortcuts. You have to suffer in training; I believe very much if I do not die in training then I will not race well. The race is short, but the practice is long. If you feel tired one morning, then you can skip the session, but try later in the day, maybe you will be fresher then; do not just cancel the day. Or even go out and play with a soccer ball, which may turn out to be a good training session. Personally, I do not see a point in racing unless you have died in training. Every day at 6:00 a.m., start with sit-ups and press-ups; if you do not have a strong core then you cannot hold form when you get tired in the race. I never ran longer than one hour twenty—what is the point; I was a middle distance-runner competing for 13 minutes maximum. Train in blocks. I would take eight weeks off running after the European track season. Then begin with easy jogging, a little bit each day, slowly building. If you are racing indoors, as I often did, then you must begin in October, but for those running cross country the end of October is fine. You must know when your competition will be, what date. Then build up slowly to it with hard training using fartlek. When you are eight weeks from the event you are aiming for, it is time to begin track work, but make it hard.

Stephen Cheruiyot Cherono (Saif Saaeed Shaheen)

Date of birth:	October 15, 1982
Birthplace:	Kamelilo village, Keiyo
Height/Weight:	174 centimeters, 58 kilograms now, but 55 kilograms race weight
Personal best:	1500m–3:33.51
	2000m–5:03.06
	3000m–7:34.67
	5000m–12:48.81
	2000m steeplechase–5:14.53
	3000m steeplechase–7:53.63
Longest run:	30K
Toughest Session	4 x 1600m, 3:56, 3:55, 3:57, 3:59, with one lap jog recovery
Honors won:	1999 World Youth, 2000m steeplechase champion
	2002 Commonwealth Games, steeplechase champion
	2002 African Championships, steeplechase bronze
	2003 and 2005 IAAF World Championships, steeplechase champion
	2006 IAAF World Indoor Championships, silver 3000m
	World Senior, Junior, and Youth steeplechase record

In the mid 1990's, a slim young Kenyan would often stand on the corner of the road in Iten village opposite the Matatu stage. Amongst a crowd of others, he was usually dressed in no noticeable fashion, normally in a sun-bleached black T-shirt. He was not running, just standing and watching. However, there was something about this young man that made you notice him, something even then, as an ordinary civilian, that made him stand out from the rest, of the crowd. He was not a champion runner then; he did not even own

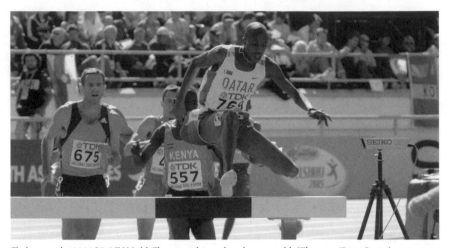

Shaheen at the 2005 IAAF World Championships, where he won gold. (*Flanagan/PrettySporty*)

a pair of running shoes, but there was a profound aura around Cherono.

Today he is probably the wealthiest man in Iten, but the road to success was a long, bumpy, arduous one paid for by his own sweat and toil.

"After high school in 1999, I became a runner as my education ended. I didn't get money for university," he says. In fact, after three years at a secondary boarding school, the money ran out and Stephen had to leave to attend a school close to his home in Sergoit. Cherono grew up in a running family. "I remember at breakfast the elder brothers telling me, 'You'll never make it, you'll never beat me.' They told me to forget about track and field, especially Christopher." Young Stephen was simply silent. "'You are not a good athlete,' I was told. Every time I train, I have that in my mind, which is the worst thing someone can tell you." Stephen was not a standout athlete in Kaplamai Primary, or at the Marakwet High School, and he could have used the encouragement. He could have used assistance, too, but that was not forthcoming. "They [his brothers] still regard themselves as the best. Maybe if I run 7:45 for the steeplechase, I'll get some respect in the family," he says throwing his hands in the air.

The athletic breakthrough came when Stephen, after running well at some local meets, was selected to run the World Youth Games 2000m steeplechase in Poland. "I won in 5:31:48. After that I went to [London] Crystal Palace and ran a two-miler [8:18.80], then a 1500 in Malmo [3:41.08], and then in Zurich I ran 8:19:12." Cherono had made his mark on the international scene.

The following year, 2000, Cherono was invited to join the Kim McDonald group in Australia. However, shortly after running a pre-season 3:40 1500m, he got sick. "I got typhoid; no money to treat myself. Nobody bothered what was going on. So of course I did not go."

The trip was delayed until the following year. "And I had to prove myself with five time-trial runs first." When Stephen finally got to Melbourne, Australia, "It was hell;

Kim's program was very hard. We ran in 35-degrees Celsius in the middle of the day and were told we must do the sessions. The sessions were very, very tough. I even ran my 800-meter PR in training. We were told to run an 800 fast before the session started, the leader ran a 1:44 and I did a 1:46.1; yes, that hard." Cherono endured sessions like 20 x 400 in 57 seconds with a minute rest, but he was not performing well (racing times like 8:25-8:30). "It was crazy; I was concentrating on speed, not endurance, yet it was only January!"

Cherono got an invitation to Europe, where he found he had an excellent base of speed, recording a "very easy" 3:37 1500m, yet he ran a disappointing 8:26 steeplechase in Lille, France. Cherono returned to Kenya. "I trained all endurance, one hour ten, one hour twenty of running, no speed work at all," he recalls. He wanted to come back and race, but his manager at the time asked, "How will you pay?" Luckily, Stephen had a thousand dollars left from a sports contract, thus he was able to procure his own ticket, so he requested that he be entered in the Zurich meet, but was told, "You are not fit to run there." "It reminded me of what my brothers used to say. I said, 'fine, I am useless,' knowing I would show them." Cherono flew to Europe at his own expense. "In the first race I ran 3:37 alone in Newcastle with no pacemaker. Kim McDonald then realized I could run fast, and he sent me to Brussels." Three days later, Stephen became the first man under 20 years old to run sub 8:00 for the steeplechase when he stopped the clock at a stunning 7:58:66. "Kim asked, 'What did you do?' I told him his program was not good for me. Anyone can write a program, as I know myself, but I know my weaknesses. I work on myself, so I do not follow a program. I coached myself for a year."

In 2002, management problems arose. "I started with an 8:15 steeple in Milan, then I flew to America. I was at the airport waiting for a ride from 4:00 a.m. to 11:30 a.m., and nobody came, so I used my last few cents to phone London and was directed to the race hotel in Portland. I arrived at noon, twenty minutes to change, no breakfast or dinner, I drank some water and set off to pace [Brahim] Boulami 'til the last 200 meters, I still ran 8:05 and I knew I was very strong." Cherono was annoyed at the lack of respect bestowed upon him. Intolerably, it happened again soon after: "I was left in the Athens airport from 3:00 p.m. 'til noon the next day!" He switched management teams and came back to Kenya for training before returning to Europe to clock some fast races. He also won his first senior title, a Commonwealth Games gold in the steeplechase, in a time of 8:19.41. Kenyans, all within a half second of each other, swept the podium. Ezekiel Kemboi took the silver in 8:19.78, Stephen's elder brother, Abraham, took the bronze 8:19.85.

At this time, the only man able to challenge Stephen's supremacy was the Moroccan Boulami. "We all knew he was cheating [which was later proven to be true when the Moroccan tested positive for erythropoietin]. Wilson Boit and I were asking for him to be drug tested, but they seemed to be ignoring him on purpose." The two ran Zurich and Boulami won by about 20m. "I was way behind and running 8:05, I said to myself 'I don't want to race anymore,' and came home."

At this time, Stephen had an injury problem on the right out side of his foot. Despite being at the top of his game, there was no medical support offered. "We pay for the injury nobody supports with treatment. Whatever you do, you have to pay. Nobody is helping, why why why?"

In 2003, Stephen shocked the athletic world, in a story that transcended the sporting press. The saga began back in 2001, when Stephen talked to a retired Qatari athlete who told him about the benefits of competing for the Arab state: "I started the paperwork but just kept quiet," he recalls. Stephen notes with interest how prior to the day he revealed his new citizenship he was virtually ignored by the press and the athletics federation. "I think I was ranked about twentieth in the world and just 'another Kenyan.'" In Zurich, his first race under the maroon-and-white flag of his new country, Qatar, he won the steeple-chase in a world-leading 8:02.48. Asia had a new continental record. Two weeks later, the country got its first track and field gold medal, in the steeplechase at the Paris World Championships.

"The tension was very high in Paris. I was unbeaten in my last five or six races, but Ezekiel had nearly beaten me [by 1/100th of a second] in Zurich. I knew there would be Kenyan team tactics. I nearly burned myself; the pace for the first kilometer was 2:34. I had to take it from the second kilometer, 5:18, and I had to burn him [Kemboi] up, that was my tactic. But I was not happy winning on that day as I came to the homestretch with someone close by, you should leave someone much farther behind. Not satisfied. I like it with a three-, four-, five-seconds [gap], that is healthy." Cherono took the title in 8:04.39 to Kemboi's 8:05.11. It was the first time since 1987 that Kenya had not won the steeplechase at the World Championships, and the only time since that year that Kenya had just one representative standing on the medal podium

In 2004, Stephen was just hoping, not expecting, that he would be cleared for the Athens Olympics. "I just waited, I had no high hopes." It was not to be. the Kenyan Federation blocked Cherono's participation. In Kenya, and in the Kenyan press, were there not only objections being voiced for his citizenship switch but his rivals were going to the press to doubt his potential. "I heard bad talk about me. I thought, 'Why say this?' And if someone talks bad about me, I take it as a challenge. They were saying 'Shaheen can never get the [world] record, he can never beat that time,' so I thought 'Let me go and show them I can win something.'" Show them he did! Cherono started his campaign to get the world record in Paris, but cold, cold weather thwarted his chances, and he ran 8:05. Then to Athens, Greece, where Stephen ran an 8:00 flat. The Brussels Grand Prix came a week after the Olympics. "Everyone was tired. Not me."

Bottling up the frustration of not being able to prove himself in Athens, he ran like a leopard and destroyed a world-class field, making Olympians look like schoolboys. Frenchman Vincent Le Dauphin did a great job of pulling the field through the first kilometer in 2:36.13 before Kipkirui Misoi took over. The paced dropped, so just before the 2000m mark (5:18.09) Cherono was forced to take over. He ran the final kilometer in 2:35.45, clocking 7:53.63, a new world record and nearly a straightaway clear of Paul Kipsiele Koech, who although running a world-class 8:02.07 for second, may as well have been on a different planet.

"I did not run my best; I was celebrating as with 200 meters to go I knew I had the record. I was waving; it could have been sub-7:50 if I had pushed."

Stephen Cherono's Training Methodology

Monday	6 AM	60 min. full speed. It is not easy as I wear a skin suit and a full tracksuit. I do not train easy on this run, even if I am sick. I prefer to sleep for another hour rather than jog easy.
	10AM	Do not go for long runs, or you will think you are in good shape. Warm up, then 10 x 60m hill at full speed, 15 min. cool down.
	PM	30 min. very easy
Tuesday	6 AM	Same as Monday
	10 AM	Rest
	PM	30 min. easy
Wednesday	6 AM	1:30 at high speed
Thursday	6 AM	Same as Monday
	10 AM	Rest
	PM	30 min. easy
Friday		Repeat Thursday
Saturday	AM	Fartlek, 60 min. variations, when in good shape 2 min. hard, 1 easy for 30 min., then 1 min. hard, 1 min.e easy to make up one hour. If I start up the season then 10-, 8-, 6-, 4-, and 2-min. efforts with a 2-min. recovery after each effort.
	PM	Rest
Sunday		Nothing.

Comments

This program runs from November 'til March. From the end of track season (early September) until the end of October, I rest, no running whatsoever. The program then changes in April, when full-speed runs become medium-speed. On Tuesdays then I run track, and Wednesday's run is reduced to 60 minutes. Thursday morning now becomes a track workout.

My body is not balanced [but] the worst thing in the world is exercises. I would prefer to run for ten hours before doing an hour of exercise. I hate stretching, I do no stretching, and I hate gyms. I do pure running. For long runs it is difficult to get someone to pace, so I had the idea of two bicycles one on each side to help; I saw this in Europe with an athlete. I used to hate fartlek, but what I like is interval training. I used to go to Kamariny but it got too crowded, so now I use Chepkoilel at 6:15 a.m. for training. I do not have many regular training partners, they can train with me for one day or two... but if you train with me you are not going out to town following training, you have to rest and stay home, sleep. You leave your car at home when you come to train. But most runners now want to go out to town [Eldoret] following the training and that is not for me. No distraction. No email, no nothing, so you can focus just on training.

Do I train with my brothers? We stay at the same home, we cook together, and we can train together for a week. Then after that everyone goes his own way.

How do I know when I am ready to run a sub-8:00 steeplechase? I run the tough session [see above] one month before doing so. In the final week, on Tuesday, I run the last hard session for a Saturday race. I warm up with 45 minutes jogging, I am careful to go slow so no lactic accumulates, then straight into it." The "it" being another than any other human has come remotely close to, sublime sub-8:00 steeplechase win, and Stephen has done this more times than any other human has come remotely close to doing. Best Advice: From Renato Canova: "Money is not important; the last thing to consider is money. Believe in yourself. You will do it, you must believe in yourself."

Stephen's Take on Becoming Qatari

Nobody is against me in Kenya. Athletes tell me it is the right decision. Now, finally there is change in the sport; the federation is looking at its problems. Before nobody cared about sportsmen. The problem with athletics in Kenya is you have a lot of bulls, if this one gets old; you just get a new one. In Qatar they offered support in many ways; medical, housing, financial bonuses, like most federations do, but not in Kenya. It's a business decision, and what is wrong with that?

Moreover, as the dust is settling on the tracks, people are finding out the answer to that is absolutely nothing.

Jeruto Kiptum

Date of birth:	December 12, 1981
Birthplace:	Metkei, Keiyo District
Height/Weight:	5'8", 57 kg.
Coach:	Self
Personal bests:	800, 2:04.0
	1500, 4:08.6
	3000m, 9:01:90
	3000m steeplechase, 9:23:35
	5000, 15:32
Honors:	2004 African Championships
	2005 World Steeplechase, silver medalist
	2006 African Champion steeplechase, bronze medalist
Toughest session:	5 x 1000 in 2:54 with 2-min recovery
Favorite Session:	10 x 400 in 58-59 seconds

"Many times I went without," recalls Kiptum, who started to run in 1998. "Food was not always there." As a schoolgirl, she ran just for recreation at a primary school in Kapcheputuk. Her walking custom began much earlier. "We lived in a grass hut, and I would often travel up to 10K walking around looking for jobs to get food for the family. We had a big family, three sisters and four brothers. Hungry mouths." The goodness, she reflects, is that today the suffering made her truly appreciate the "something little I have" and to put that "something" to proper use.

Running certainly came naturally to Jeruto. "I did not train, but I won competitions at school. In my first year of running I was picked for the national junior cross country team to run in Marrakech in 1998." The coaches did not expect much of the newcomer and she was told to act as the team pacemaker. "Draw the pace out, go to the front always and keep the pace hot," she was told. Kiptum went to the lead, as instructed, and nearly stole the race, earning a silver individual medal, and a team silver as well.

Soon after that, she quit running so she could fully concentrate on her studies. Following graduation from the all-star school Sing'ore, she joined the Armed Forces and enrolled in boot camp Army training. As soon as she resumed running, the world-class results returned. "Running for me was easy then, the training only today is hard."

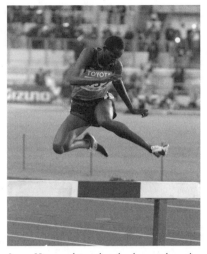

Jeruto Kiptum claims that she does not have the most eloquent hurdling styles, but it seems to work! (*Flanagan/Prettysporty*)

A big breakthrough came in 2006 when Jeruto beat the world record-holder and 2005 world champion, Uganda's Dorcus Inzikuru. "I saw it was only a result of hard work and hard training. This encourages me to keep up with my efforts." Inzikuru, in turn, complimented Jeruto. "She is very powerful and a big fighter. It is hard to race against Jeruto."

Jeruto's Training Schedule

Monday   AM   Hill repeats. 15 x 600-800m at a moderate pace

            PM   Jog to a field and run diagonals to remove the stiffness from the hill work

Tuesday   AM   Track, Intervals. Begin with 2000m repeats, easy jog mixing with 1200's and 1000's for endurance. The closer the race season gets, the more the distance is reduced to repeats of 8 x 600m, or 6 x 400m and 4 x 200m at full speed with a 60-sec. recovery for maximum speed development

            PM   Stretching and 30 min.

Wednesday   AM   40-50 min. of moderate speed, followed by 10 x 100m strides run again at a moderate, not full out pace.

            PM   Rest

Thursday   AM   One hour at 60-70 percent effort

            PM   40 –min. easy and 10 x 100m strides

Friday   AM   Track; 40 min. of running 200m with 200m recovery jog, or if far from the race 5 x 1200m trying to pass the 1K mark in close to 3 min.

            PM   40 min. easy jog

Saturday   AM One session, a long run of 70 min. run at a moderate pace.
Sunday   Rest day

Comments:

I know my strengths, so I must work hard on my weaknesses. I can maintain a fast pace, and I can finish, but I have very poor hurdling form. If I can not improve it then it may be best I turn to the 5000 meters. Right now, I think I have a great program for the 3000 meters. Kiptum trains with men—two groups—a strong pack for when she is in shape, and a lesser-talented group when she is in base training. "I never want my training sessions to get competitive; that is why I don't train with women," she reasons.

She includes a lot of hill work, especially in the early season. When beginning the program in October, after a month of rest, Jeruto runs six times a week for 70 minutes of easy long runs, either at 6:00 a.m. or 10:00 a.m. depending on the weather, for two weeks. She then adds fartlek—alternating 2 minutes hard, 2 minutes slow running, once a week for two weeks. Then hill work is added twice a week. If the legs feel too stiff, Jeruto is quick to switch back to plain easy runs to maintain a feeling of strong running with fresh legs. Track work begins in January, and the year's focus is on the summer's track season.

Ezekiel Cheboi Kemboi

Date of birth: May 25, 1982
Birthplace: Kabomo area, near Matira, Marakwet
Height/Weight: 5'5" 51 kg
Coach: "Moses (Kiptanui) was my first coach, and then Paul Ereng and
                    Joseph Ngure. Now self-coached"
Personal bests: 3000m, 7:57.11
                    3000m steeplechase, 8:02.49
Honors Won: 2001 African Junior Championships, steeplechase champion
                    2002 Commonwealth Games, silver
                    2002 African Championships, steeplechase, bronze
                    2006 Commonwealth Games, gold
                    2003, 2005, 2007 World Championships, steeplechase, silver
                    2003 All-Africa Games, steeplechase, gold
                    2004 Olympic Games, steeplechase champion

In school, Kemboi ran competitions "Just for fun, as a hobby," he remembers. "I heard about all the big-name Kenyans, but I did not think I would become a runner myself. I was more interested in soccer, playing in primary the years 1990-1992." However, after finishing at Kapsowar secondary school, Kemboi decided, as he loved track athletics, that he would try to become a serious athlete. The local athletes of his district were great steeplechasers, so Kemboi selected this discipline for his event. He sought out advice from a local hero, Moses Kiptanui.

His first race, a small Athletics Kenya meet in Kakamega in April of 2001, was a resounding success. "No one was at the meet that was good or very fast, so I got the win, I think just under nine minutes," he modestly recalls.

Kemboi was selected to represent Kenya at the African Junior Championships, and he returned from Mauritius with the gold medal. The following year he plucked two more Championships medals and lowered his personal record to a world-class 8:06:65. "I arrived quickly!" Kemboi now jokes. In 2003 he had to play second fiddle to the rising star of fellow Kenyan Stephen Cherono, losing in an enthralling battle of sport and patriotism at the Paris World Championships by less than a second. A strong rivalry was sparked between the two, with Ezekiel not mincing his words about what he thought of Stephen's defection to Qatar.

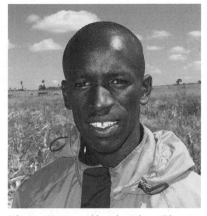

The one Kenyan gold at the Athens Olympics belonged to Ezekiel Kemboi. Not only does Kemboi volunteer to help at all the Shoe4Africa races, but he is the first to arrive and the last to leave. A great ambassador for the cause. (*Author*)

Ezekiel's crowning moment would come the following year, at the 2004 Olympic Games. "Training for the Olympics was tough. The last three months were very bad. Hard hard, hard work," he says. After winning the trials and being sure of a spot in the Kenyan team, Kemboi was relentless in his focus on one goal, to win the gold and avenge his loss at the World Championships.

"I did lots of sleeping every afternoon because the training was so hard. It was days full of pain." Nothing comes easy, and Ezekiel was fully prepared to pay the price. He recalls track sessions that left him faint and dizzy.

The result in Athens was perfect, for Kemboi and Kenya, as he led a clean sweep of the medals to win the gold in 8:05:81; a hair's breadth outside the Olympic record. "I ran the heats and finished second; the next day I jogged thirty minutes and ate and slept, that was all, the next day I did the same, only adding some exercises." On August 24th, Kemboi went to the start line with no team tactics at all. "I was only ready to run my best race ever. After all the hard training I did, the race was easy."

Training for an Olympic Gold

Monday	AM	Long run 1:20:0
	PM	40 min. jog before exercises
Tuesday	AM	Speed work (track), 6 x 400m at 55 sec. with 45 sec. rest, then 2 min. jog and 4 x 200 in 25 sec. with 30 sec. rest; "that is it"
	PM	Optional jogging depending on how you felt
Wednesday	AM	In a tempo run, I do 5 x 1K, at 2:45 sec., with 1:00 rest
	PM	Rest
Thursday	AM	Hill work: 3 x 5 200m hills in 33 sec. And jog down the hill recovery with 3:00 to remove the lactic.
	PM	Compulsory 45 min jog

Friday	AM	Track, 2 x 1000 (2:30), 2 x 800 (2:00), 2 x 600 (1:30:)
		and 2 x 400 (00:58) all with 2 min. rest.
	PM	30-40 min. of easy jogging
Saturday	10 AM	Progressive long run of 1:20–1:30. 20 minutes warm-up,
		then from there up to the hour hard and fast.
		After one hour still "hot" but gently coming down.
Sunday:		Rest day

Christopher "Jogoo" Koskei Cherono

"If you have a clear vision, you will have a good harvest"

William Cherono Kiptarus and Felista Sanieko sure had fast genes; the history of the fastest steeplechasing siblings in the world began on August 14, 1974, in a small trading post close to the road that leads to the town of Moiben.

Their first-born child became inspired after reading about Kenyan athletic success in the press. Their second born, Abraham Cherono, won a medal at the Commonwealth games, their next born, Stephen Cherono, is the current world record holder, and there are four more siblings now in hard training!

"I remember in 1992 seeing Henry Rono, Peter Rono, and Moses Tanui in the newspapers. I thought that I would like to be like them and be traveling to Europe. So I decided to train to become an athlete, so I, too, would get to go over there." And so started the illustrious career of Chris Koskei Cherono, one of the most charismatic characters ever to clear the barriers in the running arenas. His defining moment came in 1999, winning the world steeplechase championships in Sevilla.

Chris's Pearls of Wisdom

"If you have a competition on the weekend then take it easy after Tuesday. Do something but just endurance easy running. On Friday, I would do exercises and very little running."

"A favorite session was 4 x 1200m, running laps of 60, 60, and 58 with a 3-minute jog recovery. I would get my brothers to pace me laps of this."

"For long runs I used to train with Ismael Kirui when he was the World 5000m Champion."

"For shorter repeats I used 800m runners David Lelei and Kenneth Kimutich to pace me over the last 150 meters of my repeats to practice on my kick."

"I would do a time trial of 1500m with 800m runners once a week. If I hit 3:40 then I knew I was in shape."

"Nowadays, I see a marathon runner pacing a marathon runner. Why? Use a faster man always if you want to improve!"

"The important thing is discipline. If you do not have it, then it follows, you will not be a good athlete."

"Follow the program; if you do not and jump it or reduce it, you will not survive."

"The coach is the main person who will help you to excel."

"The biggest mistake I see is runners refusing to stay in the camp and wanting to go to town; you cannot; you must stay in the camp and be disciplined."

5000 Meters and 10,000 Meters

National Records–5000m

Daniel Komen, 12:39.74, 1997 (then, WR)
Eliud Kipchoge, 12:52.61, 2003 (WJR)
Vivian Cheruiyot, 14:22.51, 2007

National Records–10,000m

Paul Tergat, 26:27.85, 1997 WR
Samuel Wanjiru, 26:41.75, 2005 WJR
Linet Masai, 30:26:50 2008 WJR

Olympic Medals 5000m: John Ngugi, 1988, gold; Kip Keino 1968, silver, Paul Bitok, 1992 and 1996; Pauline Konga, 1996, Isabella Ochichi, 2004, Eliud Kipchoge, 2004, Eliud Kipchoge, 2008, silver; Naftali Temu, 1968, Edwin Cheruiyot Soi, 2008, bronze.
Olympic Medals 10,000m: Naftali Temu, 1968, gold; Richard Chelimo, 1992, silver; Paul Tergat, 1996 and 2000; Mike Musyoki, 1984, bronze; Kipkemboi Kimeli, 1988; Micah Kogo, 2008, bronze.
World Championship Medals 5000m: Yobes Ondieki 1991, Ismael Kirui, 1993–95, Daniel Komen, 1997, Richard Limo, 2001, Eliud Kipchoge, 2003, Benjamin Limo, 2005, gold; Benjamin Limo, 1999, Edith Masai, 2003, Vivian Cheruiyot, 2007, Eliud Kipchoge, 2007, silver; Shem Kororia, 1995, Tom Nyariki, 1997, John Kibowen, 2001, Priscah Jepleting Cherono, 2007, bronze.
World Championship Medals 10,000m: Paul Kipkoech, 1987, Moses Tanui, 1991; Sally Barsosio, 1997, Charles Kamathi, 2001, gold; Tanui, 1993; Tergat, 1997–99, silver; Barsosio 1993, Tegla Loroupe, 1995, 1999, Moses Mosop, 2005, Martim Mathathi, 2007, bronze.

Training for the 5000m and 10,000m

Moses Tanui can be called upon as an authority on distance running, with a World Championship 10,000m gold medal in his cabinet! He advises, "When training for the 5000 and 10,000 speed has to be remembered." Here's a sample training week:

Monday	One session of easy running and one of intervals, 5 x 2000m with 3:00 jog rest. Finish the session, as with all interval sessions, running 5 x 200m flat-out to keep your finishing speed in order.
Tuesday	One session of easy running and another of medium-to-hard running of over 60 minutes.
Wednesday	One session of easy running and one of intervals, 20 x 400m with 1:00–2:00 min jog rest, plus the 5 x 200m for speed.
Thursday	Two sessions of about one hour each, one easy and the other at a medium pace.
Friday	The same as above

Saturday　　One session of easy running and one of intervals. Could be 10 x 1000m with 2:00–3:00 min jog rest, and the 5 x 200m

Sunday　　Long run in the morning around 1:30:00

The times for the above intervals are of course individual, but though the effort should not be full speed, the athlete should finish the sessions tired out.

Ismael Kirui, world 5000m champion of 1993 and 1995, sees little difference in his training for cross country and track running. "As long as the training is hard, it does not matter too much what kind of training you do."

Yobes Ondieki, an athlete from Kisii District, had an outstanding range in distance running: 1500m, 3:34.36; 1 mile, 3:55.32; 2000m, 5:01.6; 3000m, 7:34.18, 5000m, 13:01.82, 10,000m, 26:58.38 and half-marathon, 61:41. Ondieki, the first man in ten years to defeat Morocco's Said Aouita over 5000m, is best remembered for his world record 10,000m and his world title 5000m in 1991.

Ondieki's reputation among the Kenyans was that of a tough trainer. Patrick Sang and Richard Chelimo told tales of such extremes as two track sessions per day. Ondieki never neglected pure speed in his training. A tough session for Yobes? "10 times 200 meters in 22 to 24 seconds with a short rest." And for the afternoon session? "10 times 800 meters at 10 meters race speed with 30 seconds rest or less."

A believer in high-altitude training, Yobes based himself in Albuquerque, New Mexico (1600m). In the 1991 season, in which Ondieki ran his personal-best 5000m time, he trained at home in Kenya and in Davos, Switzerland (1560m). "I prepared well, but I didn't underestimate anyone. I knew I had to be ready for anything because I didn't know how well the others had prepared themselves." He says. Running 13:01.82 in Zurich, Yobes realized he'd hit top form. Instead of his customary method of continuing hard training, he backed off, reduced the work load, and "took it easy." The result was a World Championship title in Tokyo.

Daniel Komen claimed that intensity is the key word. He aimed to make his training sessions harder and harder, believing there are no limits. Working off a two-minute jog recovery, Komen ran such workouts as 4 x 1 mile, the first run in 4:10 and the last close to 4:00. The training paid off in 1996, as Komen lopped an amazing four and a half seconds off Noureddine Morceli's "tough" 3000m record. Komen, who admitted to being "stunned" with the result, then planned to attack the 5000m record. His 12:45.09 in 1996 came close; it was the second fastest in history. He got the record in 1997 with his 12:39:74.

Sally Jelagat Barsosio

Date of birth:　　March 21, 1978

Birthplace:　　Kapchebelel, Keiyo tribe

Height/weight:　　5' 5" (165 cm), 98 lbs. (44-45 kg.)

Training Sessions:　　Two per day; two quality sessions during the cross country season, three in the track season.

Favorite session:	Morning run, distance
Hardest session:	Fartlek
Long run:	"I have now built up to 1:20:0, though up until 1997, it was little more than 50 min."
Honors won:	1992 World Junior Championships 10,000, 3rd place
	1993 (3rd place) and 1997 World 10,000m Champion
	1993 (3rd place) and 1994 World Cross Country junior champion
	1995 African Games 10,000m champion, 1995
	1995 (3rd place) and 1997 (5th place) World Cross Country; 1996 (10th place) and 2004 (17th place) Olympic Games 10,000m finalist
	1997 Grand Prix 5000m champion
	1998 African Championships, 5000m, 2nd place
	1998 World road relay team, 2nd place
Personal bests:	1500m, 4.13.11
	2000m, 5:39.4
	3000m, 8:35.89
	5000m, 14:46.71
	10,000m, 31:15.38
	Half marathon, 72:05

"I run to be a champion." Each night, after the Kenyan Broadcasting Company has aired the daily news, the sports are shown. A young, lithe Kalenjin girl is seen smiling in disbelief as she jogs around a filled-to-capacity stadium, enjoying the rapturous applause on her victory lap. It is footage from a dream that came true.

As a young girl, Sally Barsosio admired the achievements of Kenya's first female World Championships track medalist and wished one day to be a champion. Susan Sirma's bronze in the Tokyo 3000 in 1991 motivated Barsosio to train harder than most would dare to imagine. After only two years she equaled Sirma's feat with a bronze in the 1993 Stuttgart World Championships 10,000m. However, it was not enough for Sally.

"I wanted to be the best. I run to be a champion," she said. She persevered, and then, in 1997, her chance came in the Athens World Championships 10, 000m.

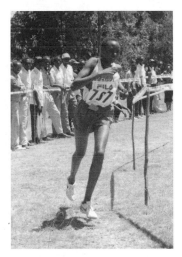

Sally always gave 110% in any competition she ran, here winning the Eldoret Discovery in 1996. (*Author*)

"With five laps to go, I knew I could win. I could not believe how strong I was feeling. Before the race, with Wami, Ribeiro, and the Chinese, I was aiming for the bronze because I knew those girls were strong." On her training for this event she adds, "It was good because the schedule that helped me win this gold medal [see below] I made myself in Form One at school [at 15 years old]." In winning the World Championships, Barsosio ran a now-surpassed world junior 10,000m record of 31:32.92. (Sadly, Sally's earlier time of 31:15.38 from the 1993 Worlds was not ratified as a junior record as no drug test was administered in those days.)

The most surprised person in Athens was Barsosio herself. "It took me three whole days before I could believe it. Imagine, I was walking round not really believing I had won!" A radiant smile full of with all those pleasant memories appears on her young face.

Success indeed came at the highest level. "I have no training secrets; I just run and train hard. It is here for anyone to see. . . others can follow it," she charitably offers. But be warned by the following story.

A few years ago when Sally was training for the Athens World Championships 10,000m, she was running on the soft dirt roads on the outskirts of Eldoret. As she was heavily wrapped in a large shapeless sweat suit and woolly hat, Sally's sex was indeterminate from afar. A group of male Fila runners trailed her at a distance, trying to close on the "unknown" athlete but making little headway. Comments flew that we must be chasing a new upcoming champion.

Kilometer after kilometer rolled by, and it was a good half-hour before the world-class runners overhauled Barsosio. They were shocked into silence as they realized the runner they had had so much trouble hunting down was a woman.

Remembering this with laughter, Mark Yatich exclaims, "She was running with the speed of a man, and I do not think she knew we were following. We were killing ourselves but she kept on pushing herself more and more." Yatich shares the Bix 7-mile course record with John Korir and has run a 61-minute half-marathon.

Comments

"The morning run is the *must*," Sally emphasizes with an iron conviction. "And when I am in Europe it is a must that I also go to the track." However she adds that after the groundwork that she will have undertaken in Kenya at 2400m altitude, the sessions are somewhat "easy" for her. "To have discipline is very important," she continues. "No one does the training for you; it is you!" If Barsosio feels she has slipped out of racing form, she tries to enter a lot of 1500s in small school track meets, aiming to run them in 4:20 or so (on dirt tracks at altitude) to gain the necessary speed. Hills are one of the keys of Barsosio's training plan. Her racing tactics are akin to those of many Kenyan athletes; start fast and run faster still. Often in local competitions, even with victory assured, she wrings out each ounce of energy from her small frame, and how she flies.

The Barsosio diet is typical of most Kenyan athletes. She has recently invested in a large coop of hens, and thus fresh eggs appear at each meal.

"I have no secrets. I just train as hard as I can manage each day. And I pray to God."

Training week

Used in the buildup to the World Championships gold.

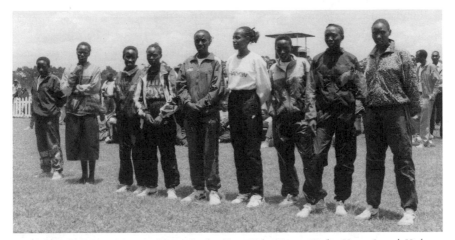

Female legends of Kenya. Margaret Okayo, Caroline Tarus, Helen Kimutai, Pauline Konga, Lornah Kiplagat, Jane Ngotho, Naomi Mugo, Rose Cheruiyot, and Sally Barsosio. (Author)

Monday	Long run, up to 1:20:0 (less in 1997, approx. 50-60 min.)
Tuesday	Speed work—10 min. hard tempo, 10 min. up a slight hill, cool down.
Wednesday	Fartlek workout of 50 min.
Thursday	Hill work 40-50 min. of hard hill climbing
Friday	Long run, as Monday.
Saturday	Medium-speed tempo run
Sunday	Rest day

All the above sessions are preceded by a pre-breakfast morning run of 40-50 minutes.

Track Training—A week at Nyahururu

Monday	Hill work, 50 min.
Tuesday	Medium-tempo speed run of 40 min.
Wednesday	Track. For example, 10 x 400m at 70-74 sec. with 1 min. rest.
Thursday	Long run, a 1:20:00 steady run
Friday	Track. For example, 20 x 200m or 4 x 800m, with jog rests of equal distance
Saturday	Medium-tempo speed run
Sunday	Hill repetitions

All the above sessions are preceded by a pre-breakfast morning run of 40-50 minutes.

Sally raises an interesting point when she dispels another myth of Kenyan running. "Some people think just because the men train in large groups they run so well. But we women also are running well and we are isolated; we train alone."

A couple of weeks prior to the 2000 World Cross Country Championships, Sally was switched, for tactical team reasons, from the long event to the short; the result was an eighth-place finish. "That was very bad. I had not prepared my speed, only my stamina. In Kenya this can happen. When I am racing I like to know the event I am going to run so I can do the training. But what can I say? Other athletes do not understand the problems we face [in Kenya]."

Augustine Kiprono Choge

Date of birth:	January 21, 1987
Birthplace:	Kipsigak, Nandi
Height/Weight	5'8" 163 lbs.
Honors won:	2003 World Youth 3000m Champion
	2004 World Junior 5000m Champion
	2005 World Junior Cross Country Champion
	2006 Commonwealth Games 5000m Champion.
Personal best:	800m, 1:48.7
	1500m, 3:32.48
	3000m, 7:28.78
	5000m, 12:53.66
	10,000m, 29:06.5 (a)
Tough Session:	4 x 400m in 55 sec. with 90 sec. rest

Life was full of hardships for young Augustine growing up. "My parents didn't go to school, and they enjoyed the local brew. There was often no food when I was younger, a tough situation. However, it gives the athlete encouragement to reflect on these times, and how you worked through them. Like I used to run to primary and back, 8 kilometers each way out of hardship, but this of course helped me too...." That foundation made Choge one of the world's top 5000m runners and one of the most exciting prospects for Kenya's future. Little did he know it back then.

Choge was a footballer in primary school, and when he joined Kabikwen secondary, like all students, Choge had to run. He did commendably and a teacher took him aside and told him to concentrate on athletics. While running in the provincial championships, he met Isaac Songok, who suggested to Brother Colm that Augustine should come to the camp. An invitation was extended. In December of 2002, Choge was learning a lot at the camp. "I didn't know about hill work, speed, or fartlek. Brother Colm's videos [of athletics] inspired me. I was sitting in the dining room with athletes like Viola [Kibiwott], who had won the World Juniors. It was very inspiring for me."

In the camp's dining room, there is a wall of—pictures of all the alumni who have lived or trained at St. Patrick's. You see Olympians Kip and Charles Cheruiyot, Peter Rono, Matthew Birir, Wilson Boit Kipketer, Wilson Kipketer, and so many more. Brother Colm stood in front of the wall and spoke to the group as Choge listened wide-eyed. "All you see who are on the wall have passed through here. They ate at the tables where you are eating; they ate the same food." Choge, starry-eyed, left the camp determined to become a world-class athlete.

In 2003, Choge ran cross country meets and placed second in the jackpot series to Eliud Kipchoge, who would win the World Championships 5000m in Paris, later the same year. Choge was selected to run the 800m, 1500m, and 3000m in the East African youth championships, and after winning all three (1:49:7, 3:43.7, and 8:04:2), he won the world youth 3000m in Canada.

In 2004 after leaving school, Choge moved to St. Patrick's. The result was a new world junior 5000m champion that summer. The next year, "I did good; I went to France to run the World Junior Cross Country Championships." "Good" meant first place. "Good" was also a new track PR of 12:53:66 for the 5000m; not bad for an 18-year-old.

In 2006, the Commonwealth Games were held in Australia. The favorite was the Aussie, Craig Mottram, a charismatic runner who

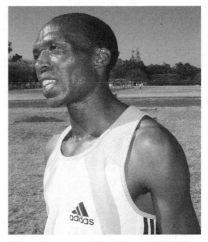

The Commonwealth Games Champion Augustine Kiprono Choge used positive thinking to turn a partisan Australian crowd to his advantage. (*Author*)

was fast becoming a legend for being able to take on the best of the Africans. Choge loved the atmosphere of the partisan 'Aussie crowd. "They cheered for Australia, but I took all the energies." He went to the line thinking of the words of his manager, James Templeton. "You have nothing to fear, you are okay. Focus only on yourself. Do not think of them. Try your best to win." Choge, like many times before, did just that setting a new Commonwealth Games record of 12:56.41.

Comments

In the 5000 meters, after the pacemakers drop out, pay attention. You must focus; someone can drop the pace, you may be sleeping, and a gap will open. Paul Tergat told us, "Nothing comes easy, so train hard. If you are supposed to be in the training camp, then be there."

In the race, if the pace drops, also be ready to push unless you have big confidence in your sprint. Also, if there is rain and you cannot go to the track, for example, then instead of canceling the session try to replicate it by going to a flat road or something; always try to do something. Doing intervals, for example, 4 x 400 meters in 58 to 55 seconds with 90 seconds rest. Do not push; just see how the body moves. We often do fartlek with Brother Colm blowing the horn on his car. Sometimes uphill, sometimes downhill we push.

Athletics is no longer just about running. It is more scientific these days. There is a lot of work, not just running. For instance, stretching. There must be a smooth response to the way you move. How your legs move, tempo, alignment, timing, not only running.

Training Plan

Monday	6 AM	40 min. easy easy (this can be 8-minute miling or slower)
	10 AM	30 min. high speed
	4 PM	35 min. easy and exercises
Tuesday	6 AM	45 min. easy
	10 AM	Exercises
	4 PM	Rest
Wednesday	6 AM	40 min. easy
	10AM	40 min. of running diagonal strides on a grass field
	4PM	30 min. run and exercises
Thursday	6 AM	30 min. easy
	10 AM	Fartlek. 45 min. of 3 min. hard, 3 min. easy, or 3 min. hard, 2 min. easy. Alternatively, running in front of Brother Colm's car and doing "horn" fartlek with ever-changing bursts of speed.
	PM	Rest
Friday	AM	45 min. easy
	10 AM	High Speed 30 min.
	4 PM	Rest
Saturday	6 AM	40 50 min.
	10 AM	45 min. easy
	PM	Exercises
Sunday	AM	1:20

Best Advice

"Try to follow what your coach tells you. Whilst training it will not be easy, but persevere. What you plan may happen, or not, but do not be discouraged." *From Wilson Kipketer*: "Eat well the day before a race; go to sleep early and rise early. Stretch a little before a light run 40 minutes before the race. Concentrate and do not be distracted by any noise or anything around you. After the race is time for enjoying."

Isaac Kiprono Songok

Date of birth:	March 23, 1984
Height/Weight:	5'4" 54 kg.
Birthplace:	Kaptel, Nandi
Personal best:	1500m, 3:30.99
	1 mile, 3:54.56
	2000m, 4:56.86
	3000m, 7:28.72
	5000m, 12:48.66
Honors won:	2001 World Youth 1500m Champion
	World Cross Country Championships, 1996, silver; 1995, bronze

Kilometers per week: 110

Tough session: 4 x 400 (55 –sec.), 5 x 200 (24 sec.), with 2 min. rests

Favorite sessions: 600m and 400m repeats

Songok began running in primary school, in
1999, he won both the 2000m steeplechase
and 5000m championships. "In 1994 I was
selected to represent the class at school; I won
for my class, then for the school. I kept on winning up to the district level. I was running free,
using barefoot with no training specifics. In
1995 I got to provincial level, and in 1996 I was
at national level."

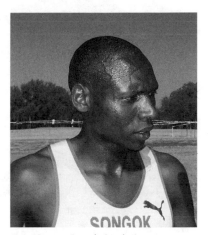

There was a slight setback in 1997 as
Songok was not training well, and not having
luck at the steeplechase. "I was not jumping
well," he remembers.

Isaac Kiprono Songok. (*Author*)

Brother Colm spotted Isaac at the 2000
World Juniors trials, when the 16-year-old flew
to a barefooted 13:37 at altitude. Colm gave
young Isaac some counsel. "My advice to him
was to move to the 1500m, I wanted him to develop his speed." Songok took the suggestion and the following year he had a 3:35 PR and a convincing win at the World Youth
Games. As a senior he is one of the world's best.

Training Week:

Monday	6 AM	40 min. easy easy (this can be 8-minute miling or slower)
	10 AM	30 min. high speed
	4 PM	35 min. easy and exercises
Tuesday	6 AM	45 min. easy
	10 AM	Exercises
	4 PM	Rest
Wednesday	6 AM	40 min. easy
	10 AM	40 min. of running diagonal strides on a grass field
	4 PM	30 min. run and exercises
Thursday	6 AM	30 min. easy
	10 AM	Fartlek. 45 min. of 3 min. hard, 3 min. easy, or 3 min. hard, 2 min. easy. Alternatively, running in front of Brother Colm's car and doing "horn" fartlek with ever-changing bursts of speed.
	PM	Rest
Friday	AM	45 min. easy
	10 AM	High Speed 30 min.
	4 PM	Rest

Saturday	6 AM	40 50 min.
	10 AM	45 min. easy
	PM	Exercises
Sunday	AM	1:20:00

Comments

"I believe in my kick. In training I use 200 meters and 300 meters repeats for finishing speed, and I remember my training in a race. If you are only good in lapping, you can not win a medal." Songok never runs intervals longer than 1000m, and three days before any major competition he takes it easy and jogs.

Benjamin Kipkoech Limo

Date of birth:	August 23, 1974
Birthplace	Chepkong'ony, Keiyo tribe but Uasin Gishu district
Height/Weight:	5'10" 63-65kgs. ("At 64, I am dangerous; if I go below 63 I am very weak and have no kick; I need muscles to drive the body.")
Personal bests:	1500m, 3:37.59
	3000m, 7:28.67
	5000m, 12:54.99
	10,000m, 27:42.43
	10K road, 28:00
Honors won:	World Cross Country Championships 4K—1999, gold, 2001, bronze; and 2003
	IAAF World Championships 5000m—2005, gold; 1999, silver
	2001 Military Games 5000m, gold
	Commonwealth Games 5000m—2002, silver; 2006, bronze
	2002 African Championships 5000m, silver

"I used to run at school, I loved to run. Everyone at school had to run, but I found it easy to run with the older boys; this was back in 1982-83. So when I was in Standard Five, I started competitions." In those days, Ben did not even know about international competitions or the possibilities of making athletics a career. However, that changed in 1987 after he listened to the radio. "We started to hear about athletics and everyone wanted to represent Kenya." The problem for Ben was time management. He had no time for training, and it was less than two miles to school, so the only opportunities arose when his father sent him to the shops, or on chores that involved going somewhere, instead of jobs on the *shamba*. So Ben ran when he could.

In 1988, Ben heard about the Olympics and was fascinated. "I wanted to go; every Kenyan who was on the radio news was getting a medal, so I thought everyone who went to the Olympics got a medal. I thought, 'Great, I want to go too and get a medal.'"

In Chabara secondary, running barefoot, Ben was now running all distances—the 400m, 1500m, the relays. He liked the longer distances, but because of his quick speed he was included in the shorter events when representing the school. A move due to the cold of the Marakwet area took Limo to Lelboinet to finish his schooling. "I learned that most of the successful runners had enrolled in the Army, so I joined up, on July 17, 1994."

"Things were not as I expected," explained Limo, who had to spend the next year in Army enrollment training. It was only in April of 1996 that he could resume full training. Having no running shoes, Limo went to the Kikomba market in Nairobi and bought a pair of used shoes. They cost him dearly, more than 2,000 shillings. "Much, much more than I could afford, in fact I kept those shoes right up 'til 1998, when I got a pair for making the national team."

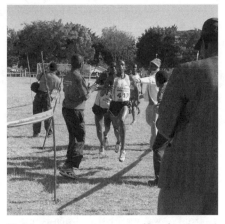

Training partners, room mates, and best friends, until on the battle field. Choge just nips Songok at the Kabarak cross-country December 2006. (*Author*)

Training for the 1997 season, Limo noticed the improvement. He was inspired by the international results of Ismael Kirui and Joseph Kibor, who had been in rival schools. Kirui offered Ben some important advice that year. "Ismael told me that the IAAF was adding a new race to the cross country championships, a 4K race. Ismael told me I should run this event, as I was fast." Ben took the advice and finished third in the national trial race after placing eighth in the Armed Forces Championships. "The coach, James Kibet, noted how I was improving and I was selected." Limo thought Marrakech was local; he was yet to get a passport. The trip was an arduous, typical team-Kenya one—Nairobi to Zurich, to Brussels, to Casablanca, finally to Marrakech. Hungry and tired, he arrived with a new friend, John Kibowen. "He inspired me; after a disappointing 1996, he did wonders in 1997. I thought, 'Whatever he does [in the race] I'll be behind him, on his heels.'" Limo ran with Kibowen and was at the front until the last 500m, when three teammates rushed by him. Still, fourth place in his first international race, and that being the World Championships, was no mean feat.

Limo came back to Kenya and joined the KIM camp. "I decided I wanted to leave the 1500m and try the 3000. In 1997, I had run 4:07 for the 1500 in Eldoret, so I doubled the time and thought that would 8:14 be an okay finishing time." In Limo's first 3000m, he showed his inexperience. "I ran in lane two on the shoulder of Moses Kiptanui. After five laps I was finished, but I hung on for an 8:05, at altitude, not bad I thought. It gave me encouragement. No more 1500's for me."

Selected to represent Kenya in the World Road Relays Limo, won team gold, and he won his 5K leg, "So with this result I decided to say goodbye to the 3K and become a 5000-meter runner. When I returned to Kenya I ran the Armed Forces 5000." In June of 1998, Limo ran a debut 13:29 at altitude, finishing third behind two renowned champions, Tom Nyariki and Paul Koech. Soon after that, he went to Europe and ran a superb

13:07:38 at the Rome Grand Prix. However, shortly afterward, a left calf-muscle pull curtailed his season.

Limo showed his professional attitude in 1999. He went to Spain to compete in some cross country races to gain experience running in European mud (less glutinous than Kenyan), as he had heard the conditions at the Belfast World Cross would be muddy. The homework paid dividends. Limo was triumphant in the big race. "It was great win, a stepping stone, but it was not the max, I also wanted success on the track, to be a champion there."

On the track, at that summer's World Championships, Limo was delegated as the sacrificial Kenyan to push the pace. As the race progressed into its later stages, Limo admits to feeling "burned in the legs and the lungs." Slipping back, he was suffering and soon no longer leading but running behind teammate Daniel Komen. A group of Moroccans ran in front. "I was maybe sixth when Komen called to me, 'Where are you? You go!' So the last 600m I kicked hard, hard, and managed to finish second. With 300 meters to go I shouted back to Komen, 'You can go too!' but we were tired; the last two laps were 59 and 58 seconds." It was a great year for Limo, who ran under 13:00 four times, ran a 7:28.67 3000m to win in Monaco, and finished the year with silver and gold individual World Championship medals.

Limo's disappointment of 2000 was not in making the Olympic team. His previous winter had been injury-riddled. "We were six in the Olympic trial race, then three of us fell down, and 1, 2, 3 had gone." Despite the setback, Limo went to Europe and ran 12:55.82 for the 5000m. It seems incredible that a runner of that caliber was not able to make his national team.

Back in Kenya, Ben was watching the Olympics on TV with his younger brother, who was still in school. The brother had stomach aches, so Limo rushed him to hospital; tests revealed nothing. "The next morning I returned with some clothes for him, and he was gone." Devastated by his brother's death, Limo immediately stopped training. That was the end of that season for Ben.

In 2001, Limo returned to place third at the World Cross Country Championships, though despite running 13:24 for 5000m at altitude in Nairobi, he did not qualify for the Kenyan team for the world track championships. Instead he went on a racing rampage, competing 16 times on the tracks of Europe, "Too, too many, I came home, I was over racing." He had again run some great times, including yet another sub 13:00 5000m.

A fever kept Ben out of the following year's cross country season, so he came to America to do some road races. "I thought, 'Let me get my endurance this way instead.'" It worked. Limo returned to find himself in fantastic form, and he won a few Grand Prix meets, then went to the Commonwealth Games. "It was a direct final, and the problem there is that you get a lot of inexperienced people pushing, and I fell over. I thought, "Should I get up?' Well, we had to work as a team, so I got up. But I no longer felt in the race." In a photo finish, Limo lost to Sammy Kipketer, 13:13.51 to 13:13.57.

In 2003, Limo again ran well in the World Cross, winning a bronze medal, but he was not satisfied with the rest of the year. He thought it might be time for a reassessment. In

2004, he moved from his base in Kaptagat to Iten, and picked up a knee injury. He flew to Europe, ran badly (13:31 in Rome), and called it quits. "I had not rested since 1988, and my body needed a break. I did some rethinking. I still was chasing what I did not have. I needed success on the track."

When Limo resumed training four months later, he had gained a lot of weight. "At first I was not able to break three minutes for the 1000, then after a week I was down to 2:55. This gave me the encouragement to look ahead to Helsinki." He ran the cross country trials and finished eighth, but an administration mistake put Joseph Kosgei in that position. Rather than complain Limo decided perhaps it was best to prepare for the track instead and forget cross country. For speed, he entered some local 1500m races. "I got third at Kakamega in 3:40, so I knew I was back to shape. I had wanted sub-3:50, so I knew I was coming. I was training too much so when I came for competition it was easy." An example: Limo was supposed to run 16 x 300m in 45 seconds with 45 seconds of recovery, but he was hitting 41 versus 42's.

He went to the world championship trials and had a photo finish with Isaac Songok, running 13:11 at Kasarani Stadium in Nairobi. The federation limited Limo to running just three races before the championships. "I wanted more because I did not know if I had good speed. So I worked hard in training for speed, doing 2K repeats, using five people to help with the pace," he says.

Training before the championships in Stockholm, Limo had a lot on his mind. His wife was due to give birth. "I called and wished her well, and I said that I was now on the road to the World Championships and would be leaving Sweden." When Limo got off the plane on Monday in Finland, he checked his text messages. There was a text from home. "I Ii Dad, God has blessed us with a baby." Elated, Limo won in a sprint finish. His dream had come true; a World Championship's title on the track.

The following year, Limo took a bronze medal at the Commonwealth Games. Again, he finished his season by running a sub-13:00 5000m, something he has achieved in all but one of the last eight years of summer track!

Training to Win a World 5000m Title

Monday	6 AM	60 min. easy pace "to 'take out the hangover,' as it is a surprise for the body to run again after a day's rest."
	4 PM	40 min. easy. Exercises
Tuesday	6 AM	50 min. medium up
	10 AM	Speed fartlek* or intervals. Something longer like 2 x 1200 (3:09), 2 x 800 (2:00), 2 x 600 (1:28).
	4 PM	40 min. easy, drink water and get rest. Must relax in the day.
Wednesday	6 AM	A long, progressive, long run of 1:15:0 to 1:20:0. After 50 min. though, do not add any more speed or you will kill your track speed.
	4 PM	Jog, or even relax in the evening
Thursday	6 AM	Tempo work, 1K or 2K at a constant speed, or at 10 AM intervals.
	PM	Easy jog

Friday	AM	Something very light, 50-60 minutes.
	10 AM	Jog 30 min. then 50 min. of exercises and stretching
	4 PM	Recovery, very light 30 min.
Saturday	6 AM	Long and easy, 70 min.
Sunday		"I never train on a Sunday unless I am in the national team camp. This way it gives me a day to get relaxed in the mind."

*10 min. hard, 2 min. easy, 5 min. hard, 3-easy, x 2; then 4 hard, 2 hard, 1 hard all with 2 min. recoveries, then lastly 10 x 1 min. hard, 1 min. easy.

Comments

Every morning, sit-ups, press-ups, not less than 30. When doing intervals be progressive, increase the pace as you run. When I run 5 x 1000, I start with 2:40 and end with 2:35. As the race approaches, run 600 meter repeats and lower with a high speed. I use 58-seconds per-lap pace for the 600 to sharpen my speed. Focus on one race and you will perform well.

Sylvia "Sleepy" Jebiwott Kibet

Date of birth:	March 28, 1984
Birthplace:	Kapchorwa Keiyo District
Height/Weight:	164 cm. 44 kg.
Personal best:	1500m, 4:10.07 (4:07:46 indoors)
	3000m, 8:40:09 (8:41:82 indoors)
	5000m, 14:57.37
	10,000m, 31:39.34,
	10K, 31:44
	Half marathon, 1:11:37
Honors won:	2006 African Games, 5000m, bronze
	1999 World Juniors, 1500m, silver

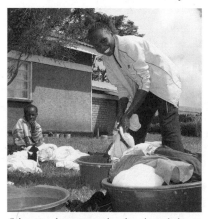

Sylvia spends a morning hand washing clothes in Irene Kwambai's garden. (*Author*)

Never "Sleepy" when it comes to the race day, Sylvia has awesome speed. Seeing her soar and sashay along the dirt roads of Iten is an eye-opener; she has gears beyond the gears.

"When I started running, I got sent to Uganda for the East African Championships in 1998. They gave me running shoes and a tracksuit, and this was inspiring, and kept me interested in athletics. When I ran the following year in Poland, I got money too. I thought, 'Wow, I like athletics!'"

Sylvia is amongst the new breed of Kenyan women; she excelled at the junior level, retired from athletics, gave birth on January 4, 2005, to Jepkosgei, then in November of that year started running again. Barely a month later she placed eighth at the Iten Shoe4Africa 10K, and was back at the forefront of Kenyan running, just missing a place on the 2006 World Cross Country championships team in the spring.

In August 2006, in a close tactical battle, she took a bronze medal in 15:57.14 at the hotly contested African Games in Mauritius, just a second behind the world record-holder, Meseret Defar, who ran 15:56.00, and World Champion Tirunesh Dibaba, who ran 15:56.04. Kibet's sterling comeback was complete. A year later she would miss a medal at the World Championships by an agonizing 5/100ths of a second! In 2008, after winning the prestigious IAAF Berlin Grand Prix, she was selected to run at the Beijing Olympics, where she placed fourth.

Pre-Competition Training Block

Monday:	AM	70 min. steady
	PM	40 min. easy
Tuesday	10 AM	30 min. easy, 45 min. steady to fast
		then 10 x 1 min. fast, 1 min. slow, then a cool down.
	PM	Washing clothes all afternoon at Irene Kwambai's house.
Wednesday:	10 AM	15K fast run on the Pound Loop
	PM	Easy 45 min.
Thursday:		Two easy runs of 40 to 60 min.
Friday	10 AM	Intervals, 2 x 2000m, 1200m, 800m, 600m, 400m
		untimed with 90 –sec. rest
	PM	Easy jogging 40 min.
Saturday	AM	60 min. steady
	PM	45 easy
Sunday	Rest day	
Monday	AM	60 min. steady
	PM	Hill work. 50 –min.s compromising of 90-, 60-, 30-, and 15-sec. sprints, with a jog of the same distance run as recovery. On Helen's Hill.

In-Season Training Week

Monday:	AM	60 min. steady
	PM	30 min. easy
Tuesday:	AM	45 to 60 min. easy to steady run
	PM	Track 10 x 400m, 60 sec., with a minute standing rest
Wednesday	AM	One run of 60 min. medium speed
Thursday	AM	Track, 5 x 1000m, 2:50, 2 min. rest
Friday		Travel to competition
Saturday		Compete
Sunday	AM	Easy 60 mins

Comments

In 2006, at the Berlin Grand Prix 5000m, Sylvia was running and fearing the last lap. "When you race the Dibaba sisters of Ethiopia, you know it will be painful." She ran a stunning 60-second final lap but finished only sixth. "That is what you have to train for today in running track if you want to succeed. The Ethiopian ladies can run 56 seconds, so you must train for speed. Run lots of speed, start with road or cross country races in the spring, and then focus solely on the track throughout the summer."

Daniel Kipngetich Komen

Date of birth:	May 17, 1976
Birthplace:	Keiyo District
Height/weight:	5'7" (170cm), 121 lbs. (55 kg.)
Favorite session:	Morning steady run.
Sessions per day:	Two mostly; can be three.
Miles per week:	120
Hardest session:	Track workout, 4 x 1 mile, the last mile as close as possible to 4 min. flat
Length of long run:	Up to 2 hr.
Personal best:	1500m, 3:29.46
	Mile, 3:46.38
	2000m, 4:51.30
	3000m, 7:20.67 (3000 indoor, 7:24.90)
	2 miles, 7:58.61
	3000m steeplechase, 8:54.5
	5000m, 12:39.74 (5000 indoor, 12:51.48)
	10,000m, 27:38:32
	10K (road), 27:46
	Half marathon, 64:52
Honors won:	1994 World junior champion, 5000m and 10,000m
	1997 World Champion 5000m
	1998 Commonwealth Games champion, 5000m
	1998 African Championships, 5000m, gold
	1998 World Cup 5000m champion
	1998 World Cross Country Championships, 4K, 2nd
World records:	3000m, 2 miles, 5000m, indoor 3000m and 5000m.

In the early 1950s they said a man could not run faster than four minutes for one mile. Those theorists would have scoffed at the thought of back-to-back four-minute miles, but then again, they had not seen the Tartan-tearing stride of Daniel Komen. He became the first and still today the only runner ever to blaze back-to-back miles under four minutes per mile when he recorded 7:58.61 in 1997!

After an outstanding junior career, Komen first appeared in the senior ranks when he won a place on the 1994 Commonwealth 10,000m team. Lameck Aguta, who eventually won that race, recalls: "Komen was a junior, and it was his job to set the pace. We told him to go fast fast, and he did! I think the first 800 was 1:57; nobody went with him, and he was no pacemaker!" Komen's opening lap was 57.5, which gave him an immediate 100m lead!

A year later, with more even laps, Komen helped pace Moses Kiptanui to a new world 5000m record in Rome. The young runner was so nervous that he didn't sleep the whole night before the race. The result for him was a world junior record of 12:56.15. These results were just a preview of what the world would see the following year.

Komen began to dominate the 5000m in 1996, and most pundits expected the Kalenjin runner to win the Olympic title. But the unexpected happened; Komen did not even make the Kenyan Olympic team, finishing fourth in the Kenyan trials.

Perhaps running with pent-up frustration, Komen dominated the post-Olympic season, running an exhilarating 3000m in Rieti, slashing more than four seconds from the old world record.

The following year (1997), Komen easily took the World Championship 5000m gold. After an "easy" 3000m, Komen injected a couple of laps worthy of a 1500m final. "I watched the race as I ran on the big stadium screen. I was ready that day, he says." Although the field closed in the final lap, Komen had the situation well under control, knowing they could not catch him.

A world 5000m record followed, and more records after that. Some have been lost, some remain, even at ths writing.

Training Week

Monday	AM	Morning run at moderate speed, 1:10:00
	PM	Afternoon run 40 min. normal speed
Tuesday	AM	Hard speed 30 min. with 20 min. warm-up
	PM	40-50 min.
Wednesday	6 AM	45 min. easy
	10 AM	Track, 6 x 1000m at 2:30 with 60 sec. rest
Thursday	AM	Steady morning run of around one hour.
	PM	30 min. easy.
Friday	AM	45 min. steady.
	PM	Hill work, usually interval running of around 20 repeats.
Saturday	AM	Long run 1:40:00

Variations of Track Workouts (Altitude!)

Time trials of 3000m or 1500m.

1 x 1600 (4:10), 1 x 1200m (2:55), 1x800 (1:56), 1 x 400 (55), twice.

15 x 400m @ 56-57 seconds with 45 sec rest jog.

45 min of running diagonals on the infield.

12 x 800m @ 2:01-03 with 200m jog rest.

The Marathon

National Record	Paul Tergat, 2:04:55, 2003 (then, WR)
	Catherine Ndereba, 2:18: 47, 2001 (then, WR)
Half-marathon NR	Samuel Wanjiru, 58:35, 2007 (current WR)
	Mary Jepkosgei Keitany, 66:48, 2007
	(Susan Chepkemei has run 65:44, though the time is not accepted by the IAAF as the Lisbon course had a net drop of 70M.)
Olympic Medals	Samuel Kamau Wanjiru, 2008, Gold
	Douglas Wakiihuri, 1988, silver
	Eric Wainaina, 1996, bronze; 2000, silver
	Joyce Chepchumba, 2000, bronze
	Catherine Ndereba, 2004, silver
	Catherine Ndereba, 2008, silver
World Champions	Douglas Wakiihuri, 1987
	Catherine Ndereba, 2003, 2007
	Luke Kibet, 2007

Since 1991, Kenyan men have won every Boston Marathon except two. In the 1996 race, there were seven Kenyans in the top eight positions! In the 14 editions of the IAAF World Half-Marathon Championships from 1992 to 2005, Kenyan men won nine individuals titles, twice taking a clean sweep, (1995 and 1997), and won eight team titles. Although the Kenyan women were less dominant, taking only three individual medals, they did collect a commendable ten of the 42 individual medals over the history of the event and claimed four team titles.

Bill Rodgers, a four-time winner of both the New York City and Boston marathons, was *the* road racer back in the 1970s and 1980s. "The Legend" reminiscences about his Kenyan duels. "I remember racing against a Kenyan runner for the first time in 1974 at the Charleston Distance Classic in West Virginia. I was very pleased to defeat a top runner like Jeff Galloway that day, and be not too far behind second place John Vitale, my old University of Connecticut and track rival, and now a friend. John was edged out by a man called Philip Ndoo, who had gone to college in the United States. A few years later, I raced against one of the finest distance runners of all time in a famous half-marathon called San Blas in Coamo, Puerto Rico in 1978. His name is Henry Rono, and at the time, he held the world records at 3K, 5K, steeplechase, and 10K. I was ranked one of the top marathoners in the world that year, and I felt we would have a super duel meeting each other half way from our best race distances, and I was right! We ran neck and neck until the final half-mile and Henry sprinted for the finish. I followed ten seconds later. During the 1970s and 1980s, I raced against other top Kenyans, like the legend Joe Nzau and Wilson Waigwa. I can say that every Kenyan runner I ever met was like the salt of the earth; very friendly and low key, humorous, and very, very determined to win. I just love that attitude! Run forever, Kenya!"

Kenya has had less success in the marathon at the Olympics and World Championships than it has had in distance events on the track or in major city marathons. The reason can be traced to economics. When you are an African marathoner, money has to be a main consideration.

"If you over-race, you won't last at the top," explains Cosmas Ndeti. The race must pay if athletics is your career. Major sponsorships do not exist for Kenyan runners. If a Western athlete were to win the Olympic marathon, the sponsorship money would be substantial, but a Kenyan would probably receive nothing apart from a bonus from his shoe sponsor, if he had a bonus clause in his contract.

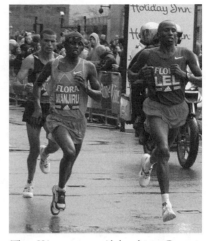

The Kenyan way. Abderrahim Goumri, Morroco, (2:05:30), Sammy Wanjiru (2:05:25), and Martin Lel (2:05:15), turn the 2008 London marathon into a street race. (*Urban Bettag*)

Competing in a major city marathon, a top runner—regardless of origin—can command an appearance fee, and earn prize money and shoe-company bonus money. "Boston was my jackpot!" laughed Moses Tanui, after collecting $100,000 in April of 1996. Add to that figure appearance money and the bonus received from Fila sportswear and it totals a staggering amount for any athlete, let alone an African.

There are no Olympic training grants in Kenya, and there is no appearance money for the Olympics or World Championships. Since it is exceedingly difficult to run more than two world-class marathons in a year, the top runner must choose his races with his finances in mind. All of the members of the Moi Air Base marathon squad admitted that winning Boston or New York is their dream achievement. The prize money at Boston is the same whatever country you come from; that is about the closest Kenyan athletes get to equality.

Despite the major championship "shortfall," Kenya has still accumulated seven Olympic medals in the marathon in the last 20 years, a record superior to many "running" nations. The first came quite unexpectedly from Douglas Wakiihuri, a virtually unknown Kenyan who lived in Japan. The Kikuyu tribesman, born at sea level on the Kenyan East Coast, had gone to Japan in 1983 as an 18-year-old to train with Kiyoshi Nakamura, the famous coach who had brought Toshihiko Seko into the marathon limelight.

Wakiihuri debuted in 1986 with a 2:16 and progressed the next year to 2:13, hardly harbingers of a gold medal at the World Championships in Rome. He trained in Sweden and warmed up with a win at the capital's Stockholmsloppet, half-marathon running 61:40 before traveling to Italy. At the World Championships he dueled with Ahmed Salah of Djibouti, then the second-fastest marathoner in history, eventually striding away to win the top place on the podium.

As an Olympic favorite in Seoul in 1988, he again battled with Salah, but this time there was a stronger runner—Gelindo Bordin of Italy (the third-place finisher in Rome). Wakiihuri had to be content with the Olympic silver medal. Sixteen months later, he won the Commonwealth Games marathon in Auckland in 2:10:27. Then, after an absence on the world stage, Wakiihuri made a golden comeback in 1995, winning the Marathon World Cup in Athens.

Wakiihuri trained hard with three-hour-long runs, followed by a mid-day session in the gym, and then an easy one-hour run around five o'clock. "The day after this session, I would take it easy with only one 15-kilometer run and a two-hour gym session," Wakiihuri related.

Kenyans have been labeled the free spirits of running. They run with their hearts, not their heads, some observers claim. It is true that it is not uncommon to see a Kenyan marathoner set off at breakneck speed, only to drop out or start walking later on. The self-belief that Kenyans have in themselves is unmatched, however, and their enthusiasm is understandable. Wilson Kiptum, a little-known runner training in Kapsabet, said, "I heard that [Sammy] Lelei ran very well in Berlin [2:07:02, the second-fastest marathon ever at the time]. I know I can run faster than Lelei; if somebody takes me to a race with Lelei running, he will not beat me. I'll stick with him until the end; I don't care what pace he runs." This from a runner who had yet to beat 31 minutes for 10,000m!

The easygoing Kenyan attitude is exemplified in the three stories below of how these Kenyans fell into world-class marathon running.

Stephen "Baba" Kiagora, the runner-up at the 2006 ING New York City marathon, on his introduction to running:

I was running first for just enjoying. I ran from Meru to Isolo, which is about 90K in jeans—no running clothes, my legs were raw. After the soles of my shoes were worn through, I got so many blisters. These were not running shoes. I tried to run home, but I could not, I had to take the bus. I was sitting there finished on the back seat. I ran from Nanyuki to Nyeri, which is longer. When I arrived I drank five sodas at once. I was so thirsty. All this running was not for training, it was just that I liked to run places. So after enjoying these runs I said to myself why don't I do this as a job.

Hosea Kiprop Rotich of Kapsabet was a defender in Kapsabet United village football team, and then he decided that team sports were not for him. He bought a pair of running shoes and began training. After two years, he entered the 2006 Nairobi Marathon in 2006, "I thought it would be nice to be top ten," he says. Rotich surprised even himself. "I ran 2:10:17 and won by three minutes." How did he train for that race? "I had a friend Simon Wangai, who was following a plan from El-Mostafa [Catherine Ndereba's coach]. So I took this plan; it worked." Rotich has since improved to 2:07:24.

Philip Manyim was a world-class steeplechase pacemaker. "I paced everyone, like Shaheen and Boulami, the last two world record-holders." However, in Switzerland in 2004, Philip decided he had had enough of making other people's names, and it was time to earn his own merits. "So I went from the steeplechase to the marathon. No training, I just said to my manager, 'Let me try.' In August I was racing three kilometers and by

October it was up to 42 kilometers." After running in the lead for 90 minutes, Manyim faded to 13th place, in 2:18:17. "Renato Canova said 'See how it goes, and if it is tough, then don't hang with the leaders. Well I tried, but I was so tired!'" Within one year, at the real Berlin Marathon, Philip, who was encouraged by his debut, took his first marathon win, recording 2:07:41!

Training Week
"This is the program I used for Berlin."

Monday	AM	1hr 20-mins medium speed
	PM	60-mins Easy
Tuesday	AM	Speedwork, 5k, 4k, 3k speed with 1k recovery jog on a dirt road
	PM	40 mins easy run
Wednesday	AM	90-mins long run, "this we do steady, not timed, but not slow"
	PM	60 "Easy, easy pace"
Thursday	AM	Speedwork, can be fartlek, like 2' hard 1' easy for 20-times
	PM	40-mins easy run
Friday	AM	80-minutes with long hills, pushing on the climbing part
	PM	faster running on some short 80-100m hills
Saturday	AM	30-38 kilometers long run. (30, 35, 38 on a three-week cycle)
Sunday	AM	60-minutes easy, and then rest for the day."

Armed Forces marathon training

Many of Kenya's top athletes are affiliated with the Armed Forces and train with other runners at the camp to achieve remarkable results, for instance, Jackson Kipng'ok's 2:08:08 in 1994. Athletes not in the service can also join the camp runners for training. William Musyoki, who lives a few kilometers from the N'gong faction, frequently links up with the military for marathon training. The group ordinarily will have no fewer than 15 fit full-time athletes. At the Laikipia Air Base there were about 40 marathoners in the fall of 1996, and thus the training sessions were always competitive and never taken easy. The strong get stronger and the weak wilt!

Each morning of the training week below, a 40- to 70-minute run is taken on a "how you feel" basis (at about 6 a.m).

Monday	Noon	35 40K long run.
	PM	Exercises and strolling.
Tuesday	Noon	Intervals, 5 x 1000m
	PM	Jog 40 to 60 min. or 2 min rest, strolling.
Wednesday	Noon	90 min. steady
	PM	Jog 40-60 min.; 30 min, full speed).
Thursday	Noon	Hills, 2 x 27 min.
	PM	Jog, plus exercises continuous uphill or rest; running.
Friday	Noon	Same as Wednesday noon
	PM	"How you feel."

Saturday   Noon   Tempo/fartlek run
                PM   Rest; full speed, 15K
Sunday   Day of rest

Eric Kimaiyo is a typical Kenyan marathon success story. Living away from the city up in the Cherangani Hills, Kimaiyo trained primarily with long-distance runs, some up to 50 kilometers, and most completed at a steady to good speed. No high-tech methods, no complicated training schedules. Each day was like the previous day—endurance running. This led Kimaiyo to a 2:10 marathon. "I just decided that I would try to become a runner, so I ran. It was that simple," laughed Kimaiyo, discussing his scientific approach to training. Kimaiyo would end his career with a 2:07:43 before dedicating his time to opening an athletics training camp at Kapsait, Kenya.

Paul Kiprop Kirui won the world half-marathon championships back in 2004, and then decided to move up to the marathon. In 2005 he ran what he deemed a disastrous 2:11:28 at the Milan event. When he returned to Kenya, some of his training partners suggested that Kirui, who is the brother to Willy, Ismael, and the late Richard Chelimo, should return to his specialty distance, where he has run 60:18. However, Kirui reasoned that it took time for the body to fully adapt to the marathon program. He continued his plan of increased long runs and using tempo runs instead of interval sessions. The next year, his 2:06:43, placing second in the Rotterdam Marathon, was the fifth-fastest performance of the year.

Wincatherine "Catherine" Nyambura Ndereba

Date of birth: July 21, 1972
Birthplace: Gatunganga, Nyeri
Height/Weight: 5'2", 98 lbs.
Miles per week: 90-100; last year, 80-90
Length of long run: 3 hrs. longest
Hardest session: 7 x 2K track
Personal bests: 5000m, 15:27.84
                       5K road, 15:09
                       10K road, 31:02
                       Half-marathon, 67:54
                       Marathon, 2:18:47
Honors won: 1999 World Half-marathon, 3rd
                       1999 New York Marathon, 2nd
                       2000, 2001, 2004, 2005 Boston Marathon champion
                       2000, 2001 Chicago Marathon champion
                       2003, 2007 World Marathon champion
                       2004, 2008 Olympics, silver medal

Catherine Ndereba, a Kikuyu, has the enviable record of finishing on the podium in 16 of her 18 marathon races, and as taking a medal in every Olympic/world championship event she has entered—an incredible, unique achievement.

Catherine was not an exceptional junior athlete when she grew up in Nyeri. She ran competently in school, yet did not set any records or make headline news. Her coach, Stephen Mwaniki, saw talent and advised Catherine to stick with athletics after schooling. Catherine had wanted to be a schoolteacher, but Stephen recommended that she to join the Prisons as his wife had done. This way, he reasoned, Catherine could continue with her sport. Following graduation in 1995, Ndereba burst onto the scene by making the Kenyan national team. she went to Seoul to run in a Road Relays competition. The following year, she was in the United States winning more road races than you could shake a stick at.

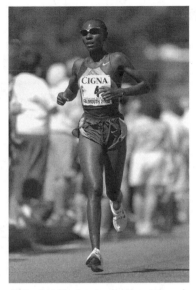

Catherine Ndereba wins the Cigna Falmouth Road Race in 2006. (*Parker Morse*)

Says Lisa Buster, Catherine's manager, "Catherine is special. She has immense focus and discipline. Last year, two weeks before the Osaka Marathon, she was helping plan her sister's wedding. In the morning she had a track workout, then she drove for two hours to help with the arrangements in Nyeri. She changed from the tracksuit to Catherine the lady, as she had to meet the Minister. By six o'clock all the jobs were done, and we had to drive back two hours to Nairobi. But Catherine still had another hour's training run to do. So she changed again, and set off soon after, running down the road with us trailing behind her in the car, using the headlamps so she could see where to go, as it was dark by then. That's Catherine."

Ndereba barely missed qualification for the 1996 Kenyan Olympic team at the 10,000m distance. In 1997, she was absent from the running scene as she took maternity leave to give birth to her daughter Jane. "I did not run at this time, I took a lot of time off; I don't believe in training through a pregnancy, it is not the healthy way, I think." Ndereba was back in 1998 with vengeance, named the top road racer on the U.S. circuit by the world's leading running magazines, *Runner's World* and *Running Times*.

A move to the marathon in 1999 (6th 2:28:27) proved to be fortuitous; the distance was made for her. She also collected the bronze medal at the world half-marathon championships, and the team gold, in Palermo, Italy. By winning Boston, slated as the Kenyan Olympic Marathon trials in 2000, Catherine was a hot favorite for the Olympic title; except that the selection committee was out to lunch, and somehow she was omitted from the team. It was a travesty. A livid Ndereba toed the line in Chicago in the fall of 2000 and ran the then fifth fastest time ever, 2:21:33, each stride powered by the hours of preparation that had been saved for her run for gold in Sydney. A woman in her prime denied by politics, Catherine still scowls about the issue seven years later. Following Chicago, she said, "They will not dare to leave me home for Athens."

To establish and demonstrate her position as the world's number one she decided she needed the world record for her resumé. Not a problem. Her coach, El-Mostafa Nechchadi, picks up the story.

We looked at the 2:20 barrier and said, 'Okay, let's be the first to run under it. We knew Catherine could do it physically. This is the training necessary, let's do it.' By the timing of the gods, Naoko Takahashi ran 2:19:46 on September 30th, and on October 7th, just one week later, Catherine put her plan into action.

A 70:14 for the first half, then a 68:33 second half smashed the Japanese woman's week-old record as Catherine finished in 2:18:47. It was no fluke the following year, after a season of winning road races both in the USA and Japan that she clocked another sub-2:20 (2:19:26) again at Chicago, albeit behind Paula Radcliffe's new world best of 2:17:18. The following year, Ndereba again ran a sub-2:20, in London (2:19:55), before attacking the World Championships in Paris. At those prestigious games, she took gold in 2:23:55. "I was praying hard to close the race and come to the finish line. It was a very special day for me."

As an experiment, Catherine jumped into the New York City Marathon, putting together a scant three-week training program, with a two-week taper that would leave most athletes shuddering with self-doubts. "I wanted to see if I could do three marathons in a year." The result was a rare loss as Catherine recorded the second fastest time ever on the New York roads: 2:23:03. Fellow Kenyan Margaret Okayo had to run a course record of 2:22:31 to defeat the legend.

When Catherine pulls out these smooth performances she looks a picture of perfection running along at five-minute miles. She reveals that as she is zooming down the roads she often sings a little Swahili song, the gist of the repeated line being, "If we keep on praying, our God is able to do whatever we ask in his name."

Being the defending world champion and having won Boston in the spring, Ndereba was told she would be traveling to Athens for the 2004 Olympic Games. Despite running with a torn hamstring, meaning she could not execute her usual late attacking surge in the race, Ndereba maintained her medal-winning record in a major championships by taking the silver. Under the circumstances, she was delighted. "To win an Olympic medal has been a dream of mine for so, so long, I cannot tell you."

In 2005, she again took a medal at the World Championships Marathon, this time silver, against her nemesis, Paul Radcliffe, arguably the greatest-ever women's distance runner.

The following year, 2006, saw a "warm up" win on a wintry day in Osaka. "It was so cold! I thought it was cold when I set the world record in Chicago, but this time it was even colder. Imagine, I ran the whole way and did not even sweat!" The win was only 89 days before Boston, and thus the organizers, who maintain a 90-day no-racing rule, kept her from the start line. Sportingly, Catherine jumped up and down on her sofa at home, yelling and screaming for Rita Jeptoo to win the race, which she did. "A Kenyan won! A Kenyan won!" Catherine exclaimed.

In the fall of that year, Catherine was enticed to try for that elusive New York win she so desired. A bathroom issue made for an atypical race for the Kikuyu woman, who ran with stomach cramps for the full distance. She did, however, make the podium, placing third in 2:26:58. A true champion she smiled, never once mentioned an excuse, and congratulated all the other runners at the press conference following the race, demonstrating even in the face of defeat, she is a winner.

In 2007, Catherine was locked out of the big spring marathons; sometimes it does not pay to be a consistent champion. In the summer, this time under extreme heat and humidity, she returned to Osaka to contest her third World Championships marathon. Running a tactical race, Catherine made a late move to defeat the best the world had to offer and collect her second title as marathon champion of the world; no other woman in history has two golds, and silver; she also has a bronze from her four World Championship appearances.

Moreover, Catherine is one of those lovable athletes who walks with grace even beyond her amazing athletic achievements. Athletes, by the nature of the sport, tend to be selfish individuals. However, once in a while a world champion like Catherine comes along who transcends the standard. In 2003, she was the reigning world marathon champion, moments away from running her second New York City Marathon. The other elite women were a collective bag of nerves, sitting staring at the wall in the cafeteria that acts as a pre-race holding area, rubbing the last dab of liniment into their legs. Some chattered nervously. It was a chorus of "Me, me, me." At the far side of the room, smiling, cool as the proverbial cucumber, and with her unmitigated attention spent upon tending to the needs of her blind friend Helen Cherono, was "Catherine the Great." This had been Catherine's focus for the past three days, as Helen had turned up unexpectedly from South Carolina, sans accommodation, and asked to room with Catherine at the elite race headquarters hotel.

A little more than two and a half hours after this event, Ndereba was standing by the Tavern on the Green restaurant having run the second-fastest New York Marathon ever, 2:23:03. Her first words, after graciously praising the winner, Margaret Okayo and thanking her for honoring Kenya, were, "Has Helen been okay whilst I have been running?"

Whenever Catherine leaves for Kenya, she carries a large shipment of Shoe4Africa equipment for the athletes back home. She does not complain when the big sacks of shoes arrive. In fact, she smiles while deciding which worthy athlete will be getting what. These short stories speak volumes for why Catherine, for many of us, rises above the title of The Great.

Whilst working on the New York Road Runner's Audio Guide project in the fall of 2006, Catherine revealed her thoughts on racing:

You know me, I don't have a tactic, and I normally start the race and see how I feel. I do not run anybody else's race. When the gun goes I must evaluate with my own body and see. Then as the race develops, I run accordingly. So you can say that I do not have a set tactic for any race. Along the way, I am monitoring my form and running entirely to how I feel, not what the other runners are doing. If I feel good in the final miles then I will start to push from about three miles out.

When I am in the last few miles I am just concentrating on getting to the finish line and how nice it will be to be there. The legs feel tired for sure, but that is for everybody.

When Catherine is in Boston Marathon training, the specifics begin in December and January. Most of the runs are easy runs of 75-90 minutes, building a base. Wind-sprints, 8 x 150m at 80 percent effort are used to keep the speed intact, and hill intervals of 400m build strength. The long run is every ten days. After a month, speed work is introduced on the track, typically:

20 x 400 at 67-69 sec. with 1 min. rest.

Pyramid intervals: 800, 1200, 1600, 1200, 800

Fartlek: 1 min., 2 min., 3 min., 2 min., 1 min. hard with 1 min. rest.

The mileage will now peak at around 100 miles per week.

"I had bad experiences with very high mileage, so my general training plan is balanced more towards quality," indicates coach Nechchadi. There are two out-and-out speed sessions per week, and the rest of the runs are kept below the 85 percent effort level. The long run is goal-specific. For marathon training the run takes up to 2.5 hours and is run slowly (the longest is three hours), though when the training is for the 10K, it is reduced by an hour. The goal is only to spend the time on the feet. Fartlek sessions are a key ingredient. Apart from the above track sessions, Ndereba also runs a 1 minute fast, 1 minute slow run that totals 40 minutes.

When preparing for 10,000m, Ndereba lowers the mileage to 80-90 per week and runs the intervals faster, with a longer recovery. Thus 65-second 400m runs with 90 seconds rest instead of 67-69 seconds with 60 seconds rest.

Some 5K and 10K road races are run to sharpen racing tactics, and, as noted above, the bi-weekly long run peaks at 1:30:00.

Training Week (Boston 2000)

Monday	AM	75 min. easy
	PM	40 min. easy.
Tuesday	AM	40 min. easy
	PM	Track 800m, 1200m, 1600m, 1200m
Wednesday	PM	60 min. easy.
Thursday	AM	40 min. easy
	PM	7 x 2K
Friday	AM	40 min.
	PM	40 min.
Saturday	AM	40 min.
	PM	Fartlek.
Sunday	Rest day; no running for religious reasons	

Comments

I do races to just see where I am, not really to try and win the races. That is not important. But following the race I can look [at the result] and see what needs to be done. Well, if I run a half-marathon and go under 1:10, then I know all is great, but if it is a minute or two slower, then I add more speed work to the plan. Concentrate on your running; do not do other business in marathon training. I would fall apart thinking about both. Better to do running now and business later after the running career. In the last two weeks before a marathon taper with the mileage, but continue with speed work, doing some fast short intervals, but no long runs at all. I don't like to be rushed on the race morning as I get confused, so don't rush anything.

The day before a race, Catherine will go for an easy jog, and go home for lunch. She will eat a plate of pasta, go back to the hotel room, and drink water to hydrate. In the evening, she has a good pasta meal before going to bed at 8:00 p.m. The next morning, between 9:00 and 10:00 a.m. (for a noon start), she will have just bread and tea, [Kenyan Chai with large amounts of milk and sugar added]. She then stretches a bit before very lightly jogging for 15-20 minutes, nothing more.

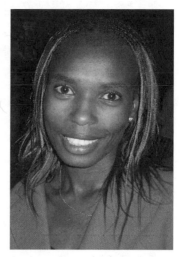

Rita Jeptoo Sitienei. (*Author*)

I don't want to disappoint myself by saying I am going to do this. It is just for me to see how it develops on the day. Like with training every day you go out and do your best, I like to see the race as just another of those days. The weather is for everybody, and as it is nothing we can control, then there is no use in worrying about it. I don't mind whatever it is.

Rita Jeptoo Sitienei

Date of birth:	February 15, 1981
Place of Birth:	Moiben district, Uasin Gishu district
Height/Weight:	5"7", 44 kg.
Coach:	Renato Canova
Personal Records:	5000m, 15:56.90
	5K, 15:58, 10K, 31:12
	15K, 47:31
	20K, 1:03:47
	Half -maraton, 67:05
	Maraton, 2:23:38
Honors Won:	2006 Boston Marathon Champion
	2004 Milan and Stockholm Marathon, Champion
	2006 World Road Running 20K championships, bronze
	Kenyan National Marathon, Cross Country
	and 20K team member

10K into the 2004 Stockholm Marathon, Rita Jeptoo pushed away from the field. "I remember there were lots of people cheering and I felt good." After two hours and thirty-five minutes, Rita had won her first marathon, and second place was more than a mile behind. "I was inspired by Tegla Loroupe to do distance. Nobody told me to go to the marathon; I decided just to try it. I was not pushing more than seeing what the event was about."

Life had been hard for Rita. She choose athletics after dropping out of school. "My family could not afford the school fees, so I had to decide what to do. I ran in Kapcheplangat primary; I had done well, so I knew I could run."

At first Jeptoo had ran cross country, the move to the marathon was a fortuitous one. After Stockholm, she won Milan in 2:28:11, and then in 2005 was selected to represent Kenya at the Helsinki World Championships after placing third in April's Turin marathon. The big breakthrough came in April the following year. On Saturday night, at 6:00 p.m., she was the very last elite athlete to arrive in Boston for the marathon. "My passport had been lost in Milan, and I thought I was not going to make it," she says. The organizers had put her down as a scratch. She ran in the lead pack, and between miles 23 and 24 she put in a devastating 5:06 mile to overwhelm her last opponent, Latvia's Jelena Prokopcuka. Following the race, Rita explained, "All things went well, I trained very well for here. It is my first big-city marathon. My coach told me, "Go run very well, because you can."

Training Schedule

Sunday: 1 hr. moderate (14K)

Monday: 45 min. easy + 5 circuits for strength endurance, type A, rec. 5:00 (15K)
               1 hr. moderate (14K)

Tuesday: 1 hr. moderate (14K)
               20 min. easy + 10k in 36:44 (14k)

Wednesday: 1 hr. 10 min. progressive run (17K)
               45:00 easy + 10 x 80m sprint uphill (12k)

Thursday: 1 hr. 8 min with short variations of speed (17K)
               53 min moderate (13K)

Friday: 1 hr. 14 min. moderate (18K)
               1 hr. easy (13K)

Saturday   45 min. moderate (11K)
               47 min. moderate (11K)

Week 1: 183K

Sunday: 1 hr. 39 min. moderate (av. 4:00 p/K) (25K)

Monday: 1 hr 8 min. with short variations of speed (17K)
               1 hr. moderate (14K)

Tuesday: 46 min. progressive run + 10 x 200m climbing, hard, recover 4:00 (13K)
               1 hr. 14 min. moderate (18K)

Wednesday: 52 min. easy run (11K)
               44 min. easy run (10K)

Thursday: 8K in 30 min. 36 sec. + 8 x 1000 (track) recover 200m in 1:15,
               in 3:20, 3:18, 3:19, 3:21, 3:17, 3:18, 3:19, 3:09 (17.5K)
               8K in 29:44 + 10K in 34:02 (18K)

Friday:	1 hr. moderate (13.5K)
	58 min. moderate (13K)
Saturday:	36 min. easy + 6 circuits for strength endurance,
	type A, recover 5:00 (14K)
	1 hr. moderate (14K)

Week 2: 198K

Sunday:	1 hr. 48min. moderate (av. 4:00 p/K) (27K)
Monday:	1 hr. moderate (14K)
	1 hr. 2 min. with short variations (15K)
Tuesday:	33 min. easy + 7 x 7 min. at marathon pace recover 4:00 moderate
	(totally 1 hr. 13 min.) + 8 min. easy (29K)
	42 min. easy run (9K)
Wednesday:	1 hr. moderate (14K)
	1 hr. easy (13K)
Thursday:	1 hr. 2 min. moderate (15K)
	42 min. easy + 15 x 80m sprint uphill (11K)
Friday:	24 min. easy + 20K at 3 hr. 40 min. pace in 73:36
	41 min. easy (9K)
Saturday:	1 hr. with short variations (14K)
	47 min. easy (10K)

Week 3: 205K

Sunday:	30K in 1 hr. 57 min. 44 sec. with last 5K climbing
	(21:12 + 19:48 + 19:22 + 18:56 + 18:42 + 19:44)
Monday:	1 hr. 8 min. easy (16K)
	1 hr. 2 min. with short variations (14K)
Tuesday:	44 min. moderate + 8K in 29:36 (av. 3:41)
	1 hr. easy run (13K)
Wednesday:	1 hr. 22 min. progressive run (21K)
	1 hr. 15 min. moderate (19K)
Thursday:	32 min. easy + 7 circuits for strength endurance,
	type A, recover 5:00 (14K)
	42 min. easy (9K)
Friday:	53 min. easy run (12K)
	53 min. with short variations (12K)
Saturday:	42 min. easy (10K)
	36 min. easy (8K)

Week 4: 196K

Sunday:	18 min. warm-up + 33K in 2 hr. 44 min. on hilly course
	(Eldoret, Iten, climbing for 250m of difference in altitude)
Monday:	40 min. easy (9K)
	40 min. easy (9K)

Tuesday: 1 hr. 14 min. with short variations (18K)

              1 hr. 3 min. progressive run (16K)

Analysis of January 2006:

Kilometer 870 (average: 28K per day)

Training Sessions: 57

Sessions for strength endurance: 3

Sessions with short/medium hills: 3

Sessions of long run: 4

Sessions of specific marathon endurance: 1

Special blocks: 1

Sessions for aerobic power: 3

Comments

Make the long longs progressive, speed up along the way. I always stretch, after every training run I do. Before Boston 2006, I trained in Iten where it is very hilly, so in Boston the hills did not feel like anything at all. I changed the location in 2007 and did not run so well, but it was also so cold I never started feeling good. I was also hitting my PR in the half one month before, so maybe I had worked too hard on the speed. (I note: due to a mix up, Rita was not following her usual program from February onward until the 2007 Boston).

Martin Kiptolo Lel

Date of birth: October 29, 1978

Place of birth: Kimgingich, Nandi

Height/Weight: 175 cm., 56 kg.

Coach: Claudio Berardelli

Personal bests: 10K road, 27:25

                      Half marathon, 59:42

                      Marathon, 2:05:15

Honors won: 2005, 2007, 2008 London Marathon

                      2003 and 2007 ING New York City Marathon Champion

                      2003 World Half-Marathon Champion

Martin Lel owns a nice, comfortable gray Toyota 4X4, but you will hardly ever find him driving the car; that pleasure is left to all his friends, who constantly need help and rides from here to there. As his car is perpetually being "borrowed" Martin crams himself inside the 30-cent communal Kenyan Peugeot taxis that squeeze twelve into a six-seater capacity when riding around town, or between Eldoret and the training camp in Kaptagat. He never complains, and adds with a smile, "If I need the car, I can always find it!"

As a young boy, Lel would follow his father from village to village, walking for up to five hours, as his father preached the bible, "He has preached since 1967 'til now. It is in my heart that I know the blessing came from him for my running success. God gave me the talent to assist him with my running," says Martin. Today the local church gives thanks for its refurbishments. The entire day of Christmas, Martin was either in church, at home feeding his many needy neighbors, or arranging for his car to go and pick up people, like the old lady who lives down the valley who needed to be taken to the clinic for an injection that afternoon. Like a friend notes of Martin, "Often he does not go home, instead he stays at the running camp, because at his house there is also a line of people needing assistance and money, and Martin has a reputation never to say no."

Years ago, at the Kimngeru primary school, Lel was encouraged by his teachers to run. "I was running and enjoying, not yet exploiting my talents," he recalls. At second-

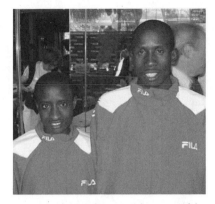

Margaret Okayo and Martin Lel, winners of the 2003 ING New York City Marathon. (*Author*)

ary school at the Chemuswa Nandi School, his athletic talent started to shine—luckily, because the family was very, very poor, and it took a sports-sympathetic teacher to keep Lel, who could not afford the school fees, at the school. "I was beating everyone, my games teacher was confused about what I should run, because whatever distance I ran I won at."

In 1998, Lel left the school and went to work at the family grocery store to earn funds for the family's needs. The word "store" does not properly convey the business; it was more of a hut selling necessities. "I started very early because at 8:00 a.m. I had to be selling goods. I had to cycle 8K to look for goods to sell. Even lunchtime was difficult; there was no time in the day for me to train. I would finish and be back at home at 9:00 p.m." The world nearly lost one of its greatest marathon talents to a small family shop. His brothers knew his potential and encouraged Lel to keep on training whenever he could make the time.

There was a half marathon race in nearby Eldoret in January of 2001 on a hot Saturday morning—the Discovery Race, a concept Moses Tanui had begun a decade ago to unearth new talent. Lel traveled on a communal taxi bus to the start, and he finished a credible fifteenth. "My neighbor Noah Bor tried to convince Dr. Rosa, who was in charge of selecting the Fila team then, to take me as an athlete. Rosa agreed." Unfortunately, the family did not; they wanted Lel as a valuable work hand. Noah's brother, Simon, a 2:08 marathon runner, brought the family five sacks of maize to try to persuade the Lels to let Martin go to the training camp. After some further deals involving livestock and Martin agreeing to weed maize on the weekends to earn money to buy his younger sister school books, he was released by his parents to begin arduous training.

In January of 2002, the hard work began, and in March, with an injury, Lel went to Italy to compete; "I ran 15 races and 12 times I was on the podium. I returned home to Kenya, and my family did not first believe, they were very pleased to see me and hear of the successes."

All the races had been between 10K and 21.1K but Dr. Rosa told the Nandi, "You are fit to run a marathon." However, Martin was not convinced, thinking it was too hard. Again, Simon came to the rescue and told Martin, "You can survive, it is not that bad." Lel tried Prague but did not finish due to the injury. He had been concerned, due to the shoe problem that had bothered him earlier in the year, that the marathon event was not for him. However, as the injury cleared up he was able to train with full force for the long event, and in the fall of 2002, he placed second at the Venice Marathon, running 2:10:02, coming in behind fellow Kenyan David Makori who ran, 2:08:49.

Things only got better for Lel. In the following year he was selected to run for his country for the first time, and he repaid the selectors with a world title at the IAAF World Half-Marathon Championships. A month later, he took a win at New York. "I was afraid at New York, I was running easy but thinking I should have respect for the other runners, that something might happen, but with 800 meter to go I knew I was going to win, so I pushed off. That race made me a top marathon runner. You know, runners like Ezekiel Bitok, and Paul Tergat give me courage. What am I lacking if these guys are 35 and 40 years old and still running good and I am only 27? I can achieve many things."

In 2005, Lel won the London Marathon with a devastating kick late in the race, (using 4:38 24th mile) to distance himself from a star-studded field. The following year, he was edged out by two seconds by compatriot Felix Limo. "I was confident of my finish, I really do not know what happened," explained Martin after the race. In 2007, Martin had one promise, "I will be alert this time, and I will be ready for Felix!" True to his word, Martin won the event in 2:07:41, running incredibly even 10K splits of 30:12, 30:10, 30:19, and 30:32.

Training

Monday	AM	70 –min. progressive run
	PM	70 min. and 15 x 20-second diagonal sprints
Tuesday	AM	13 x 2-min. fast, 1 min. slow
	PM	50 min. moderate pace
Wednesday	AM	70 min. medium
	PM	1 hr. medium speed
Thursday	AM	16K up hill steady run
	PM	Easy 40 min.
Friday	AM	70 min. easy to steady
	PM	55 min. easy
Saturday	AM	10 x 1k in 2 hr. 50 min. with 90 sec. recovery jog
	PM	50 min. easy
Sunday	AM	1 hr. 30 min. recovery run
Monday	AM	Xmas day, no running
Tuesday	AM	60 min. steady
	PM	50 min. moderate pace
Wednesday	AM	60 min. medium
	PM	1 hr. medium speed with some fast bursts

Thursday	AM	70 min. with 20 x 1 min. fast, 1 min. slow
	PM	Rest
Friday	AM	70 min. easy to steady
	PM	5 min. easy
Saturday	AM	50 min. tempo
	PM	50 min. easy
Sunday	AM	2 hr. easy

Comment

In my mind, to sprint at the end of a marathon because that is what I practice for in training runs, so it becomes automatic. You need to be disciplined and listen to the coach.

Work toward excellence and the maximum. We have a good morale in the training
group, and what can we not do if the team all works together?

The Week Before Running a 2:06 Marathon

Monday:	AM	1 hr
	PM	30 min. in the afternoon
Tuesday:	Same as Monday	
Wednesday:	AM	10 x 1 min. fast, 1 min. slow
	PM	30 min. jog
Thursday:	Travel day.	
Friday:	AM	Easy 40 min.
Saturday:	AM	30 min. jog.
Sunday:	6 AM	Breakfast. Tea with lots of sugar and milk. Bread, jam, and a sports drink with maltodextrin. (Martin never seems to be able to get his bottles in a race so ends up drinking water, though his bottle are prepared with minerals and maltodextrin should he ever catch one.)

Coach Claudio Berardelli on Lel Winning the London Marathon, April 2007

The training began in December following the recovery from an injury. At the end of
January, he ran a 38K very hilly course in the Nandi Hills in 2:08. However, just before
going to Puerto Rico for the World's Best 10K he discovered a stomach problem that gave
him a couple of week's problems. Although he did not stop training, we did have to cancel Lisbon. Three weeks to go and his form was remarkable; he ran the 38K loop in 2:10,
but the last 5K was run in 14:18 with a slightly uphill last kilometer covered in 2: 40.
Nobody at the Kapsabet Camp was able to keep Martin within their sights.

After the runner-up spot in 2006, there was a change in the training. "We introduced
more training runs at a steady-state speed close to Martin's marathon speed." The incre-
ments begun at 16K, then to 18K, and up to the half-marathon distance. "On the day of
the half–marathon, Martin was still so-so with his stomach problems," recalls the coach.
Nevertheless, he ran 65:10. James Kwambai [who would be the runner-up at Boston] finished in 64:16. On Sunday, a week before London, Martin ran 2 x 5000m on a road with
a few undulations, 14:16 and 14:07 with a 3:00 rest.

Although Lel lost by a couple of seconds to Felix Limo in London in 2006, he did not think it necessary to work on his finishing speed for the 2007 event. Claudio explains. "It was not the problem of a kick [why he lost], it was more that we had to set his mind to be very focused in every single situation, from the start to the finishing line." He continues, "Martin is psychologically very strong. One of the most professional runners I have ever worked with. He never refused any advice from me and he was really taking care of his lifestyle. The days before the race I could see he was feeling the effects of the race but he was not at all nervous, just confident."

Richard Kobe Yatich (Mubarak Hassan Shami)

Date of birth:	December 1, 1980
Place of birth:	Kaboskie, Kerio Valley, Tugen
Height/Weight:	5'8", 50-51 kg.
Coach:	Renato Canova
Miles per week:	130
Personal best:	10K road, 27:59
	15K, 42:43
	Half-marathon, 61:09
	Marathon, 2:07:19
Honors won:	2006 World Half Marathon Championships, silver
	2006 Asian Games, silver
	Marathon Champion: 2005 Vienna, 2005 Venice,
	2006 Prague, 2007 Paris
	2007 World Championships Marathon, silver

In hot and humid weather conditions of 23 Celsius, Richard ran with a pack of runners at the front of the Asian Games Championships in Doha. He glanced at his watch. "I saw we passed halfway in 69 minutes. I thought, 'That's a woman's time, too slow, let me go,' and I kicked away from the group." Yatich ran a negative split—62:52 for the second half-beating the runner-up, Bahrain's Khalid Kamal Taseen, by nearly three minutes. In 2 hours 12 minutes 44 seconds, Qatar won its first marathon gold medal. In Qatar Yatich was heralded as a national hero. The man had come a long way since his early days as a youthful cattle herder in the highlands of Kenya.

"I believe I was born to run, I was very fast. I grew up chasing animals." The first problem for Yatich was that he was extremely poor and could not afford to attend school. Every day life was a constant struggle, as his very existence was perched on the poverty line. Certainly he did not have money to enter any races; thus being recognized was a problem, as he never appeared in any race result. "In the year 2000, I jumped in a race and I was unofficially number six. I knew I was good because I was beating a lot of experienced people."

Richard's brother, who he had earlier supported, now started selling bread to support Richard and bought his brother a pair of precious training shoes and a tracksuit. Yatich tried out for the army but was not employed, despite being promised a commission. Then

in 2002, help came from 1992 Olympic
Champion Matthew Birir, who had been assisting Yatich,.."[One time] he gave me a pair of shoes
and said, 'This is the last pair I will give you until
you make it, and go abroad!'"

Matthew Birir recalls, "When I met Richard
and he asked me for assistance I was not interested to know his running results, I wanted to see
what kind of person he was." In Yatich, Birir discovered a driven soul. Richard wanted badly to
succeed through running, and Birir saw that he
was over-training, giving himself no recovery.
"Peace of mind, rest and proper diet was
required." He came and stayed at my parents
home, sleeping, eating, and training under my
direction for a few [three] years."

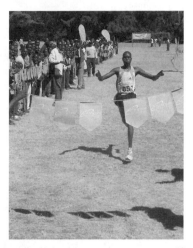

Richard Yatich wins the Baringo Half
Marathon. (*Author*)

Yatich entered a race where he knew a prominent manager was attending. "I was asked by this
manager, 'What do you run?' and I told him I could run anything, any distance. He
laughed at me and said that he would return in three months and that I should concentrate on one distance. He told me, 'You can't call yourself an 'everything runner, that is
ridiculous!'"

The manager never came back for Yatich. In 2003, another manager told him if he
placed in the top 25 of a certain race, he would get help. Richard did and that manager
disappeared. Yatich did not give up.

The big break came at Paul Tergat's half-marathon in Baringo. Yatich ran a course
record of 61 minutes. "I was introduced to another manager, called Gianni Demadonna.
He told me it is impossible to run 61-minutes in Kenya. So I continued training, just
believing in myself." Finally, a minor manager took Yatich to Belgium, where he ran low-
key races. "I told the manager, 'Get me big races and I can do well.'" Yatich was then
entered in the high profile Seven Hills Road Race in Holland. True to his word, he bolted from the gun and immediately opened a gap that was never closed. In winning the race,
he beat high-profile names like Fabiano Joseph and Paul Tergat (albeit Tergat was running on tired legs six weeks after his marathon world record, fulfilling a commitment).
Yatich was no longer worrying about collecting shillings as a cattle herder. He was recruited by the country of Qatar, something he talks about in a veiled manner. "They have paid
me the bonuses for my medal, but I am yet to get the promised salary." For a man who
lived his childhood on the edge of penury, the promise of a lifelong salary far outweighed
the colors of the Kenyan flag. "Of course, for the money, I went. In Kenya, if you have
problems they simply replace you with another runner. I have lived in poverty and nobody
helped me then; I know I have to help myself. That is why I run, and because I was born
to run." Few would disagree.

Plan for the Paris Marathon

Sunday	44 min. moderate + 12k in 37:09
Monday	1 hr. 6 min. moderate
	52 min. easy
Tuesday	38K in 2:09:10 (hilly course)
Wednesday	1 hr. 3 min. moderate
	56 min. with short variations of speed
Thursday	Travel Eldama Ravine - Nairobi - Mombasa
	47 min. easy
Friday	52 min. easy
	44 min. easy
Saturday	Mombasa: World Cross Country Championship, 7th place
Sunday	Travel Mombasa - Nairobi (Rest)
	Monday Travel Nairobi - Eldama Ravine
	1 hr. moderate
Tuesday	1 hr. 12 min. moderate
	1 hr. with short variations of speed
Wednesday	1 hr. 8 min. progressive run
	54 min. easy regeneration
Thursday	28 min. easy + 4 x 5K recovery
	1K in 14:53 / 3:33 - 15:03 / 3:44 - 15:15 / 4:02 - 15:44
	(tired after Mombasa)
	36 min. easy regeneration
Friday	1 hr. 8 min. moderate
	1 hr. 2 min. with short variations of speed
Saturday	1 hr. 18 min. progressive run
	47 min. easy + 13 x 100m sprint climbing
Sun	44 min. easy + 6k at 3:08
	1 hr. moderate
Monday	18 min. warm-up + 35K
	(Ziwa, going up with 300m of difference in altitude, from 2,000 to 2,300m in 1:58:24, last 5K in 18:44, still tired in his legs)
	Note: "Going back home he had a car accident, with a strong impact between his chest and the steering wheel. Strong pains when breathing. I feared a rib infraction; fortunately it wasn't and the pain was due to the impact only."—Renato
Tuesday	Rest
Wednesday	43 min. easy
Thursday	48 min. easy
Friday	1 hr. 2 min. easy
Saturday	1 hr. 8 min. progressive run
	48 min. easy + 6K in 18:41

Sunday	1 hr. 41 min. moderate (28K)
	Monday 1 hr. 3 min. moderate
	1 hr. 6 min. with short variations of speed
Tuesday	42 min. easy + 5K in 15:08
	48 min. easy + 5K in 14:46
Wednesday	1 hr. 16 min. moderate
	Travel Eldama Ravine - Nairobi
Thursday	Travel Nairobi - Paris
	40 min. easy
Friday	37 min. easy
	36 min. easy
Saturday	44 min. easy
Sunday	Paris Marathon, 2:07:19 (NR) winner

Circuits

> 120m bounding (flat)
> 300m running fast (flat)
> 20 sagittal splits on the place
> 60m sprint climbing
> 40m skipping climbing
> 60m sprint climbing
> 40m heels-to-buttocks climbing
> 60m sprint uphill
> 40m bounding climbing
> 100m sprint climbing
> 10 squat-jumps on the place

Comments

"I don't like to run less than 32-35 kilometers per day." Yatich does not like too much speed work. "It is the quick way for me to get hurt, and I don't need it. That is why my running program is mainly just runs for endurance." When off-plan (before the Baringo victory), the morning is typically a 25-kilometer run and the evening a 10-kilometer run. Hill work, 15 x 80m fast sprints, is done once a week. "I have never gone beyond 15 x 110 meters in hill work," he says. A track session was 4 x 5000m with 2-1/2-minutes jog recovery runs in 15:52, 15:48, 15:38, and 14:52. "On this session I can go crazy and run the last one as fast as 14:18." Another session is 25 x 400 in 68 seconds with 30 seconds rest. Or 10 x 1000m in 3:02 to 2:50 with a one-minute rest, then 5 x 400 in 65 seconds, still using the minute's rest, and to finish, a fast 1500m. There are no rest days, but on Sunday Yatich trains only once. When he runs long, it is typically 35 kilometers and run at a fair clip. He is very careful not to dip below 49.5 kg. or he knows he will perform badly, feeling weak. "I can get *too* thin!"

Felix Kipchoge Limo

Date of birth:	August 22, 1980
Place of birth:	Chepketemon, Nandi
Height/Weight:	5'6", 58 kg. (60 kg. in the off-season).
Mileage:	High 220K per week; low 150K per week
Sessions per day:	"This depends on the program, if it calls for over two hours of running, 140 minutes, I will run only once, but 120 minutes or under, then it will be two sessions.
Toughest session:	2000m on the track "tough to run even pace for five loops."
Longest Run:	40K, only once, usually 38K
	"Often I start the program with a long run to tell the body 'something' is coming up."
Personal best:	3000m, 7:40
	10,000m, 27:04:52
	10K, 27:39
	20K, 58:34
	Half-marathon, 61:15
	Marathon, 2:06:14
Honors won:	2001 World Best 15K
	2004 Berlin Marathon, winner of 2004 Rotterdam, 2005 Chicago, 2006 London Marathons

"Running 2:06 has a lot to do with running fast also in training." When Felix went to school, he walked 2K to primary and 7K to secondary school. "Only if I was late did I run." Felix was more interested in schooling. He ran in physical education class knowing that he had a talent, and wished that he could use it for a scholarship to study in the United States. He wrote to a number of universities, but none responded, thus his learning was put on "suspend" mode.

In 1997, he joined a group of athletes in the Nandi Hills to train for cross. In November of 1998, Global Sports Management spotted Felix and brought him to Europe. "I tried hard, and I ran 42:38 for the 15K, it was my big introduction," recalls Limo. Next up, in August 2000, was a 10,000m on the track in Brussels; he ran a stunning 27:04:52. However, Felix decided not to concentrate on the track. "I was slow in the 3K and 5K, and as there are only two or three 10,000s in a year, I decided [financially] to look to the roads." In addition, Felix already had plans for the longer distances and noted, "I did not feel that I could exploit my talent the best on the track surface." The following year, at the Seven Hills 15K in Holland, Felix set a world's best of 41:29 defeating the legendary Haile Gebrselassie.

In 2003, he attempted the marathon in Amsterdam. "I was fearing, losing power at 38 to 40K. I was running listening to myself, 'when will the power lose.' Near 40K the manager Jos Hermens told me 'You can win it.' I got inspired, but then he went to William [Kipsang who would win the race, and who was also managed by Jos] and told him too,

'You can win it.' And he did [laughing], but all in all it was a good start."

Felix recorded a sublime 2:06:42 debut. "The time I was thinking was 2:07-08. It seems, though, the training that I was doing was for 2:06." The marathon world had a new star.

Felix does not like to predict his future, or what he will achieve in athletics. "It leads to disappointment, like in 2006 when I was preparing to defend in Chicago." A spinal injury forced him to withdraw from the competition. Then there was the issue of the Olympics in 2004. "I was told the fastest spring marathon of 2004 would get a place on the team. Felix duly ran that time, 2:06:14, and then lost the spot to a man who ran about five minutes slower."

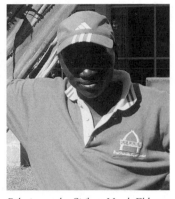

Relaxing at the Sirikwa Hotel, Eldoret, Felix is one of the most admired marathon runners on the circuit today, both as a competitor and as a gentleman. (*Author*)

Training for a 2:06 Marathon

Monday	AM	60 min. minimum easy running
	PM	As above
Tuesday*	AM	Fartlek, not less than 15K of 3 -min. hard, 1 min. easy
	PM	Easy running; distance does not matter
Wednesday	Same as Monday	
Thursday	AM	Longest run, 38K,
		starting the program at 30K and working up.
	PM	Rest
Friday	Same as Monday	
Saturday	AM	Speed; if ran 38K on Thursday,
		then 1 min. hard, 1 min. easy, if 30K then 2 min. hard,
		1 min. easy, for at least 15K.
Sunday	"Sleeping! I am a Christian so I must go to church on that day."	

*Can also be hill work. Felix runs a warm-up for 30 minutes, then goes up a 200m hill and down the other, before turning and running back continuously for a total run of two hours. Another speed session four weeks before a 2:06 marathon: 15 x 1000m "We ran the intervals in 2:50 except for the last five, which I did in 2:45." (2800m altitude, dirt running track!)

The effort levels: Long runs are done at 60-70 percent effort, the same effort as easy runs. Intervals are run at 80 percent intensity. "If you run at 100 percent you will pay during the race."

Before London 2006

Monday	37 min. easy
Tuesday	Very light speed work of 12 x 400 "just to keep the body moving."
Wednesday	One hour easy and traveled to London

Thursday	40 min. easy
Friday	Same as Thursday
Saturday	40 min. "with some strides to see how I felt"
Sunday	Breakfast of spaghetti with a white sauce, and tea.

In the race, water every 5K (Felix estimated he drank a total of 2-3 liters, something he practices on his long runs). First place 2:06:39. "I was happy all the big guys were there. Even happier when the press ignored me before the race and I could sit in my hotel room conserving energy."

Racing Tactics

I have to monitor my opponents. If you think of other things, you lose the grip on the race. You count the number of people, you calculate who normally dies, who is weak. I know most of my competitors. For instance, Gebrselassie has shown he is often weak in the last three kilometers, unless it is a time trial, he is good when he controls the field knowing the race is set up for him, but in a field like London where he has to race other runners he is yet to win in the marathon. Martin Lel is fast in the finish and a very hard competitor to beat.

Comments

"Those people who run for money will never achieve. Run to be your best at running, and then the money will come. Do at least four long runs over 34K." Felix also does several 30K runs in the 12-week marathon program. On the track, he rarely runs short intervals, 400m is the shortest he will do, and then he does a mega-dose of 25-repeats with a scant 200m recovery jog. Following a marathon, he rests for one month; total rest. Then he begins running using the gym, "For one month I strengthen all parts of the body, all over to make the body strong. Using only light weights." On stretching: "I am stretching; it is part of the treatment to reduce the risk of injury. I stretch after the morning run. Sometimes after the evening run too, in a non-specific way." Limo sleeps according to what is on the television, he also likes to read to relax in the evenings. On diet: "Just typical Kenyan foods. I eat nothing special." And on Patrick Sang: "Sang was a consistent man [in competition], that I admire and wish to emulate. He told me to listen to my body. Concentrate on quality, not quantity, and plan to maintain, not always to try and increase your training."

"The goodness with marathons is you focus on one race; it is easy to plan and organize as you know the exact date. I run just four races per year, two important marathons, then two test races in full training of between 10 miles and a half-marathon, three to four weeks before the marathon. I am even happy if these test races go poorly as it usually means I am training well. They are never done at maximum effort, just to tell me where my body is in regards to training."

Felix is stoically against drugs in the sport. "Aiy, it is better to have two shillings and your good health than to take drugs and be sick tomorrow. I am not interested; better to have a little clean money than cheat. You will not have a good career with cheating. Cheaters are never good people."

Moses Tanui

Date of birth	August 20, 1965
Birthplace:	Sugoi, 20km from Eldoret. Nandi tribesman.
Height/weight:	5'7" (171 cm.), 123 lbs (56 kg.)
Training sessions:	Usually two per day.
Hard session:	Hill run, dirt road 22K, starting at 1300m altitude, finishing at 2700m. 1 hr. 30 min.
Km per week:	200-240 in half-marathon training
	210-250 in marathon training
Personal bests:	1500m, 3:41.8; 2000m, 5:03.7; 3000m, 7:39.63; 5000m, 13:17.80; 10,000m, 27:18.32; half-marathon, 59:47, marathon, 2:06:16
Honors won:	1989 African Championships 5000m, third; 10,000m, second
	1990 Commonwealth Games 10,000m, second
	World Championships, 10,000m, 1991, first; 1993, second
	1995 World Half-Marathon Champion
	1990 World Cross Country Championships;
	1991, second; 1993, fourth
	1999 Kenyan marathon record, 2:06:16
	Boston Marathon, 1995, second; 1996, first; 1997, fifth;
	1998, first; 2000, third
	2000 Chicago Marathon, third

In a world of convenience and support, we often forget the simplicities like an actual ride to the competition, or a pair of running shoes, or even a pair of anything to put on your feet. A young Moses Tanui had very little of anything growing up in the way of material possessions. When he first began competing, barefoot of course, in the mid-1980s, it was not uncommon for the boy to walk half a day to get to a race. "I had no money to take a ride, what option did I have?" he asks with a wry smile.

The first time Moses appeared in black-and-white print, it was in 1986, for a 14:45.0 5000m Military Championship race in Nairobi; he placed fourth in his heat. Not a precursor that he would finish 18th in the World Cross Country Championships ten months later.

There were more improvements in 1988, when Tanui placed sixth at the World Cross, won the national 10,000m championships, and showed amazing versatility by winning a 1500m silver medal at the East African Championships. Tanui takes up the story.

I was at Kasarani doing a track work-out early in the morning, 25 x 400m. The finals were being held later that morning. The Kenyan officials were complaining they had no one to run with Kip Cheruiyot [1500m Olympian] in the championships for Kenya, and I said, "I am here!" Moses mimes with arms flapping. They let Tanui run, and Kip barely held him off for the gold, winning by just a tenth of a second in, 3:41.7. Moses also ran in the 1988 Olympics for the team, placing eighth in the 10,000m with a 27:13.23.

Tanui would win world titles on the track and the road, and he twice placed second in the World Cross Country Championships, making him the closest male ever to that elusive trifecta of championships on all surfaces, which was one of his many goals. Only the marathon distance remained to be conquered.

He left the track for the roads in 1993 after losing his 10,000m world title to a young Haile Gebrselassie. Lap after lap the Ethiopian runner dogged Moses and trod on his heels. Lap after lap Tanui turned shook his arm at the Ethiopian, asking him to please keep his distance. Tanui waved to the officials, but nobody took action. Then the inevitable happened. With more than a lap remaining, Gebrselassie pulled the entire shoe from Tanui's foot with his spiked shoe. Immediately Gebrselassie sprinted by, and although Moses closed with a bare left foot and a 56.1-second last lap, it was only enough for silver, 27:46.02 to 27:46.54. Speculating, one could easily say the encumbrance of one missing shoe cost Tanui the gold. "That was enough to take me to the roads," Moses sighs. Still to this day, no Kenyan has ever won more national 10,000m titles than the four Tanui took home.

Moses was more than just a great runner, he was forever helping the local community of runners. His kitchen was abuzz, feeding twenty or thirty runners with fried eggs and other food as they came by each day. His vehicles were always ferrying runners to races or training site. "When you are brought up in an extended family, you think wider, and helping others is part of the process. They are like your sisters and brothers," he says.

Turning to the Marathon

What would drive this man to push his body to the extremes of pain over twenty-six miles? After all, his financial future was assured, he had been winning signature races for nearly a decade. His name was known and was secure in history as the first man to run a half-marathon under the hour, and he was feared, as a competitor, on the starting line of any race he entered, with a staggering array of world-class times ranging from the 1500m (3:41 at altitude, see above) to 13.1 miles (59:47).

Tanui had had a couple of cracks at the marathon, and had finished a creditable third at Boston in 1995 behind the flamboyant Cosmas Ndeti, yet he had not displayed the talent many knew he was capable of showing at the classic distance. In his first marathon, in New York 1993, Moses was in third place up until the 39th kilometer before fading to tenth and a 2:15:36 time. His race at Boston 1995 was the first marathon he was happy with, but perchance a fellow Kenyan's remarks about a slow winning time in 1995 being the result of a "weak" field in the post-race press conference fueled Moses' desire to win the Centennial Boston.

Tanui, despite living thousands of miles away and submerged in a radically different foreign culture, knew the relevance of winning this Boston. "This is the marathon to win, the hundredth," he would say in the winter of 1995/1996 when solidifying his torturous training regimen with extra runs, extra speed workouts, less rest, and more effort.

The Start of the Flood

Tanui trained with the Fila team for the centennial Boston. The team was his initiative and inspiration; the Nandi tribesman created and built the team from the ground up. In 1991, under the brand name of K-Way, the team, using standard supermarket Superga shoes, started out as team-Tanui, a solo act. About a year, later Fila took over the reins. Tanui remembers, "Fila were not a running manufacturer in those days, but they saw the results, like my wins in Milano, and realized the opportunities. I was running a lot in Italy; I was winning a lot, too."

After his world championships win on the track in Japan in 1991, Tanui became a sought-after athlete. An Asics representative approached the Kenyan in his Tokyo hotel room offering a sponsorship. Tanui, however, recalled when he had approached Asics in 1987. "They told me, 'you are a national athlete, but not an international athlete!' [despite being at the Olympic Kenyan national team standard]. So when they returned in 1991 I said, 'Don't you recognize me? I am still the same person! Goodbye!'" Tanui felt a certain loyalty to the Italian connection, and his ambition was to build his own successful squad, albeit with shoddy shoes. "The shoes were [laughing] a little bit. . . basic. Then, luckily, Fila started developing and listening to our ideas."

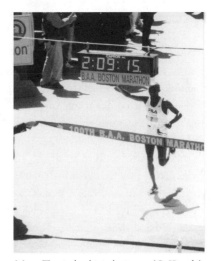

Moses Tanui takes his jackpot race. (C. *Kinuthi*)

With Kenyans today on the podium of virtually every major marathon in the world, it is easy to forget that pre-1995 these East Africans were not the marathon marvels they are nowadays. American stats guru Ken Young notes, "In 1995, there were just 81 sub-2:20 marathoners, and a decade later a staggering 478." Incredible growth that obviously can not *all* be attributed to just one man, but to underestimate Tanui's immense influence would be wrong and dismissive of the truth. The man was a born leader, even when in the midst of his severest training program he would be coach, mentor, and advisor to a troop of three dozen athletes that followed his footsteps each training day, like disciples after their professor.

It was a link effect; the plan that Tanui passed on to Joshua Chebet was given to ten of Chebet's friends, and soon most of Kenya was on the Tanui diet of marathon training. "I developed a training plan, and stopped the runners from doing crazy things like going for five-hour training runs. You should have seen what Eric Kimaiyo was doing when I found him and Chelang'a...ooh!" Moses drifts off into tales of over-training and under-eating.

The Jackpot Race

The 1996 Boston Marathon had 38,708 starters, a record to this day, and an exceptional elite field; it was a win that every elite athlete wanted on his or her resumé. Moses, who won in 2:09:15, employed a policy of patience before pushing strongly in the final stages to distance himself from his competitors and take the then-richest ever marathon purse of $100,000. At the halfway point, a deluge of African legs raced along at world-record pace, led by Ndeti, who was hoping to capture his fourth successive title. A Kamba tribesman, Ndeti had proclaimed that God was going to assist him to not only a win, but also to set a world record. Once past the Newton Hills, however, Cosmas' star faded as Lameck Aguta (eventually fourth in 2:10:03, he would win the following year's Boston) accelerated. "That day I was ready, but I did not count on the others being even more ready. Moses was unstoppable." remembers Lameck. At mile 23, Moses injected a 4:49 mile, and that sealed the race. A protégé of Moses', Ezekiel Bitok, placed second in 2:09:26, with Ndeti third in 2:09:51. The Kenyans swept the top five places with Sammy Lelei taking that fifth spot in 2:10:09. Incredibly, three of the top eight (Yego, eighth, Tangus, seventh, and Bitok, second) were Tanui-trained and schooled. "Bitok had been dropped by Kim McDonald's group for not being fast enough, so I took him to my program to see what he could do. He came second." Tanui said with a grin.

Arriving back in Eldoret, Moses opened his suitcase of worn running clothes, and a winner's medal—a unicorn with a diamond stuck in the mythical horse's eye—fell out of his suitcase on the living room floor. Picking the medal up and holding it in his hands, Tanui exclaimed, "This race was my jackpot."

Three years later, after more success and another Boston win, Tanui set the Kenyan record at the marathon, running 2:06:16 at Chicago. A mistake in seeing the course markers caused Tanui to surge at 30K thinking it was 35K. Many reporters on the day believed that with a more conservative pace, Tanui would have held on to the world record pace that Khalid Khannounchi, who had hung back on the surge, maintained. In the following Olympic year, Tanui ran the trials for the Kenyan marathon squad at Boston. The top three were to be selected. Moses placed third, second Kenyan after Elijah Lagat. A month after his selection he somehow was removed from the team, a move that broke his spirit. He continued to run for another four years, running a 2:10 marathon in 2004, though never got back the fighting heart his fellow Kenyans feared when he stepped to the starting line of any distance race.

Moses Tanui Today

A large silver luxury Mercedes pulls into the driveway of the Great Rift Valley Gymnasium and "Grand Prix" Restaurant building, having been driven a short distance down the road from a huge mansion in the fashionable Kapsoya area of Eldoret. Moses climbs out smiling, one hand holding his cell phone. "It's Lagat, he's coming into town," he says of Elijah, a man who beat Moses to the finish tape on Boylston Street in 2000 by a mere three seconds. He strides across the tiled floor of his pseudo–Indian-palace office building, built in the colonial style of the Imperialists of 1952, and orders food from the restaurant that he has installed on the ground floor. There is also a bar on the building's first floor, and Tanui has been tending it of late. "Looking for good staff is tough," he mutters, after explaining that he was tending the bar until 3:00 a.m. last night, and before mentioning that his gym instructor just ran off with over $300 of his money.

Upstairs in his airy office, with pictures of him setting world records on the walls and meeting world dignitaries such as American presidents, he explains his future. "Next door

I have all the gym rooms. Downstairs I want to make an internet café next to the restaurant, and in the compound build some lodgings for athletes to come and board when training in Eldoret." The complex will become an athlete's compound, and with the boss being a wealth of knowledge, its lodgers will be spoilt for advice, and training routes and partners. "Eldoret really is the perfect place for training, and I have so many connections here. . ." he adds with modesty, as in the running world Moses is the mayor of Eldoret.

Moses is also the ambassador for the Shoe4Africa program, a mentor to half the up-and-coming athletes in the town, and constantly called upon as a VIP for special occasions. His position as liaison to the legends is witnessed by the constant stream of athletes who keep stopping by his building. The only non-runners are his family members. "I can't get my children interested in running!" he exclaims as two kids, Kiprotich and Kiptoo, looking somewhat Western with slight paunches, enter the café and head for the sodas. "They are not as hungry as I was when I was a boy."

As Elijah Lagat arrives, so do the plates of food; it appears that his restaurant day staff also need to be re-organized as the food is not what was actually ordered. "This is Africa!" is Moses' retort as he waves a chicken wing in the air. Then he launches into his thoughts on an article in the day's press attacking the results of Kenyan Athletics. "We need to have the athletes in one camp and to have the coaches working together. We need discipline and why not find that here? If the federation has sense, they will see that Eldoret is the place to base a team, and then we can have togetherness and beat the Ethiopians. That is the only thing they have over us."

There are many prominent Kenyan athletes who would like to see Tanui heading the training of the national team, and if he could do what he already has done, it would be a winning formula, Italian style.

Comments

"Know your own weaknesses." By trying the marathon distance, Moses knew that he had to work on his strength in the final 5K. Anyone who witnessed the final 5K at Boston in 1996 could see he had done his homework! "Run races at your own pace. . . when training for a big race, don't disrupt the training with other races." Moses's philosophy on the marathon buildup is somewhat unusual. He believes in just a month buildup. Of course, the runner will have trained normally prior to this month, but not at marathon intensity and volume.

During cross country season, Tanui always raced and trained for that surface, believing that the strength gained there will hold him in good stead for the roads. "Good tactics in the marathon are to hang to the back of the lead pack for the first 20K so you keep out of trouble and have no problems at the water stations. In the second half you must be in touch because somebody can make a break to the finish."

In April of 1996, the Kenyan Amateur Athletic Association held a track meet at Eldoret's Kipchoge Keino Stadium. Deplorably, the organizers forgot, or had not intended, to purchase prizes for the many participating athletes. Tanui, who was present as a spectator, immediately drove into town and purchased prizes for the athletes—just one example of his generosity and assistance to the young athletes of his nation.

Training: February/March 1996, a month before the Boston Marathon

February 21	AM	70 min.
	PM	60 min.
February 22	AM	110 min.
February 23	AM	70 min.
	PM	60 min.
February 24	AM	25 min. warm-up, 10 x 1K
	PM	60 min. 2 min recovery.
February 25	AM	Hill session, 22K uphill.
February 26	AM	70 min.
	PM	60 min.
February 27	AM	120 min.
February 28	AM	30 min. warm-up, 20 x
	PM	60 min. 60 min. fast, 60 min. slow
February 29	AM	60 min.
	PM	60 min.
March 1	AM	30 min. warm-up, 4 x 3K
	PM	60 min. 3 min. recovery.
March 2	AM	60 min.
	PM	60 min.
March 3	AM	38K run in 2:15.
March 4	AM	70 min.
	PM	50 min.
March 5	AM	25 min. warm-up, 25 x 1 min fast, 1 min slow.
March 6	AM	Hill work, 22K in 1:28.
March 7	AM	70 min.
	PM	70 min.
March 8	AM	25 min warm-up, 4 x 3K
	PM	60 min. 3 min. recovery.
March 9	AM	70 min.
	PM	60 min.
March 10	AM	38km run in 2:15.
March 11	AM	60 min
	PM	50 min.
March 12	AM	25 min. warm-up, 12 x 1K
	PM	50 min. 2 min. recovery.
March 13	AM	70 min.
	PM	60 min.
March 14	AM	Half-marathon. Fast
March 15	AM	60 min.
	PM	60 min.
March 16	AM	30K run in 2 hr.

March 17	AM	70 min.
March 18	AM	25 min. warm-up, 6 x 2K
	PM	50 min. 2 min recovery
March 19	AM	70 min.
	PM	60 min.
March 20	AM	100 min.
March 21	AM	70 min.
	PM	60 min.
March 22	AM	25 min warm-up, 5 x 3K
	PM	50 min. 2 min. recovery.
March 23	AM	70 min.
	PM	60 min.
March 24	AM	38km run in 2:15
March 25	AM	70 min.
March 26	AM	25 min warm-up, 25 x
	PM	60 min. 1 min. fast, 1 min. slow

When the schedule called for two runs of about one hour per day, Tanui would run medium pace for one, easy for the other. The training surface was dirt roads and the altitude around 2000m.

This marathon schedule works! Four runners out of the top eight in the 1996 Boston Marathon followed it. The slowest of the four recorded 2:10:49.

For half-marathon training, Tanui believes in some slight modifications—reducing the mileage a bit and more emphasis on speed work. For adaptation, therefore, the structure would remain the same, the long runs shortened and the speed sessions run at increased pace.

"The important training is my hill session; this builds up my strength. In the training period I run this session twice a week, but if I have a competition then I run the hill just once." His hill training is legendary among the athletes of the Eldoret region. As you have seen, the hill is long: 20K! And it starts at 1300m and gains another 1400m of altitude before the end! "I run this alone mostly; my driver drops me at the start and picks me up at the finish," he said. Tanui took a little under an hour and a half to complete the climb. "Yes, it is hard, but very good training; after running here you fear no hill!"

Before his victorious run at Boston in 1996, Moses took the last week easy. The last long run had taken place two weeks earlier.

Monday	60 min. steady.
Tuesday	50 min. easy, extra stretching.
Wednesday	50 min. of jogging, extra stretching.
Thursday	40 min. of light running and stretching.
Friday	50 min. of easy jogging, stretching.
Saturday	40 min. of easy jogging, stretching.
Sunday	Complete rest.
Monday	Boston Marathon, first in 2:09:16

After finishing the race he rested one week before resuming training for the Olympic 10,000m. Lamentably, a leg injury forced him to drop out of the Kenyan trials after 15 laps. "I had been nursing a tendon ligament injury since Boston. The blistering pace worsened it," said Tanui.

Tegla Loroupe

Date of birth:	May 9, 1973
Birthplace:	Kapsait, West Pokot District.
Height/weight:	5'1/4" (153cm), 88 lbs. (40 kg.)
Training sessions	Two per day
Favorite session:	"Speed work of all kinds."
Tough session:	"Speed work!"
Hardest session:	30 x 400m run in 78 sec.
Km per week	160-170
Personal bests:	1500m, 4:29.39
	3000m, 8:33.36
	5000m, 14:45.95
	10,000m, 30:32.03
	15km, 48:30
	10 miles, 52:17
	Half-marathon, 67:12
	Marathon, 2:20:43.
Honors won:	1993 World Championships 10,000m, 4th
	1994 and 1998 Goodwill Games 10,000m, 1st.
	1995, 1999 World Championships 10,000m, 3rd
	1996 Olympics: 10,000m, 6th
	1997, 1998, 1999 World Half-marathon champion
	1998, 1999 World Marathon record
	1994, 1995 New York Marathon champion
	2000 London Marathon champion
	2000 Olympics: 10,000m, 5th; Marathon, 13th

The spearheading of the Kenyan women's challenge in distance running was Tegla Chepkite Loroupe. The diminutive Kenyan's winsome smile and dancing eyes have made her a darling of the press and public, and her commitment and steel-hard training have brought her success on road and track. Loroupe was born high up in the Kapsait area, West Pokot District. She was one of 22 siblings ("My father, Abraham, had four wives,") and ran about four miles to Kapsait primary school each day. "There was no power [electricity] or water in Kapsait, so we traveled everywhere by foot. I was training better to be a runner than many runners train. Even my mother, Mary Lotuma, can run fast, and she has never tried to be *in* running. She would travel 40 kilometers when younger, on foot, visiting relatives."

Running school races, she noticed her talent for fast running. After finishing at Nasokol Girls School, she enrolled at the Rift Valley College of Science and Technology, where she was discovered by one of Kenya's longest serving coaches, John Macharia. Tecla Chemabwai, who was a teacher at the college became Tegla's biggest influence.

Tegla made an immense impact on marathon running in her first try at the event, winning the 1994 New York Marathon. She had been concentrating on the 10,000m and cross country prior to 1994, and her win at New York started her on a new, profitable career.

In 1995, Loroupe returned to contest New York again. The week before her departure for the States, she received the sorrowful news that her sister Albina had died due to a stomach hemorrhage back in Kenya. Tegla stopped training and yearned to return directly home to her family. In accordance with her sister's wishes, however, she reluctantly competed at New York. "When I was running, I could see her still smiling, looking happy."

Crossing the finish line first, Tegla burst into tears, releasing the emotions that had welled up inside her the entire previous week. It was an amazing performance—a 2:28:06 clocking on a very windy day. One of Tegla's victims was world champion Manuela Machado of Portugal, who finished two and a half minutes behind her.

The warm weather in August at Goteborg (site of Machado's World Championships victory) would certainly have suited Tegla better than the cold and wind of New York, but Tegla opted for New York (in November), a city she loves. She has won other road races there. "Coming to New York is like going home; I have so many lovely friends over there," recalled Tegla at her European base in Germany.

Three straight New York triumphs were not to be. Tegla started the 1996 race "all guns blazing." Unfortunately she ran out of ammunition, and misjudging the pace, faded badly, finishing seventh.

Tegla was baffled. The explanation came a few days later. A doctor with New York Road Runners, Lewis G. Maharam, MD, FACSM, discovered problems with Tegla's spine; a stress fracture was the culprit.

In 1998, she returned with a vengeance, shattering the world marathon record, first in Rotterdam in 1998 (2:20:47) and then in Berlin the next year, four seconds faster.

At the 2000 Olympics in Sydney, after winning the prestigious London Marathon that spring, she placed 13th in the marathon, and six days later, fifth in the 10,000m.

Although still competing to this day, Tegla's horizons have broadened. In 2003, she founded the Tegla Loroupe Peace Foundation, a mission aiming to end tribal violence and cattle rustling in her home district. In 2006, she was named a United Nations Ambassador of Sport by Kofi Annan.

Comments

Tegla, like the majority of Kenyans, sees the positive side of training with others. While staying in Germany, she lives with a group of Kenyan athletes, many from her home district. Before the New York Marathon in 1996, she trained with Joyce Chepchumba, who was to finish third in New York and earlier in the year was runner-up in the London Marathon. "Sometimes it is good to run alone also, to gather your thoughts," she says.

Training is monitored by how the body feels. If the muscles are tired and achy, then Tegla can run two easy sessions of 45 minutes to recover. If she feels strong, however, then the morning session is a quality workout with again 45 minutes of easy running in the evening.

The philosophy behind Tegla's marathon buildup is one of preparation with both quality and quantity. The long run, once a week, takes two and a half hours. Intervals, often twice a week, are tough—for example, 3 x 3K at marathon pace with two min jog recoveries. 15 x 1K at faster than race pace—3:18 per kilometer—is another typical session.

When asked about her training, she explained that the difference between 10,000m and marathon training is minimal. She just increases the length of her weekly long run for marathon training. Tegla trains similarly to Rose Cheruiyot and Lydia Cheromei—a lot of fast-paced tempo runs. One of Tegla's individual traits, however, is that she loves running a long hill session—a session that could be 12K or more of steady uphill running.

After completing a marathon, Tegla takes a month's rest before resuming training. The marathon buildup takes three months on average and Tegla likes to include some shorter races as sharpeners. She also feels that she is still very competitive at 10,000m. "I do not want to run too many marathons too soon. That is why I concentrated on the 10,000m at the Olympics; [it was] too soon after Boston to run another marathon." (She had finished second to Uta Pippig in that April race, winning $50,000.)

A Typical Marathon Training Week

Monday	AM	60 min. easy, 15K
	PM	60 min. easy, 15K
Tuesday	AM	90 min. normal speed
Wednesday	AM	1-2 hr. easy
	PM	60 min. easy.
Thursday	AM	Interval session
	PM	90 min. easy.
Friday	AM	75 min. easy
	PM	Jogging
Saturday	AM	2.5 hr. easy, long run
Sunday	AM	90 min. easy, until the last 30 min. (run hard)

Tegla's light-on-her-feet running action is virtually perfect for marathon running. Normally starting off behind her major competitors, Loroupe ropes them in as the kilometers unfold, her effortless stride enduring against the fatigue that attacks all.

A Boston victory still eludes her. In her first Boston (1995) she was "overtired by running too many races." She suffered stomach pains and finished ninth in a respectable 2:33. In 1996 she nearly pulled off the win, but was swallowed up in the final miles by Uta Pippig.

Boston does remain one of Tegla's important goals. She promises to practice drinking on the run, as both her Boston Marathons have given her problems collecting her bottles from the drinks tables. "Lack of practice," she says. "In Kenya I am never drinking on my long run." Don't bet against the diminutive Kenyan in a future Hopkinton-to-Boston race.

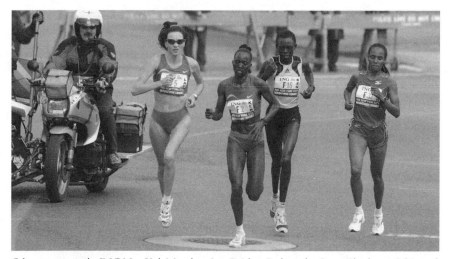

Salina running in the ING New York Marathon. L to R: Jelena Prokopcuka, Susan Chepkemei, Salina, and Derartu Tulu. (*New York Road Runners*)

Salina Jebet Kosgei

Date of birth:	November 16, 1976
Place of birth:	Simotwo, Keiyo district
Tough session:	7 x 2K in 6:50 with 90 sec. rest
Favorite session:	10 x 400m in 68-69 sec.
Longest run:	38K long run
Personal best:	800m, 2:01
	5000m, 15:01:79
	10,000m, 31:27:83
	Half marathon, 67:52
	Marathon, 2:23:22
Honors won:	2002 Commonwealth Games 10,000m Champion
	2003 Paris Marathon
	2005 Prague Marathon
	2006 Standard Charter Singapore Champion
	2006 Berlin runner up

Salina Kosgei began running in Kapkenda Girls School in 1987. The motivation was nothing more than fun, though the girl was encouraged to pursue the sport by Ank De Vlas, the headmistress, who saw talent and potential in her, "I ran 100 meters, 200 meters, and the 800 meters up to the national level at school," Salina recalls. The schoolteacher inspired Kosgei to train hard, and gave her the much-needed support a young Kenyan needed.

"Life was tough; I did a lot of work on the farm, and had to run the 7km to school. But, I persevered. With the headmistresses encouragement I believed I could make it," she says.

Her first breakthrough came in 1992 at the World Juniors in Seoul when she finished eighth in the 800m. A further improvement came when she joined the senior ranks and placed fourth, narrowly missing a medal at the same distance at the 1994 Commonwealth Games 800m. In the early 1990s, unlike many other Kenyan women, she was encouraged to run by her fiancé, Barnabas Kinyor. Kinyor won a bronze medal for Kenya at the 1990 Commonwealth Games in the 400m hurdles. He later became an 800m specialist (1:44.95), and Kosgei says, "Marrying Barnabas was good because most Kenyan women stop running after marriage, but he stopped his career to help me continue. In Kenya that is rare."

Kosgei herself could not make money in the 800m event, so slowly she started to move up in distance until her manager suggested she tried the 10,000m for a trip to compete at the 2002 Commonwealth Games in Manchester. The Kenyan team was only taking two runners for the 10,000m so Salina took a crack at the 25-lapper and qualified. In Manchester, nobody had high expectations of Kosgei whose reputation was that of an 800m runner. However, starting the last lap, the Kenyan found herself in third place and was determined to push hard to ensure a medal this time, "I thought, "Let me just go as hard as I can, and I won gold!" Her time was a Championship record of 31:27.83.

In 2003, a 16th place finish at the Paris World Championships made her realize that perchance another step up, to the marathon, was the next progression; she debuted in 2004, running 2:24:32 for the win in the same city. In 2005, placing fourth in the ING New York City Marathon convinced Salina that she could run at the highest level, and in 2006, she placed second in Berlin, running a personal best of 2:23:22.

Comments

After a marathon, she takes ten days of rest before starting up the running again. Then she runs for an hour a day for ten days before starting the program. When training for a marathon, she uses a three-month plan.

Training Plan (Used before Berlin 2006)

Monday	AM 90 min. steady	PM	30–min. easy
Tuesday	AM Track, 10 x 1000m in 3:25-30 with 60 sec. rest	PM	Easy jog, 30 min.
Wednesday	AM 70 min. easy to steady	PM	Rest
Thursday	AM Fartlek, warm up then 1 min. hard, 1-min. easy, warm down; whole session is 50-min. long	PM: easy jogging 40-minutes	
Friday:	Same as Wednesday		
Saturday	AM Long run, one week 30K, the next 35K, then the longest 38K		
Sunday	Rest day		

Best advice

"Do all the program you have been given by the coach, otherwise you are not going to make it. Run with your smart head; do not try for what is not possible. Look at your training, then see what you can achieve." Salina does not use gym work, though she stretches a couple of times per week and takes a massage occasionally. She trains exclusively in Kenya (Kapsabet) at altitude and flies directly from her home to the race without thought for altitude adjustment. "Don't attempt more than two marathons per year," she says. On diet, she has this to say, "My favorite foods are *ugali, sukuma wiki*, beans, and milk. Traditional Kenyan food."

Daniel Kipkoech Yego

"If you want to go to school then you must work for the school fees." Young Daniel was told that brutal news as a child. His mother had a liking for the local brew, and the family lived in poverty. Undeterred, Daniel collected and started selling charcoal to attend primary

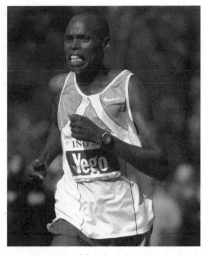

Daniel Yego placed fourth at the ING New York City Marathon in 2006, one place behind his mentor, Paul Tergat. (*Alison Wade*)

school. The funds were not sufficient, yet he prevailed: "I would bribe the teacher with charcoal to allow me to sit in the class and attend lessons. When the headmistress came to collect the school fees, I would climb through the window and run home; that is how I got through school. I loved school and wanted to be a teacher." Little Wonder Yego has succeeded in life and is known by his training partners as a very disciplined hard worker.

Daniel's Training for the New York City Marathon, 2006, with Paul Tergat and Robert Cheruiyot

Monday	AM 70 min. steady to fast	PM At least 55 min., we have a set route
Tuesday	AM 90 minutes steady, progressive ("On this day, Robert Cheruiyot was always very strong.")	PM Same as Monday
Wednesday	AM Fartlek, after a 30 min. warm up 15 x 1-minute fast, 1 min. slow ("If we run too slowly we increase up to 17 efforts. Before NYC, Titus was strongest at this session, we expected big things of him.")	PM As Monday
Thursday	AM 70 min. easy recovery run	PM Same as Monday
Friday	AM 90 min. at a medium pace	PM Same as Monday
Saturday	Midday Fast 80 –min., "Very, very hard."	
Sunday	70 min. recovery run	

The following week the group ran a 30K long run on Sunday at a fast clip and ran hill work, 25 minutes continual uphill after 35 minutes on the flat, on Monday. In New York, Yego predicted Munji would perform the best, yet he ran the worst from the group. Tergat picked up a hamstring pull two weeks before the race which left him only at 90 percent (good enough to snag third), and Yego? "I was watching only Ramaala and Rop, nobody ran their own pace, we were too slow at halfway. When the *mzungo* [Gomes of Brazil, the eventual winner] made a break, I was thinking it was not for real, *wazungos* [white people] can not run away from us. At 35K Ramaala said, "This guy is going to win!" so we tried to chase him down. Unfortunately I got something in my right eye, I dropped back to try and remove the dirt, and then Tergat and Kiagora were gone." Yego took fourth, not a result he celebrated.

Comments
Normally, stretch every day after the evening session. Use progressive distance for the long runs, from 30K the first week to 35 two weeks later, to 38K. Then return to the 30K distance for another cycle. Get lots of sleep when in hard training. Run cross country, 12K races, for speed.

Best Advice
"Maintain your running weight." When Yego was injured, prior to his breakthrough, he increased his weight by four kilos. The weight would not leave his body; "I said, 'Okay, let it be 65 then,' but after two more months when I put on lots of clothes and ran in the hot sun I came down again and found my running form."

Lornah Kiplagat

Date of birth:	May 1, 1974
Birthplace:	Kabiemit
Miles per week:	Varies but up to 225K before Boston 2000
Sessions per day:	Two usually, once on long-run days.
Favorite session:	No favorite, just loves running!
Hardest session:	5 x 5K at marathon pace, or faster, with a meager 1-min. recovery. Long run before Boston up to 3 hrs. However before Lornah ran her marathon PR she ran for 4 hrs. in a forest after getting lost!
Personal Best:	5000m, 14:51:95
	5K road, 14:47
	10,000m, 30:12:53
	10K road, 30:32,
	10 miles, 50:54
	20K, 63:56
	Half marathon, 66:25 (world record)
	Marathon, 2:22:22
Honors:	2006 World Cross Country Championship, silver
	2006 World 20K Champion

2007 World Cross Country Championship, gold
2007 10 miles, 20K and half-marathon, WR

The Early Days

Lornah Jebiwott Kiplagat's career began, inadvertently, as running for an education, a vocation that today she promotes through her professional running in a namesake foundation based in the Netherlands. Each weekday she would leave her small thatched hut with its dry caked-mud walls in the rural village of Kabiemit and glide like a gazelle across fields of thick grass and corn to run the three and a half miles to school. She would run home and back for lunch too, making each day a total of 14 miles running. "This was my groundwork (70 miles per week in her pre teen years), though I did not realize it at the time. I was meant to be a runner; I also did not know this at the time, not to help myself, but so I can take my place on earth and contribute in this world."

Lornah strides out to take her third Mini title in 2006. (*Author*)

Although Kiplagat ran to school, it was not by immediate choice. "If you were late the teacher would cane you. . . every time I walked I was late, so I learned to run there. I liked to sleep a little bit late, and I could catch up with running, so it seemed like a good idea." At the age of ten, she entered her first school races ("I would run the 3, 5, and 10K all in the same morning.".). She remembers winning most of them. It was an activity she did because she found enjoyment and excelled at the sport, not because she saw running as a means to a later career. "You can say that is why I am so behind education with my foundation. When you are young you need help and guidance, we see this as we get older."

A compelling narrative followed. Lornah, now a naturalized Dutchwoman whom I dubbed "the Simba" for her onerous training regime, left school early to go and live with an aunt. This aunt, who lived some 80 miles away in a Nakuru town famous for its pink flamingos. She happened to be an exceptional runner—Susan Sirma, Kenya's first female World Championships medalist, bronze, 3000m, Tokyo 1991—and she inspired Lornah to reach a new level of effort in her training. After a period of intense running, while supporting herself by working as a maid, she was ready to run in her first national championships.

She traveled over potholed roads for one hundred miles in a crowded Matatu taxi bus from Nakuru to the capital city, Nairobi, with a friend, to compete in the cross country nationals, held in a grass horse-racing stadium in N'gong, a place made famous by Karen Blixen, in her book, *Out of Africa*.

The night before the race, with no one to help or advise the young women, Kiplagat and her friend were forced to sleep in a restroom by the deserted N'gong racecourse. There was no accommodation offered for the girls; they had no other place to stay and at least they were able to secure the toilet door in a city with the nickname "Nai-robbery". "In those days I did not even know about hotels or what they were for," Lornah remembers. All this aside, she had no money or funds to pay for board or food. "We did not sleep so well and had no breakfast," Kiplagat says of the trip. Running barefoot, as she had all her life, she placed fifth and won a trip to the World Cross Country Championships in Stellenbosch, South Africa, where she finished 80th. However, following the nationals it was a hurried trip back to Nakuru for sustenance and a safe and sound sleep.

A year later, after first declining an offer from the late Kim McDonald, a British agent, she moved to Detmold, Germany, and was signed up by Volker Wagner, who looked after the Kenyan stars Tegla Loroupe and Joyce Chepchumba. She also was endorsed by a shoe company, as Pieter Langerhorst, who was working for that company, explains, "Another athlete whom my company sponsored said 'Sign up Lornah, she is a talent,' so I did. I remember I'd send her a pair of socks and she'd send back a thank-you note; the other runners just asked for more pairs." However, it would be another year before he met Kiplagat face to face.

Lornah thought Langerhorst was a "fat westerner", and she was pleasantly surprised when Pieter, tanned and in good shape, dropped by the hotel of her roommate Joyce Chepchumba before the 1997 London Marathon to deliver some athletic gear. The rest, as they say, is athletics history, with marriage for the couple and athletic stardom for the Simba.

There were still a few hiccups. "Take my first marathon win, Los Angeles (1997, 2:33:50). I flew to the race believing it was a half-marathon. My agent did not tell me it was a full marathon!"

Kiplagat remembers a decade ago as if it were yesterday, "That was not an easy time. For women in Kenya it was not accepted to be seen with naked thighs [bare legs] so I had to run in long pants. And this was something new for me to manage. [Women all wear skirts.] Also, people could not see me in trousers or they might think there was something wrong with me, so I ran at 4:00 a.m. in the dark. I became known as 'the Night Runner.' Luckily, I had very supportive parents."

Supportive indeed; unlike all the neighbors, daughters, Lornah was not forced into the barbaric tribal circumcision rituals, nor did she have to wash her brothers' clothes, as is still the tradition today in that region of East Africa. "Make sure you go for it, and go good!" was the advice of her late father who lived to the ripe old age of 80. Battling an oppressive, male-oriented society, Kiplagat vowed, "If I will ever get any money from this sport, then I will help others so they do not have to do what I had to do."

At the time Lornah was growing up, the men in Kenya had a role model in a charismatic, robust Nandi tribesman, Kipchoge Keino, an Olympic hero in the 1968 and 1972

Games. Lornah explains, waving her hand like she's drawing with chalk, "There was a song about him, "Kimbia kama Kipchoge Keino," run like Kipchoge Keino, and his face was on the 20-shilling bill. For the men, they had someone to be like; we had none. If you are going to be a runner then you had better be a man like Keino. Women were supposed to be the family makers, not to run. If you ran past the age of leaving school. Ah, ah, ah." She continues to tell tales of how the pioneer Kenyan female athletes would return from Europe crying, having no stanchion of support from society, family, or friends, despite being household names on the Western athletics circuit.

Kiplagat is an athlete cognizant of the need to help kids by introducing them to sports, for it is athletics that has empowered and drastically changed her own life beyond anyone's imagination. "When I started running, and it gave me so much, I knew I had to also give back. That is what I am trying to do now. Can you imagine, me? Now I can be a role model to the many young girls in Kenya." She is an immense inspiration to her 19 nephews and nieces who troop after her each step when she visits Kabiemit.

In the year 2000, the High Altitude Training Centre was opened in Iten, Kenya. Kiplagat and Langerhorst, to support the young female Kenyan athletes' athletic endeavors, funded the place. Seven years on, a gym has been added, as have rooms for about thirty athletes. A library is currently being built funded by a generous donation from Steve and Elizabeth Baskin of Atlanta, Georgia. The High Altitude Training Centre is the go-to place for athletes in Iten. The list of runners that have passed through this camp is pretty impressive: Caroline Kwambai, Linah Cheruiyot, Hilda Kibet, Kipkemboi Katui, Kimutai Kosgei, Jason Mbote and Solomon Busendich to name a scant few. Furthermore, Lornah and Pieter are both extremely instrumental in the Shoe4Africa programs that operate in Africa.

With all her philanthropic deeds, it is easy to forget that "Simba" the athlete is just as impressive with her legs! In 2006, she won her first world championship, setting a world 20K record at Debrecen, Hungary. Earlier in the year she had won silver in the World Championships Cross Country 8K behind the baby-faced assassin Tirunesh Dibaba, in Fukuoka, Japan. Lornah held the world best for the 5K until another Ethiopian, Meseret Defar, ran a couple of tenths faster in 2006. For the marathon, Lornah holds a world-class 2:22:22 PR from the Osaka Marathon 2003 and for good measure she set a new world best for 10 miles in 2006. In 2007 she became, against the odds, the World Cross Country champion, decimating the field in Mombasa to win by a clear home stretch. Later that year, she won the world half marathon championships, setting a world record in route, "that was a dream," she smiles.

The dream began three decades ago when a lithe Kenyan girl skipped over the fields with the scent of the maize and wattle trees filling her nostrils, not knowing where her future lay, but knowing she was running for something better.

Comments

"The communication between coach and athlete is very important." Says Langerhorst. "We sat together and looked very carefully at what needed to be done and asked, 'Why' to fully understand all the aspects of the training plan." More track workouts have been introduced than before, placing an emphasis on speed endurance, and consequently the records have been tumbling. Lornah keeps the recovery very short when in marathon training, even in such demanding sessions as 20 x 1000m the rest will be a scant 60 seconds. However, when in training for a 10,000 race the recovery is lengthened to allow for a more aggressive tempo.

On building up mileage: "When starting up from a rest period, I aim for 30Km per week, running three times per week. I add mileage slowly, never more than a 10 percent increase, and preferably I use 5 percent per week. This way I build up strongly."

Training Week

Monday	AM 45 min. recovery run	PM	45 min. recovery run
Tuesday	AM 45 min easy	PM	20 min. warm-up. 3x 400m (1 min. recovery), 800m (2 min. recovery), 1200 (3 min. recovery), 1600m.
Wednesday	AM 45 min. recovery	PM	60 min. recovery.
Thursday	AM 60 min. easy	PM	1 hr. 20 min. hill work, running in sand dunes
Friday	AM 45 min. recovery	PM	60 min. recovery.
Saturday	AM 60 min. easy	PM	45 min. medium
Sunday	AM Long run, 2 hrs. 10 min.		

Break-up: 20 min. easy, 30 min. medium,
20 min. fast, 20 min. easy, 20 min fast and 20 min. easy

Robert "Mwafrika" Kipkoech Cheruiyot

Date of birth:	September 26, 1978
Place of birth:	Mosoriot, Nandi
Height/Weight	6'2", 143 lbs.
Personal best:	Half-marathon, 59:21
	Marathon, 2:07:14
Honors:	2003, 2006–2008 Boston Marathon champion
	2006 Chicago Marathon champion

Robert Cheruiyot, at age 28, has the eyes of a man who has traveled far, and since he has trained with Paul Tergat for the past year we can assume that those eyes do not lie. However, those rich brown eyes have traveled much farther, farther than many could tolerate or even imagine. Robert walked on the thin line of despair and distraction, looked adversity and hardship square in the face, and by the grace of God pulled through. With a steel intensity, yet immense compassion, he took what life had offered him, and brought himself above fate's chosen path. He displayed each and every emotion that dire circumstance can lead a man to, yet emerged a champion.

Initially, life looked great for "Mwafrica"; he was elected as a head boy at Tebesson Primary School. "I was an athlete at school and good, I enjoyed running, and I liked school." Nevertheless, after Form Eight, the tide turned. "My father sold the *shamba* and disappeared; my mother remarried and then abandoned me and my brother. I was four, he was six." A piece of his heart was torn from his body, abandoned, for always. The brothers were split up, Robert going to a grandmother, Stephen going to an uncle. Stephen recalls, "It was no choice, that is how it was. I was pulled here, he was pushed there."

Another relative, a cousin on his mother's side, then helped Robert. He enrolled the boy at Kosirai High School, telling Robert he had to help with the household chores to pay his way. After two terms the cousin refused to assist further and told Robert, that he had to attend a cheaper school, Chemuswa Secondary. "I had to do all my homework at school because I was so busy being a maid when I got back home."

Food was scarce. For breakfast, Robert recalls it was Kenyan tea. "Except not the sugars, because we were so poor." The next meal would be in the

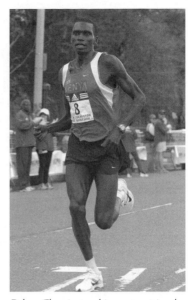

Robert Cheruiyot on his way to setting the course record at the Boston Marathon. (*Flanagan/PrettySporty*)

evening hours, *ugali* and milk or kale. "We were not alone; this is how it is for many people in Kenya, even today," He says. When school was finished, Cheruiyot was told to leave the house. "We argued and he told me to leave the house," remembers Robert with a wistful look.

Penniless and hungry, Robert walked on the fumes of his last meal from Mosoriot to Iten—a distance of 30 miles—where his brother Stephen was working as a policeman and living in the compound below St. Patrick's School on a salary of a dollar a day. Robert was hoping for financial assistance and a chance. However, over the 30-mile route, finding Stephen completely broke and in similarly ominous circumstances, Robert returned the next day.

Back in Mosoriot, Robert was at a loss. "I had nobody, nobody to care for me, no-one to look after." He wandered the town kicking the dust and staring at the ground. Those eyes were still searching for hope, because hope was free. "It was at this time I thought to end it all. Why live, nobody was together and I was all alone. I was very close to suicide."

The town of Mosoriot does not offer much in business, but Robert managed to find a job at the 786 Kinyoz barbers. "I was employed by a friend for 50-bob; it was not enough for one meal a day and a couple of cigarettes. I slept out in the night-time as I had no rent; I would sleep in the streets with the watchmen on the verandahs." They were dire and tenebrous days.

After a few months of this hardscrabble lifestyle shaving and cutting hair at the barber shop, barely eating more than a plate of cornmeal and some roadside green kale, a distant relative on his father's side named Kanus, heard of Robert's misfortunes. She took pity on Mwafrica and told him she'd assist him whilst he got back on his feet. Life turned around as Robert resumed running and soon met a man who got him an invitation to try out for the Fila team at Moses Tanui's Kaptagat Camp.

The coach, Letting, did not like Mwafrica and wanted him to leave, though Moses, who was then Kenya's most established marathon runner and owned the camp, took a liking to Robert. "He will stay," he ordered. Tanui later recalled, "Anyone could see, this man had talent, he was going to make it. He was a hard worker, very hard."

It was not an easy time in the camp for Robert; "I had problems, but I didn't tell anyone, I never tell anyone." Conditions were far from luxurious; food was often a problem, and many times the hard training was fueled by one meager meal of maize per day. "We had to share and there was never enough to go around. Imagine one loaf of bread for breakfast and maybe twenty mouths wanting it!"

At his first race, Robert placed well enough to encourage him to train harder, and to justify Tanui's conviction. One day Paul Tergat visited the athletes at the camp. Robert stared at the legend and vowed to run as Tergat did. In the large hall at Kaptagat, portraits and pictures of the great runners are pasted on the walls, and Robert stood beneath Tergat's picture for a long, long time after he left. "Imagine the next day he returned, he ran with us. After he gave me his shoes and told me to train hard. He said nothing comes without hard training."

Like an angel, had stepped from a cloud, Robert felt that the years of torment, toil, and troubles had passed. "The next day I increased my training speeds, and again the next day." The air in Kaptagat is pure; what it lacks in oxygen it gains in freshness. Cheruiyot stood outside his allotted bunkroom, a small six-by-eight-foot solitary room, and felt the chains of his youth drop from his arms. "I ran inspired, all the way to the next race."

In Kenya, it is every runner's dream to come to the front of the pack, push hard, hold off the horde of excellent athletes who will chase you to your very grave, and be discovered. At the Kencell 10Km, Robert stormed to the lead whispering his mantra, running with his faith in God. Unbelievably he won in an emphatic fashion and collected 1000 shillings on prize money; a genuine fortune. His time on that day, 28:06, was a course record, and it stands as the fastest 10K ever run on Kenyan roads. Titus Munji was second in 28:52. "He was far, far back. I couldn't even see anyone," recalled Robert, who also won a mobile phone, his first, on that day. "I went to the shop and bought shoes for 600 shillings, I got a shirt, and for 200, trousers that I used when I flew to Italy, and I bought myself food," he remembers of his first paycheck.

The Fila camp signed Robert up, and he immediately went to Italy for a series of road races ranging from 10K to the half-marathon.. There was now an undimmable brightness in those eyes as he consistently performed well.

The month after his arrival, he ran 60:06 to win the Roma-Otsia Half-Marathon in Italy. A spree of races in Italy and Switzerland earned him nearly $10,000 in six months. Not his first marathon victory, but winning Boston in 2003 gave Robert an international profile and a sizeable bank account. Since he was a child, he had had an idea of what he would do if money came his way. "I bought land, pumped water, set up everything, opened an account at a local bank, and brought my parents back together." However, the smell of success draws the hyenas, and a group of unscrupulous characters tried to lure Robert away from the sporting world. "I was smoking, I was with the wrong people, a bad crowd, and I realized I was on the road to going back to where I was," he says. The memories were clear enough in Robert's mind to jolt him back to the right path. In 2005, he asked Paul Tergat to take him back as an athlete to coach. He explains:

Paul had advised me before Boston 2003, and I won. A lot of people know Paul only as an athlete, but he is a great coach. He gives good morale. His coaching ideas are not easy to follow; there are not many people who can do his training. There is no coach like him, he never gives you the whole plan, you know in the evening there can be something different to what you are expecting. He gives you a heart like a lion.

Tergat has been coaching Cheruiyot ever since.

With that big heart, Cheruiyot has gone on to become a truly legendary marathon runner. His story of a run from a life that would have defeated most is as amazing as his running feats that headline newspapers across the globe. Mwafrica remains a humble and magnanimous man who today runs with a flame of fortune and faith in those well-traveled eyes.

Comments

"Before Boston I talked with Moses Tanui, who has always been good to me. When Moses was running, the guys in the front were very far, but Moses caught them and won. You see, you do not need to lead to win Boston. It is a big distance to go. Moses said wait, so in the race I listened to his advice and did not follow the others who ran too fast a pace. I train hill climbing, so I did not really notice the hills on the course. The downhills are harder for me. Boston is not won from out in front, but from behind with pushing. I learned this the first time I ran there."

"I started training with Tergat after we began talking about running Lisbon in 2005, when he won and I was number two, and realized we could benefit from working together in training as we share the same training ideas. As you can see from our running, it is working well. We run about 32 to 33 kilometers per day, at least. You know less than 30 kilometers per day is someone who is not quite serious yet at the distance. I am a sportsman and I have no time for my family; it is my career to run well and that must be put first. Following this race, or any marathon regardless of the result, I will rest for two weeks and go to my farm in Kapsabet. Then I return to the plan—two marathons a year—and some unimportant road races to test the form."

How to Set a Course Record at Boston

Sunday	6 AM	55-60 min. at 3:30min/K pace
	10 AM	60 min. with some surges
Monday	6 AM	70 min. at 20K
	10 AM	Hill climbing, up N'gong hill 25 mins., 60-70-min. total run
Tuesday	6 AM	55-60 min. at 3:30min/K pace
	10 AM	25K progressive to a fast pace

Wednesday	10 AM	Long run 25-30Km at 3:30-45 pace
	4 PM	40 min. easy
		("Everyday is optional to run at this time, in serious
		training it happens more than I am running at this time, but
		everyone has his own training even with the group,
		so it is individual.")
Thursday	6 AM	Same as Tuesday AM
	10 AM	Fartlek, 1 min.e hard,
		1 min. hard for 20 min.,
		first 30 min. warm-up, and after 15 min. jogging
Friday	6 AM	Same as Tuesday
	10AM	20-25km easy pace
Saturday	10 AM	Somewhat fast tempo run with the group,
		pushing from the start
Sunday		Rest day; go to church.

Margaret Okayo

Okayo currently holds both the Boston and the New York City marathon records. Her training was arduous: "In the mornings I would do about 18 to 20 kilometers of steady running, with 8 to 10 kilometers in the evening hours. I would do a lot of reading and resting in between." Okayo also uses a lot of stretching to work on keeping her stride-length long, "At least thirty minutes per day."

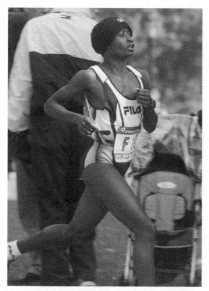

Margaret Okayo twice has broken the course record at the ING New York City Marathon. (*New York Road Runners*)

The long runs were often hilly 30K runs at a challenging pace, and most of the training would be done solo. In the three months before a marathon, she would complete at least four runs of over 35 kilometers. Okayo is not a great fan of speed work on the track, and when she did run intervals the speed would often play second fiddle to the quantity, hence her personal records at five and ten kilometers are considerably slower than most other 67-minute half-marathon runners have run for those distances. She, like Chepkemei, said she would usually do one tempo run, around 20K, and one track session, per week. As Margaret puts it, "I am pure marathon." Her diet always contains a lot of fresh vegetables and fruits when training. "You must eat fresh to stop the body from breaking down with the hard running."

Hilda Jepchumba "Airlines" Kibet

Date of Birth: March 27, 1981

Place of birth: Kapchorwa

Height/Weight: 167 cm. 44kg.

                             ("I've never been more than 46 kg. even when not training.")

Training partners: Doris Changeiywo, Sharon Tavenga, and Sleepy Sylvia.

Longest Run   2 hr. 30 min.

Personal records: 4 miles, 19:58

                             10K, 31:01

                             10,000M, 30:58:48

                             15K, 50:38

                             Half-marathon, 69:43

                             Marathon, 2:32:09

Honors: 2007 New York Half-Marathon Champion

                             2008 New York Road Runners Mini Champion

Hilda Kibet began running in 1999 after being encouraged by her younger sister Sylvia. From being an absolute beginner, she jumped right into the deep end: "I joined the last two weeks of Brother Colm's December training camp. Everyone was much faster than I was; I ran in old shoes that my sister gave me that were the wrong size, so I got big blisters. We would set off for fartlek, and I would quickly be left behind. Then later, when the runners turned and came back, I would rejoin the group, until they left me again," she smiles, remembering the early tough days. "Often I would take a short-cut. It was not easy. I was too ashamed to go for meal times; I would hide in my room." Nowadays it is she who leaves the others behind. Following the dissolution of that camp a distant cousin, Lornah Kiplagat,

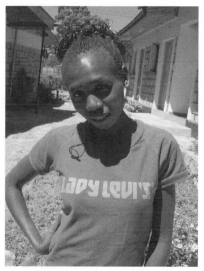

Hilda, no longer left behind on the roads of Iten. (*Author*)

invited Hilda to come and join her newly formed running of camp," she said. "'When it opens I will send for you,' and she did," recalls Kibet. In August of 2001, Hilda went to Europe for the first time. "I think I was number twenty, running a 10K in 38 minutes; I did not do very well. In fact, for the first couple of years I was struggling; perhaps I was not training very hard." Through Pieter Langerhorst's Dutch connection, Hilda enrolled at a physiotherapist school in Holland, and really only resumed her full-time athlete status after concluding her studies in 2005, when, to put it in her words, she "arrived."

At a 10K in Manchester, England, Hilda ran the eleventh-fastest time of the year, 31:46. "To date that is my favorite race; I was very focused to win on that day. I even forgot about the faster athletes in the race, like Lornah. The result was a breakthrough for me, although I had run sub-32 [31:52, Glasgow] the week before." A couple of months later, back in Holland, she ran a 4-miler in Groningen and recorded the sixth-fastest performance of all time, 19:58.

She had run in school as a child; Kenyan schools have running in the curriculum typically between May and July. "I was typically finishing second in the local secondary-school competitions," she says. She was encouraged to take athletics seriously by a schoolteacher, but she decided to concentrate first on her studies, knowing she could run later in life. Had she known, the 4K to and from school, and lunch trips back and forth, were a great foundation for training. "We had no newspapers in my village, but we heard about the great deeds people like Tegla Loroupe were doing; that was inspiring for me."

Training in Iten Before Winning the Egmond Half-Marathon, 2007

Thursday	AM	Pond Loop, 59 min. easy, 14.7K hilly loop
	PM	45 min. easy, on the tractor loop
Friday	AM	15 min. warm up. Helen's hill loop,
		4 x 5K in 18 min. on a hilly loop with 2 min. recovery
Saturday	AM	One hour easy
	PM	50 min. easy down the Kapsowar road
Sunday	AM	1 hr. 45 min run up Fluorspar (20.6K up hill dirt road
		starting at 1400m and finishing at 2770m altitude,
		a 7 percent gradient) starting at 5 min. per kilometer pace.
	PM	30 min. easy to remove the stiffness out and
		back along the straight road
Monday	AM	60 min. out and back along the Singore dirt road, easy
	PM	45 min. easy, on banana route
Tuesday	AM	2K, 1600m, 1200m, 800m speed work at Kamariny
	PM	45 min. easy
Wednesday	AM	50 min. progressive (Starting slow but winding up the pace
		to fast) past St. Patrick's
	PM	45 easy
Thursday	AM	45 min. slow, heavy rains made the roads very slippery
Friday	AM	Again the dirt roads were very muddy and slippery,
		thus switched to 30 min. down the steep tarmac road to
		Tambach, turned and 30 min. back up the hill.
	PM	50 min. easy
Saturday	AM	long run on hilly dirt roads
		20 min. easy, 45 min. medium speed pushing and then
		10 x 1 min. hard, 1 min. easy, then warm down.
		1 hr. 40 min. total
Sunday		No running, woke at 4 AM with cramps at the top of the thighs.

Massage and resting.

Monday   No pain, but taking an extra day of rest to be certain.

Tuesday   AM   60 min. normal pace, back into the training plan
                      with fresh legs

Comments

I do not have natural speed, so I want to invest in the marathon. I do mostly endurance work in my training. I never run intervals of less than three minutes. I have two hard days, one semi-hard, and three easy days of running in the week.

Benson Masya

"Training with Benson is harder than competing. When he decides to run fast in the middle of a training run, nobody can run with him!"—Friend Zablon Miano, 1993

If there was ever a Jesse James of the roads, it was Benson Masya, a road warrior who dominated the road-racing scene in the early 1990s, on both sides of the Atlantic.

Benson Masya was born on the May 14, 1970, and died on September 24, 2003 at just 33 years of age. He was the inaugural World Half-Marathon champion in 1992, a four-time winner of the Great North Run, three times the Honolulu Marathon champion, and the AIMS athlete of the year in 1992. Masya, the road bandit, left a widow, Joan, and three sons.

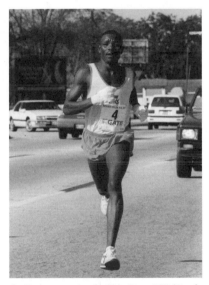

Big Benson winning the Gate River 15K. (*Randy Lefko*)

In the 1980s Masya, a former bantamweight boxer, turned to running, representing the Post Office team. It was the postal profession, not the sport, that his father wished him to pursue. "My father would beat me when he found out I had been running; he did not want me to 'play,' as he called it."

Although he had forays at the marathon distance, winning the Honolulu event thrice (1991, 1992 and 1994), it was in the shorter road races that Benson excelled. With an inferno in his soul, he won virtually every single significant road race from 5K to 21K on both sides of the pond. He carried few possessions with him in his suitcase lifestyle, which took him on a continual rocking and rolling tour of the road circuit, but a set of clippings, especially from the U.S. and British road races, were amongst his prize belongings. "Big Ben" and "King Benson" headline told stories of how he had ripped up the roads, more often than not destroying the field by over a minute. "My tactic was to set off very fast, cooking, then I would make a gap and reduce the speed, but the distance had been made," he said.

Masya squandered hundreds of thousands of dollars on a lifestyle more befitting a rock musician than an athlete. He would often bring the party to his hotel room, buying high-powered sound equipment at a local electronics store, and turning the room into a drinking den. He smoked like a proverbial devil, but continued to race like a demon, as well. Often before slumping into a drunken slumber he would reveal his sensitive side, phoning Joan back in Kenya and talking for hours, telling her how he longed for the normal family life but knew the only way for him to make a living was by using his feet.

National team member Godfrey Kiprotich recalled Benson's first raid on the U.S. roads; "I remember we had a group with the best road racers in America, and we heard about this guy Benson. He ran like a fighter, full of muscles, and right on your back. He was clipping Sammy Lelei's heels the whole run before sprinting off to win. Sammy had been the best for a long time, and then Benson just took over. He was a legend."

Masya's spirit was the epitome of the Kenyan racer. Once, after an unbeaten spell of seven months, he flew to Japan from Kenya via Britain for a half-marathon. Arriving in Japan, he was refused entry, as only one page remained unstamped in his passport. "You will have to return with a new passport!" he was told at customs. Benson turned around, flew back to Britain, flew back to Kenya, and took the communal taxi to the city center. He stood in line in Nairobi for half the day, got a new passport, took the communal bus back to the airport, and boarded an evening flight. The next morning he flew from Britain to Japan. The next day he ran the half-marathon, and lost. When he was asked about losing his unbeaten record Benson, instead of citing the obvious excuses, replied, "Ah, you can not win every day. I did my best, but someone did better. I will try harder next time."

Benson had a fighter's talent of hanging by the skin of his teeth to the training group he was running with whenever he was out of form; by the will of his mind, he could do it. His favorite training word was "cooking," which referred to the speed he liked to reach. He was a sensitive man who was humble and encouraging to runners of all levels. "I learned a lot coming to Europe. When I first came (to Europe), I knew nothing, not even to boil an egg. Running gave me the freedom to this world. I have to thank God for a lot of things in life, I was blessed." A man from Benson's tribe, Cosmas Ndeti, named King Ben as his greatest supporter and mentor, "Masya taught me a lot about running, and he encouraged me. Masya was like me, he was a winner. He did not care about times, he cared about positions."

"Fast distance runs develop the body best for road racing, most of the speed I have is from tempo runs, not intervals."—Benson Masya

Often the heavy bouts of training would only be induced by a dire lack of funds. One day in 1998 he woke penniless in the northeast quarter of Albuquerque; he had been on a party binge and had not run for two weeks. Outside his bedroom window, the soil was smothered in cigarette butts; his eyes were bloodshot and floated as he walked around the house. Sitting at the kitchen table, he searched the pages of a running magazine for a money race, asking someone to enter him; "See if you can get travel money, I need to get there," he added. Then at ten o'clock in the morning, when the tiredness had left his eyes, he slipped on his ASICS trainers and jogged to the Academy track where he ran 60 x

400m at an ever-decreasing pace, until the last few laps were a virtual crawl. Upon finishing, he duly collapsed on the grassy infield and slept for a good hour.

Two weeks later, after some more mammoth sessions including three hours of fartlek on the 365-trail in the Sandia Mountains and a rapid tempo run up the eight mile La Luz trail that starts at 7,000-ft and ends at over 10,000 feet, Benson miraculously made money by running a 28-minute 10K. Exalted with his newfound greenbacks, he abruptly stopped training again. Masya soon headed for Mexico, where his health deteriorated bad. His lifestyle curved far away from the athletic world, and a series of travels began that eventually took him back to Kenya.

In the summer of 2003, he traveled to Germany, resolute to start training for a comeback. Joyce Chepchumba recalled, "He was very, very thin and pale-looking, he had no strength, and his eyes looked very bad. He had blood under all his nails." Chepchumba gave him some running clothes and a watch to encourage Benson to begin training. Illness struck again and he was forced to return home to Kenya. Masya, a saga of rags to riches to rags, moved into the Kibera slums, unrecognizable among thousands of others who survived on pennies or less. Terminally ill, he returned to his birthplace, dying shortly afterward. The Kenyan community mourned one of its brightest stars.

The last words I heard from Benson before he died was, "I have never lost to Tergat, I have his number, I will be back to challenge the man, they will see that King Benson is not finished!" Four days after Benson died, Paul Tergat ran his defining race, the world record in the marathon.

Cross Country

The Cross Country World Championships

Senior men: 15 individual winners, 28 team golds, 1986
Senior Women: Five individual winners, 8 team gold since 1991
Junior men: 14 individual winners, 20 team gold, since 1985
Junior Women: 9 individual winners, 13 team gold, since 1991
In 1988, 1993 and 1998 Kenyan senior men swept the podium. In 1993 the men took positions 1, 2, 3, 4, 5, and 10, using none of their top three World Championship team-winning finishers from the 1992 race. In 1994, William Sigei, Helen Chepn'geno, Philip Mosima, and Sally Barsosio completed an unprecedented, and never yet repeated, sweep of individual championships.

Jackson Rutto has the honor of being the first finisher from Kenya in the World Cross country Championships. In 1981, Rutto placed 22nd. With the help of Peter Koech (24), Alfred Nyasani (25), Sammy Mogene (36), Wilson Masonic (56), and Some Muge (57), the team won the bronze medal. It was an auspicious start. Two years later, Muge, running the same time as the first two finishers, won Kenya's first individual medal, a bronze. Another two years later that was upgraded, by Paul Kipkoech, to silver. In the junior men's race, Kenya took its first individual gold, won by 18-year-old Kipkemboi Kimeli. The following year, Kenya took its first senior title, individual with

John Ngugi. With Joseph Kiptum (3), Paul Kipkoech (5), Kipsubai Koskei (7), Some Muge (8), and Andrew Masai (21) also placing well. The team won its first of eighteen consecutive championships. Since that day, Kenya has never failed to be on the podium at any World Cross Country event. The junior men took their first team gold in 1988.

The senior women took their first team title in 1991, and Helen Chepn'geno took the first individual title in 1994. The junior women won in the inaugural year of their championships, 1989, with Esther Saina (3), Ann Mwangi (4), Jane Ekimat (5), and Tegla Loroupe (28). In 1991, Lydia Cheromei gave Kenya its first individual junior women's title.

Ondoro Osoro was a prolific cross country runner for many years. In 1991, he won the World IAAF Cross Challenge and was runner-up the following year. The "secret" ingredient in Osoro's training was hard hill running. "I would run two times in the week up a long steep hill in Nakuru for about 12 kilometers." Ondoro did not take this session at an easy pace, either. "Yes, I would be sweating hard after this one!" laughed Ondoro, who has a 27:24 personal record for the 10,000m.

"Have you run in the mud yet?" asked *Simon Chemoiywo*. "It is very good, builds up good strength, makes running in Europe much easier." When the rains fall on the red dirt roads, a glutinous "honey" surface is formed. The mud clings in clumps to your shoes, making them extremely heavy. The hip muscles strain to lift the limbs. Undoubtedly, training under such conditions builds up incredible leg strength and mental mettle that truly makes the Kenyans believe that over smoother surfaces they will be unbeatable.

"It does not matter whether you run the 800 meters or the marathon, the cross country training is very important; it builds strength for all distances," says *Kip Cheruiyot*.

William Sigei looked to emulate the great John Ngugi in the early 1990s. In fact, it was a victory over Ngugi in a local 5000m race that catapulted Sigei to the forefront of Kenyan athletics. He was thereupon recruited by the Kenyan Air Force team, and his career took off. He twice won the Kenyan national cross country title (1993 and 1994) and in the same years he won the World Championships title. On the track, Sigei will always be remembered for cutting over six seconds from Yobes Ondieki's year-old 10,000m world record in Oslo, 1994. At this writing, Sigei was building a new house on a piece of land he calls "Oslo," in the town of Bomet.

"My tactic was to start very fast and maintain the pace," he says. The tactic worked; very few could match Sigei's speed endurance. Simeon Rono, a neighbor of Sigei's, remembers that Sigei would nearly always train alone. At the pace he churned out his miles, it had to be that way! "Sigei trained *very* hard; when that man is motivated, he is the best runner in Kenya," adds Rono. Sigei's favorite session was the regulated fartlek advocated by Mike Kosgei—two minutes hard with one minute easy over a 10K course. Even though the altitude exceeded 2000 meters and route was quite hilly, Sigei would run this session in about 31 minutes.

The Armed Forces use cross country training generally from November to March. Basically the schedule is carbon-copied week in, week out. The work is seen as foundation training for any type of running. A typical week:

Monday	AM	40 90 min. "how you feel"
	Mid-day	Long run, starting steady and finishing fast, 1 hr. 30 min.
	PM	40 min. easy jogging
Tuesday	AM	Same as Monday AM
	Mid-day	Fartlek, 1 hr.
	PM	Same as Monday PM
Wednesday	AM	Same as Monday AM
	Mid-day	Tempo run, 70 min., extremely hard
	PM	Same as Monday PM
Thursday	AM	Same as Monday AM
	Mid-day	Hill work, 27 min. constant uphill
	PM	Same as Monday PM
Friday	AM	Same as Monday AM
	Mid-day	Steady run, 70 min., commonly up to full speed after 20 min.
	PM	Same as Monday PM
Saturday	AM	Same as Monday AM
	Mid-day	Tempo run, 60-80 min., flat out or competition
	PM	Rest.
Sunday	Rest day.	

The training is rather similar to that of the marathon runners, who often do cross country training before beginning their marathon buildup. Stephen Langat elucidates: "After my last marathon of the year, I rest for a few weeks; then I join the cross country runners for a couple of months. Three months before the first marathon of the year I change and begin marathon preparation." The main differences is the distances covered, the cross country runners tackling lesser mileage.

Mercy Jelimo Kosgei

Date of birth:	October 10, 1989
Birthplace:	Karona, Uasin Gishu
Height/Weight:	153 cm., 40-42 kg.
Personal best:	1500m, 4:11.7
Honors won:	2005 African Junior Championships, 1500m, silver
	2006 World Junior 1500m, silver
	2006 World Junior Cross Country, bronze
	2007 World Junior Cross Country, silver

"My parents were runners, they used to encourage me, telling me one day I would become a good runner. They also would tell me about Sally Barsosio to inspire me."

Kosgei would also see athletics in the newspaper or hear news on the radio; she really wanted to be an athlete. In December 2004, she was invited to Brother Colm's training camp. "I found it so difficult; I got injuries. There were times when I was 100 meters behind in the intervals but I kept myself with encouragement saying, 'One day you'll be there.'"

In 2005, Mercy went to Tunisia for the African Juniors. She returned with a silver medal and a new-found belief. "I have arrived. I have strong belief, especially now for Beijing." Thereon, Kosgei put in more training and concentrated harder on a set of exercises she had learned at the camp. "I was introduced to pilates, drills and exercises by an Australian coach called Rob (Higley)."

World Junior Cross Country Training Schedule

Monday	6 AM	40-45 min. easy running
	10 AM	30 min. at an average speed
	4 PM	Jog 20 min. and exercises
Tuesday	6 AM	30 min. easy
	10 AM	Fartlek, 35-40 min. of 2 min. hard, 2 –min. easy
	PM	Exercises, drills, and pilates
Wednesday	6 AM	30-40 min. easy
	10 AM	Average speed 30 min. on a flat road
	4 PM	30 min. easy
Thursday	6 AM	30-40 –min. easy
	10 AM	Track* 1200m (3:30), 1000m (2:54), 800m (2:20), 600m (1:48), 400m (65 sec.) with 2 min. rest
	PM	30 min.s easy to relax the muscles
Friday	AM	30 easy
	10 AM	40 min. easy
	4 PM	Exercises
Saturday	6 AM	30 min.
	10 AM	Long run on the Sing'ore road, 1 hr. 15 min.
	PM	Rest
Sunday	AM	One 60-min. run only

*For the track season this session becomes repeats of 600m, 400m, 300m, and 150 meters

Comments

"It was my first time to participate in the world cross. I was just a little scared. When the gun went, I was fine; I was good the whole way until the last 400 meters when I was passed. But I was so, so happy." Kosgei improved on the bronze to silver in 2007.

"I never have a day of total rest. I admire Tirunesh Dibaba; she is my role model. If I have the changing speed that she does, I try very much to run relaxed and easy. I work a lot on exercises, and I try to put in more focus with the training each year I run."

John Kamau Ngugi

Date of birth:	May 10, 1962
Birthplace:	Nyahururu, Kikuyu tribe.
Height/weight:	5'10" (178 cm.), 139 lbs. (63 kg.)
Kilometers per week:	When in hard training, 1987-1992, above 240
Personal bests:	3000m, 7:45.59
	5000m, 13:11.14

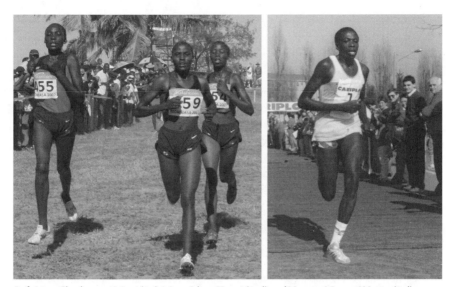

Left, Linet Chepkwemoi Masai (1st), Mercy Jelimo Kosgei (2nd), and Veronica Nyaruai Wanjiru (3rd), sweep the 2007 World Cross Country. (*Author*) John Ngugi, right, in the Cinque Mulini after winning the World Cross in 1987. Here he had to settle for second behind the late Paul Kipkoech. (*Cinque Mulini Archives*)

	10,000m, 27:11.62
	Half-marathon, 61:24
Honors:	1986–89, and 1992 World Cross Country champion
	1988 Olympic, 5000m champion
	1990 Commonwealth Games, 5000m, second (fell)
	1988 and 1989 Kenyan national, 5000m champion
	1987 All-African Games, 5000m champion
	1985 African Championships, 5000m, third
	1990 Commonwealth 10,000m record

When John Ngugi, of Ol Kalou in Nyandarua, was a child, he would run 10K daily, twice. Ngugi clocked those kilometers running to Munga Primary School in Nyandarua in the morning and home in the afternoon.

His first competition of note was the Kenyan Olympic trials in 1984, at which he finished fourth, five years after he started running competitively. "Some people encouraged me, others did not. Some people said I had a bad style," Ngugi remembered at the Mombasa World Cross Country Championships, where he was employed as a technical director. The World Cross brought Ngugi back into the limelight, as he, more than any other, had helped mold Kenya's fine name in cross country running.

In 1985, he enlisted in the Army. "It was my childhood dream to be in the Army." At first he would go to the running camps to help with the culinary responsibilities, though soon he, and others, discovered he was a much better runner than many of the athletes he was catering for each day.

The Kikuyu athlete started as a 1500m runner. When asked about his first international race, at the East and Central African Championships, in Cairo, Egypt, in 1985, he recalls this story. "The other athletes were warming up on the track and I, having no experience, presumed they were merely showing off their nice kits and shoes." Ngugi, irked by what he thought was an unnecessary show of bravado, vowed, "I'd show them who was best!" After a slow initial 800m in over two-minutes, Ngugi kicked, winning the title in 3:37.02. The trip abroad inspired him to take his training to another level. "You can say that I had the taste, and then I went for the meal."

The following year, 1986, he won the first of what would be a string of five World Cross Country titles, but, not without both a Herculean training plan and hitches along the way. In 1987, following a knee injury, Ngugi could only place 77th at the Kabarak National trials. I was not ready for the trial race, but knew I could run well at the Worlds," he says. The team threatened to strike if Ngugi was included in the squad, and Ngugi got no support from Mike Kosgei, who was then the team manager, "It was tribalism, they were all Kalenjins and did not want me on the team," explains Ngugi. James Kariuki, brother to John, recalled, "John, as a Kikuyu, was always the outsider. Now we are many runners, but in the 1980s it was all Nandi." However, Robert Ouko, in his official capacity, insisted that Ngugi would be on the team. In Warsaw, Poland, Ngugi did win, albeit after another Kenyan coach, possibly trying to sabotage Ngugi, tried to misdirect him off the course. "Two mzungo [white men] helped direct me back on course," recalls John. The following week at a smaller competition, the Cinque Mulini cross country, Ngugi finished second to Paul Kipkoech, proving that although Kipkoech may have been the better-prepared athlete, Ngugi could pull out the performance on the most important day.

It was that year that Ngugi displayed talents at the 5000m on the track, winning the African Championships in Nairobi—a victory that made Ngugi a national hero to this day. "Most Kenyans don't have a television, so for them to see a championships was a rare thing, and for me to win in a full stadium," recalled Ngugi, when flagging off a race as a Kenyan celebrity nearly thirty years later. "People still remember me for that race, more than the cross country wins."

The cross country in Auckland was another victory in 1988, and at Kilgari, where the national team trained, Ngugi started to get the reputation that marks his name with Kenyan runners to this day. He rose at 4:30 a.m. when others slept to run the first morning's training alone in the dark. He would slip back into bed and join the team at 6:00 a.m. for their run on the same course! "That's why we called him the Night Runner," jokes Joseph Cheromei.

At the Seoul Olympics, another incident sparked Ngugi's fire. "Domingos Castro told me, 'You can't run well on the track, only in the bush.' I think he was upset, he had not run well in the Cross, I think dropping out when I won one year." Coupled with the advice of Coach John Velzian (who Ngugi credits as being *the* big help), this was enough for Ngugi to take off and push hard from as early as three laps into the 12.5-lap race to open an unbridgeable gap that took him to one of the Games' most memorable winning performances. In 2007, Velzian reflected back on that day,

"Briefly what happened in the final arose very largely from his bad run semis, in which he spent almost the entire race running wide. After the race I calculated with him just how much extra he had run throughout the race and had him thoroughly understand that if he had run at the same pace in lane one he would have finished way ahead of everyone in the race. His ability to change the pace and not be unduly affected by doing so was already well known.

The plan therefore was for him to settle in comfortably and then make his move to the front group, where he would run with the pace for a couple of laps and then with six to go make his big break to the front. It was never intended that this should happen after only three laps and that he should go from last to way out front all in one move! Clearly, the intention was to run the legs off kickers like Baumann and Castro, who I was very confident would not go with him with the sudden injection of pace that I knew John could produce, but who would run him out of the medals if it came to a fast finish in the final straight.

It all sounds very simple now, but there was a lot for John, as the world's greatest cross country runner, to have to thoroughly understand for this to succeed. Especially his lap and kilometers times following the break, as well as continuing to read what was happening behind him by continuously looking at the big screen and maintaining the distance between himself and those who followed. Memories!

After winning the World Cross Country again at Stavanger, Norway, in 1989, for two years Ngugi was beset by injuries for two years that curtailed his winning streak. However, he returned to win in Boston in 1992. The extreme cold conditions could not hinder John, as he plowed through snow for the first time in his life to capture his last title."

Comments

"Never give up; just work hard." Ngugi believes that the key to success is to build the body with training loads that would scare the average athlete. "Back in 1990 we were training together and it was supposed to be an easy day, as we'd trained very hard the day before. Well, Ngugi decides to do a few kilometer repeats—he does twenty!" laughed Richard Chelimo, himself remembered as a formidable trainer. Ngugi often liked to run that bit farther than his training partners. Kosgei says, "Ngugi would get up an hour earlier than everybody else and run an extra ten kilometers." Ngugi believes in using low-key races as part of training. After finishing 108th (!) in a Kenya AAA cross country race, he smiled, "This is all part of the ongoing process of training. In Kenya I am always expected to win, but during hard training it is impossible." This reinforces Chelimo's point that when the buildup period takes place all else must be secondary, even competition.

Best advice: "Discipline, hard discipline is the answer to all running success."

Training Sample: Training for Cross Country, Kenya, Winter, the Main Day's Session

Day 1:   40-50 min. easy

Day 2:   Hill work, repeats up a steep 300m gradient

Day 3:   2 hrs. ending hard

Day 4:   10 x 1K, cross country, short rest

Day 5:   70 min. steady

Day 6:   Some form of hill work

Day 7   Fartlek or intervals (15 x 400m, short jog rest).

Day 8:   70 min. steady

Day 9:   Cross country intervals (10 x 1K, short jog rest)

Day 10:   1 hr. steady.

Day 11:   Hill work, 25 x 200m

Day 12:   1 hr., strong finish.

Day 13:   Long run, 90 min.

Day 14:   Fartlek over 15K, hilly terrain

Track Training

Quality with quantity was Ngugi's successful recipe. He believed in maintaining a large workload in the summer buildup period, often combining heavy distance runs in the morning with hard track sessions later in the day. The day's key session:

> 20-30 x 400m run in 62-65 sec., with 100m jog rest
>
> 15-20 x 1000m run in 2:40-2:50, with 200m jog rest
>
> 3 x 5000m, run under 15:00, 3 min. jog recovery
>
> 10 x 800m, run in 2 min, with an equal recovery

"This I would use to build speed." Often the "cool down" would become a tempo session. "If I felt strong then I would train hard, yes, hard!" He had no qualms about training hard the day prior to competition.

Typically Ngugi would run a session at 6:00 a.m., as with the majority of the Armed Forces team. He would cover 12-20K at a pace he would call "steady." Mere mortals would call the pace "fast." Try 1 hour 10 minutes for a 22K very hilly morning run as a warm-up for the day's main session! In the afternoon a stroll, light exercises, or a slow run would be taken at 3:00 p.m. or so.

Before each of the speed sessions a warm-up, consisting of jogging for 15 minutes and some light exercising and stretching, would be undertaken to "wake" the body. Ngugi had the ability to push his body harder and harder, even if he trained by himself.

Ngugi would often be a mere mortal himself before the training camps. Mike Kosgei remembers the period before the 1992 camp. "Let's just say Ngugi was not all that focused on running. However, when I brought him away from the town and into the camp, he focused totally on training." The result was another cross country title.

An unfortunate note to the Ngugi story is the misunderstanding over a drug test that cost him a suspension from the athletics world in 1993. It was the first year the IAAF had initiated home visits to check athletes for possible doping violations. Deplorably, no one told Ngugi, who was accustomed to giving samples at stadiums or athletics centers. Kenya is a poor country and opportunists abound. Ngugi has to arrange for guards at his general store. Suspicion of strangers is natural, especially after the experiences Ngugi has had. When the IAAF official arrived, Ngugi's explanation is that he thought him to be a fan seeking a photo or a handshake. He completely misunderstood the whole situation, which resulted in the official having to leave empty-handed.

Ngugi committed an offense under the rules of the IAAF, technically equal to an admission of taking a banned substance. Despite a number of appeals from the Kenyan federation, reinstatement came only after more than two and a half years of the suspension had been served. Ngugi lost $80,000 fighting the case. "I was promised I would get compensations of a million dollars," said Ngugi. It was a lawsuit in which everyone ended up a loser. Ngugi's weight ballooned and his conditioning during the suspension was nonexistent. "Ah, to come back in Kenya is so hard. Ngugi can return to good form, but it would take years for him to build up his form again to the level he was when he was at his best, and Ngugi is an old man now," commented William Sigei. Ten years after the fact, after many attempts, Ngugi never managed to regain the heights, and he retired from the sport.

Paul Tergat, the Caesar of the Sport

Date of birth:	June 17, 1969
Birthplace:	Riwa, Baringo
Height/weight:	5' 11-1/2" (182cm.), 130 lbs. (59kg.)
Training sessions:	Two per day. Usually the first run at 06.00 and the second at 10.00. "Like most Kenyans, I have trained three times a day, but I find two is enough."
Kilometers per week:	Not less than 200-210K
World records:	10,000m
	Half-marathon
	Marathon
	15K on the road
	20K on the road
Personal bests:	1500m, 3:45.91;
	2000m, 5:01.5
	3000m, 7:28.70
	5000m, 12:49.87
	10,000m, 26:27.85
	15K (road), 42:13
	Half-marathon, 59:17 (59:06, aided)
	Marathon, 2:04:55 (WR)
Honors:	1996 and 2000, Olympic 10,000m, silver-second
	2004 Athens Olympic Marathon, 10th
	1995-1999 World Cross Country Champion
	2000 World Cross Country Champion, 3rd
	1995 World Championships 10,000m, 3rd
	1997, 1999 Word Championships 10,000m, 2nd
	1999, 2000 World Half-Marathon Champion

The training camp of the Moi Air Base is just outside N'gong town by a couple of kilometers. The athletes stay together in Spartan living conditions, iron bunks and two dozen roommates or more per tent. The wind easily blows under the loose-fitting canvas flaps of the large Armed Forces shelters, not only bringing a chill to the air but also allowing the odd wandering creature an entry. The talk, however, is upbeat and encouraging; everyone is preparing for the day's second run, and the clock has not yet struck 8:00 a.m.

One man moves around instead of sitting on the bunks as the others do. He talks to the fringe runners whilst carrying a battered tin cup of chai, giving each athlete a word of support. "You can do it, hang with us today. You'll be flying the flag when us boys have retired." His eye wanders to the up-and-coming athletes, and he'd make them feel they belonged, pushing them to give that bit extra to the day's run.

That was a decade ago, and the standard bearer for Kenyan running remains very much the same orator today. Meet Mr. Paul Kibii Tergat.

Joshua Chelanga's description of the dialogue with Tergat, the limber Kenyan, is nothing less than sheer adulation. "I remember the early days in those tents, wanting to go home, running and thinking 'I can never make it with these guys.' And I remember Tergat telling me, 'Oh, yes you can make it.' And yes, I finally did, thanks to him; I ran 2:07:05."

The pedigree of the man is on a plane beyond superlative: five consecutive World Cross Country titles, two Olympic and three World Championships silver medals on the track (plus a bronze), two World Half-Marathon Championships, and world-record-breaking performances at the 10,000m, half-marathon,, and marathon distances. Do not ask how many World Championships medals he has, including team hardware; there are too many for counting.

The Architect Behind the Design
Dr. Gabriele Rosa, a former runner and now a coach, gets results; about that, nobody can argue. A guru whose passion transcends any personal gain; he is a man who breaks the bread with the athletes he coaches. You rarely see Rosa when the cameras are flashing, but when the sun is bubbling the tarmac, and the runners are laboriously clocking the routine miles, he is there for them. In the mid-1990s, he was always the bearded *mzungo* (white person) in the SUV, trailing the runners for hours upon hours on the dried-out dirt roads up in the Rift Valley. His window rolled down, dust in his throat, he was always quietly offering words of encouragement to the pack as they completed another long run.

Tergat met Rosa through Moses Tanui's introductions. They have been together for the full length of his career, starting in 1991, though in recent years Tergat has taken more command of his own training. Dr. Rosa has helped guide Tergat from a cross-country celebrity to a track star (still the third fastest man ever over 10,000m with his 26:27.85) and on to become the world record-holder in the marathon.

Turning to the Marathon: "It's for my family that I run."
It was not toil and talent, however, that took Tergat, from a family of 17 siblings, to the 42.2-kilometer event. It was the affection and desire to be with his kin. A few years ago, Tergat was drinking milky tea on a hot afternoon, with his children playing in the gated garden, when he revealed how much he pined for the simple things in life, like watching

his children grow up. "Life on the track is hard; you are away from home for so long. More time than you are here, home." As the last word lingered on his lips, his eyes drifted over to his wife of thirteen years, Monica Chemtai, a qualified nurse. She had studied hard in college, even after Tergat had "made it" financially, to better herself and the family.

The whole summer, Tergat, the Tugen runner, would be based in the old Gallic town of Brescia in northern Italy, along with a large group of Fila athletes. He reasoned, "If I run the marathon, then I can be here, with them," he points to where his children Ronnie and Harriet were playing "Go over just for the race, and come straight back to Kenya." With his thin hand, Tergat mimes an airplane swooping down and straight back up. "For me, Kenya is the best place in the world. For me and for my family," stresses Tergat, who became a father for the fourth time in 2006 with the arrival of another daughter to follow

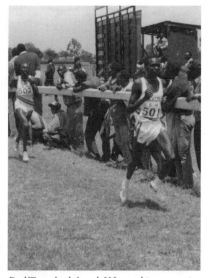

Paul Tergat leads Joseph Kibor on his way to winning the Armed Forces Cross Country title, 1996. (*Author*)

Lilly, who was born in 1999. Already at this time, most of his business interests were in Kenya, like the company he shared with Tanui, Borborei Freighters Ltd., based in Nairobi.

The marathon did not come as easy to Tergat as running success had back in 1991, a mere year after he had begun, when he was dominating the domestic races. Within one year of beginning to train, the young Kenyan had become a kingpin among his highly talented group of peers.

The story began in 1987. His late father, Kipkuna Arap Tuetok, took him on a trip to Nairobi to watch the last day's finals at the All-African Games. To say that he was inspired is an understatement. "It was a great atmosphere. I remember best the 4 x 400-meter relay. Kenya was leading, but then lost to the Nigerians [3:00.55 to 3:01.00]; we [the crowd] were very disappointed." Upon arriving home, Tergat started running. A Baringo coach of the Kongasis Athletics training camp, William K. Tomno, remembers the young Tergat. "I saw him winning the Baringo District cross country, he was good, he ran so easy. I knew he had real talent." According to Tomno, it was hard for Tergat to continue. "He had some problems, he was close to giving up in 1989." Tomno talked to a friend of his, a fellow coach called Willie Komen who worked at the Moi Air Base, and he agreed to take Tergat.

The Early Years

The town of Kabarnet, in the Baringo District, Rift Valley Province, is 265 kilometers northwest of Kenya's capital city, Nairobi. Tergat was born in the village of Riwo, just outside Kabarnet. Its inhabitants come from the Tugen tribe. The town is not noted for its abundance of elite athletes in the fashion of the more renowned and illustrious neighboring towns of Iten, Kapsabet, and Eldoret, due to the extreme heat that scorns the daytime hours. The town is best known as the birthplace of the Daniel Arap Moi, the country's longest reigning president (1978-2002).

Jackson Kipn'ogk, another of the town's running superstars and the current masters world record-holder for ten miles, says of his district, "You must struggle to run well in Kabarnet. It [the heat] will kill you. But if you make it [(pause for an "Ah"] then you *make* it."

Tergat, whose family name translates in the Kalenjin tongue to "bent neck," joined the Armed Forces Moi Air Base division in 1990 with the main objective of providing a stable income for his family. Starting workouts with the running team, he had the chance to meet with the athletes who had competed in the Olympic Games, and he was encouraged to discover they were human, just like himself. "I thought, "Why not me?" When you are in the environment, you get belief that you too can achieve." Willy Komen greatly encouraged and inspired Tergat to take athletics to the next level. Komen, who is still coaching in N'gong, recognized at once the talent of the Tugen, and Tergat today gives the coach the credit for his first drive to become a great runner, noting, "Yes, you can say it was him who started it for me."

The runner himself did pay his dues in the department of sweat, striving, and struggles; Tergat trained, and still trains, in a remorseless and relentless mode. Back in the early 1990s, he would run hill repeats until he collapsed at the mound's summit from faintness and fatigue. Simon Chemoiywo, a training partner from that era, remembers, "He would never give up. You knew he was something special, something about him was always giving more than anyone else could." In 1991, Tergat showed signs of talent as he recorded 29:46.8 for his debut 10,000m at a competition in a May race in Nairobi.

Coming to America, and the Testing Years

In 1992, Tergat was selected to represent his country at the World Cross Country Championships, to be held at Franklin Park, Boston. He had just won his first national title and had beaten many illustrious stars. Mike Kosgei, the team coach, had tipped Tergat to upset Khalid Skah, the defending champion from Morocco, who had taken the past two editions of the race from amidst a Kenyan stranglehold in the 1980s. Kosgei was rarely, if ever, wrong with his predictions and he was sure Tergat was undefeatable. At the training camp at Mount Embu, Tergat was working out like a fireball, burning each and every session. Perhaps he went a little too hard, as injury struck, and Tergat was relegated to watching the race on a television set from a hotel room in Boston. "It was the most disappointing point in my entire athletics career, even up to this day," he remembers. It was a taxing time, and the superb athlete came close to throwing in the towel and concentrating more intently on his military career.

By August of that year, he was back in competition running his first overseas race, the Amatrice-Configno event in Italy, as part of the Fila team, but he was not getting the results anticipated by his fellow athletes. "I came down in weight too quickly. Sure, I could run well, but I did not have any strength. I used to finish training sessions close to fainting." He also finished fifth at the World Half Marathon Championships, running 61:03.

Injuries hindered his progress until 1995, when he accomplished his first of what would be many World Cross Country Championships wins, at Durham in the North of England. Paul ran with the pack until Mike Kosgei waved his hand and unleashed the tall Baringo athlete's full force; Paul immediately opened up a 100m gap on the best in the world.

One month later, Tergat became only the second person to dip under the hour for the half-marathon distance. (Today no man has run under the hour more times than he has.) Later that summer, this superlative form brought him World Championships 10,000m bronze medal in Göteborg, the 27:14:70 was another personal best.

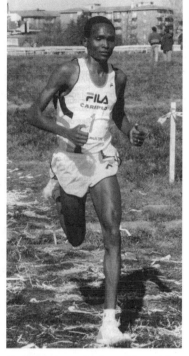

Paul Tergat is popular the world round, but especially in Italy where he has spent a good deal of his professional running career. Here he winns in 1996 at the famous Cinque Mulini cross country. (*Cinque Mulini Archives*)

The following year, even the Kenyan newspapers had conceded that the new superman of the sport, Haile Gebrselassie, would take Tergat's title when the Cross Country World Championships moved to South Africa. Haile said he wished to win on African soil, and after setting new world records at the 5000m, indoors and out, the 10,000m, and winning the World Championships 10,000m he was a hot favorite.

Meanwhile, training in the N'gong hills was a man who knew only one thing; he who trains hardest wins. "If someone beats me, then I am happy for him; he will have obviously worked harder for the result than I did," says the gracious Tergat. For Paul, the season was shaping up well, with a couple of cross country victories and a close loss to Moses Tanui, hardly a disgrace.

The national championships were Tergat's first major test. "The important race is in South Africa. It is only important for me to run a good race in the nationals. My family does not have the opportunity to see me compete often, so here is a good opportunity," he said. His family was there in force, and they expected victory. Paul did not disappoint them. He ran with the lead pack until the planned breakaway point at 8K, and then cantered home to win his third national title.

The following week was the IAAF Cross Country Challenge in Nairobi. Few foreigners bothered to come to this race. It is strenuous enough to try to run with Kenyans when they are on foreign soil, but on home ground and at altitude, it is a fruitless endeavor. The contest was one of the hardest to win, due to the fact that 60 of the best Kenyans were entered. However, Tergat won easily; he was in great form. The attention of the sportswriters started to drift south, from Addis Ababa back to Kenya.

The World Championships turned out to be a runaway for the Kenyan team. Tergat's plan was to remain with the group until the last couple of kilometers, then slip away to capture his second world title. The first 10K went in 27:57, an unbelievable pace in cross country. In the 11th kilometer, when inevitable weariness was setting in, Tergat made his move. At the same moment, a tired Gebrselassie stumbled at a log obstacle; when he looked up, Tergat was gone. The last 1500m was run in 3:45, equal to Tergat's track best! Some observers mentioned that if Gebrselassie had not tripped then maybe the result would have been different. However, cross country barriers, as in the steeplechase, are there to make the race more challenging. If you do not get over them properly, it is usually due to fatigue. Also, the stumble was a mere moment and the gap between them at the finish was 44 seconds (Gebrselassie finished 5th.)

The prestigious Stramilano half-marathon seemed a good site to exploit some of Tergat's wonderful form. Like many Kenyans in the 1990s, Paul was sponsored by Fila, the Italian sports brand. So Stramilano Italia it was. Tergat knew he would fly on the roads so he wasted no time on tactics. When the gun fired, he blasted away, covering the first 10km in 27:37 and 15km in under 42 minutes. His outstanding finishing time of 58:51 would not stand officially as the course was remeasured to be 49 meters short, equivalent perhaps to eight seconds.

The summer season was capped by Tergat's much-lauded silver medal at the 1996 Atlanta Olympics. Tergat had finished fourth, suffering from cramps, behind Josephat Machuka, Paul Koech, and William Kiptum in the Kenyan trials. His international experience and proven results, however, convinced the selectors to include him in the Olympic team.

The Olympic final saw Koech nobly handling the early work. Tergat took off with a 60-second lap with 2K remaining. That last 2K was run in 5:05, a world-class time for the distance. Gebrselassie, however, was able to out kick Tergat in the final 400m, though Paul held on very well to finish less than a second behind, 27:07.34 to 27:08:17. Gebrselassie's time was an Olympic record.

Many had predicted slow times in the distance events due to the sauna-like conditions in Atlanta. Thanks to the Kenyans, though, the results were swifter than expected. Tergat was rewarded with a new personal best, albeit for just one month. In Brussels in August, he became just the fifth man in history to break 27 minutes in the 10,000m.

Starting intensive training in November for the 1997 World Cross Country Championships, Tergat again reached superb form and raced to his third straight win. He would win five straight titles becoming the first ever man to reach such a feat.

"I can't accept to have all this pain for nothing, sacrificing myself. It is for my family I run."

The Community Runner

The green mist rose from the district known as South Africa, in the N'gong hills. Groups of three and four runners start to converge upon the Armed Forces camps. The Navy have a large contingent today, perhaps due to Paul Tergat, who has chosen to join the runners this morning. Tergat is in his "light" training mode, though he still lopes over the countryside a good 100 meters ahead of the other runners.

"Every year I have periods when I do not train so hard. This is one such time [in December]. Often with the reduced training I will not eat lunch, to keep my weight." Even at a distance, Tergat's stride, which has given him numerous world championships, allows even an untrained eye to see that this athlete is very special. Tergat's talents are mostly displayed on the roads and racing circuits of Europe, though in the last few

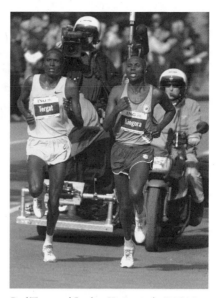

Paul Tergat and Stephen Kiagora in the ING New York City Marathon. (*Alison Wade*)

years the Tugen tribesman has branched out and now has import/export companies in Kenya, co-owns an athletics magazine, and helps with sending rookie Kenyans to foreign races.

Tergat also owns a large building in Kabarnet called the Sportsman Inn that houses offices and a café/hotel. In 2004, he was appointed an Ambassador for the World Food Program. This is an especially dear cause to Paul, who received food aid as an eight-year-old school child when at the Riwo Primary School. "I know what it means to go hungry," he says. Like the majority of rural Kenyans, life was not always easy for Tergat.

Sensitive yet bold, Tergat has managed to remain true to himself through a life starting in poverty and now full of the comforts of affluence. Recently, the Kenyan formed his own charity. In September at a hotel in Nairobi, the inception of the Paul Tergat Foundation was announced, its mission being to support children and groups from extremely deprived and destitute areas to attain nutritional support and guidance in the matters of survival. He has not forgotten how, in his formative years, hunger played a role in his own life.

Tergat's legacy will last far longer than the rich and enduring memories we have of him performing as a magnificent athlete. The Senior Sergeant shall be timeless in the history books. He is a man with a myriad of qualities. "My life is not solely dependent on running," he asserts. "I am doing many other things."

In his 2004 acceptance speech for an honorary degree bestowed upon him by the College of Bloomfield in New Jersey, he was most eloquent in summing up what he is all about. "My background introduced me to a life that demanded sheer hard work and persistent struggle, especially to get the basic necessities of daily living. We had no source of income, besides absence of arable land to till for any reasonable farming. Schools were not only distant, but lacking in facilities for any effective learning. Life was unpredictable, difficult, and hostile. Interestingly, these are the same experiences that imparted in me virtues that lead to success: hard work, determination, and the will to conquer all odds, as well as the values of honesty, respect and excellence."

There is no doubt that this latest venture of Tergat's, his Foundation, will reach great heights. A friend of the Kenyan, Wendy Abma of Ridgewood New Jersey, says, "When he has an idea or project in mind, he doesn't hand it off to someone else to see it through, he does it himself with a contagious energy."

Turning to the Marathon

It is for the money that most Kenyan runners start to run marathons, and thus it is refreshing to hear Tergat talk of the reasons why he turned to the marathon to end his illustrious career. "The most important thing to me is my family here in Kenya. If I run marathons, I will be able to spend more time with them and less time on the road traveling to meets." Indeed, in the last few years, Paul has filled nine passports with stamps from his travels around the globe.

Before his marathon debut, Paul commented, "After [Moses] Tanui first ran New York in 1993, he told me that he could not even remember his own name. I know the marathon is a very difficult event. A lot of people have just doubled my half-marathon time and added a few minutes, but you know, it is not that simple!"

Leaving cross country and track was not an easy decision. Prior to setting the marathon world record, Tergat thought his best-ever achievement was run in Brussels. "Everybody said, 'He can only run cross country, he can only run on the roads. The world record at [10,000m] was the most satisfying race I have ever run." After following the pace of countrymen past the 7K mark, Tergat went on to lower the 10,000m mark to 26:27:85 in August 1997.

Before that race Tergat trained extremely hard, completing such sessions as:

2 or 3 x 3000m with 4 min. rest, run as close to 8 min. as possible

1 x 3000m @ near to 8 min., rest 2 min.

2 x 2000m @ near to 5:20. Rest 2 min., 4 x 1000m @ 2:35 to 2:30 with 1.5 min. rest

Or:

25 x 400, starting with 60–61 sec. and moving down to 57 sec. all with 1 min. rest

Or:

Structured 10K, alternating 30 sec. fast, 30 sec. slow

These sessions, and numerous other speed workouts (up to five per week), were performed in St. Moritz, Switzerland, at an altitude of 2000m.

Throughout his career, Paul has always ran at least one half-marathon a year. This is done because he believes that the training for the half is of benefit to both track and road competitions.

Complimentary sessions would be morning runs of around 18-20K at a pace that Paul would find neither demanding nor too easy. Flexibility also plays an important role. Paul has devised a routine that fits his long slender muscles. He works religiously on the hamstrings and he is able to hoist his stretched leg to surprising heights.

Tergat's beautiful house sits at the top of a long, rocky, steep hill in a district of Zambia. As far as the eye can see there are rolling green hills. Training loops with telling names such as "The Satellite" and "Mt. Cheruiyot" are randomly selected, though Paul rarely repeats the same loop twice in one week. "It is more interesting when you vary the routes, and around here you are spoiled for choice. I usually choose the route when I begin running."

But to what does Tergat attribute his incredible longevity in athletics? "I'm a true sportsman; whatever I do I do with an interest. I love the sport and like to test my limit. Why not try to maximize if all goes well?" he asks. "One's lifestyle depends very much on success. If you like a lavish lifestyle, then I don't think this sport is for you. Don't be despondent, either, with setbacks. In 1992, with my hamstring problems [at the national training camp in Kigari], I thought my career was over. But now I have achieved all my dreams. Have patience."

The meat of his training revolves around a figure of approximately 250K per week. It used to be slightly less (210K) when racing cross country and half-marathons. Most parts of the year he does two runs per day, occasionally creeping up to three a day. "I believe for a peak in March [World Cross Country Champions] and again for the Olympics," he says. A long run is included each week, though the distance is secondary to holding a good pace. "I train mostly with the guys from the Armed Forces. I have been running a long time, so I know if I need to make any adjustments with my training."

Tergat found training for cross country the easiest, though with mud, barriers, and hills, the transition is hard when coming from a road or track season. "If I have finished a cross season, then moving to the roads or track is much easier. Though I do find track training tedious, being in the same place," he smiles, gazing across the Rift Valley and its inviting undulations.

As a matter of interest, Tergat walked only 400m to the Kapkawa School as a child. He first knew that he could be a great runner when, in 1992, he defeated John Ngugi to win a national title. However, he was quick to rightly point out, "You may have the talent, but without hard training you will never arrive in athletics."

"Ambassador" is a fitting title for this reserved, modest man. He greets all as though they were his brothers. He rarely talks of his triumphs, and he seemingly has time for everyone. When edged into talking about victories Tergat will mention that his fifth World Cross Country title at Belfast was very special. "It was an extremely muddy, slanting course, and I had to slide to negotiate the corners. Also that I was going for that unprecedented fifth title, and was a little anxious, scared, and also excited."

However, more than about victories, he likes to talk of the many positives of the sport outside the glory moments. One of the most enjoyable parts of athletics, he finds, comes from sitting with fellow runners relaxing after a race. "Many different nationalities sitting free of politics, united by athletics."

In the 2000 Olympic 10,000m, lap after lap rolled by, and still no runner made a significant move. It was a duel that had the running journalists worldwide licking their lips; Tergat vs. Haile Gebrselassie. At the last Olympics (Atlanta) and the last two World Championships (Athens, Seville), Gebrselassie had defeated Tergat in titanic clashes at the 10,000m. Would Sydney finally be Tergat's day? Further drama was added with Tergat having to run a 10,000m a month prior to the Games to convince officials in Kenya of his right to be in the Olympic Games. Another mystery was Gebrselassie in good form? Where had he been all season?

All this and more was answered in the final 250 meters of the Australian track. It was a monumental battle of less than thirty seconds, the agony etched visibly on each warrior's face, their muscles wrenched through pain barriers. It was such an intimate moment, both exquisite yet vicious, that it almost felt wrong to observe their struggle. Tergat unleashed a savage kick that would have slain all other mortal runners. To the last few meters the taller man stayed a chest ahead of the proud Ethiopian, who was in a desperate, all-out sprint of his own, willing himself forward, saying that the impossible was possible.

Gebrselassie lunged ahead in the final two strides, to win by the smallest margin ever in an Olympic 10,000m. the runners were separated by nine-hundredths of a second, closer than the 100m final! It would be the two titans final match-up on the track.

The race, however, merely enhanced the legends of both runners. When Tergat was initially selected for the 5000m event, earlier that summer, he withdrew, saying a victory at the Olympics would be hollow without Gebrselassie in the field. Imagine! Tergat will always be linked with the Ethiopian, over field and hillock Tergat ruled; the track was Gebrselassie's domain. Their battles on the roads are not over.

In 2001, with a publicized $300,000 appearance figure, Tergat ran his debut marathon in London, placing second in 2:08:15 behind the then-reigning New York champion, Morocco's Abdelkader El Mouaziz (2:07:09). For a man who had run a half-marathon in 59:06 at Lisbon in 2000, a 2:08 clocking was not quite the hoped-for success. Tergat was disappointed, and he vowed to train harder. He had relocated to Kaptagat, at a higher altitude than N'gong, as many of Kenya's leading marathon runners trained at this locale.

"Some people at this time were telling me, 'Paul, you are not a marathoner, you are too tall (5'11")to make it.'" Tergat, at 132 pounds, did not listen. "I have always believed nothing is impossible if you set your mind to it," he affirms.

At Chicago a few months later, he was outpaced by the Kenyan rabbit, Ben Kimondiu (2:08:52), taking another runner-up spot in 2:08:56. The following spring, back in London, he improved dramatically to a 2:05:48, then the third-fastest time ever recorded, but behind the day's winner, Khalid Khannouchi. Khannouchi had to break his own world record to defeat Tergat, running 2:05:38.

"This is when I knew I had the potential!" laughs Tergat, looking back on what has now been dubbed the "Clash of the Titans" (Paul's longtime friend and greatest rival, Haile Gebrselassie, was also in the field and finished third in 2:06:35). Returning to

Chicago in 2002, Tergat proved the fast time was no fluke as he nailed a 2:06:18 in fourth place.

London in 2003 had five men charging down the homestretch, with the then-reigning Olympic champion, Gezahegne Abera of Ethiopia, taking the win in 2:07:56. Tergat was again fourth (2:07:59).

Then, in the Fall of 2003, "it" happened. The "it" was what almost every sports journalist had speculated upon since Tergat broke the hour for the first time in the half-marathon back in Milan in 1995: his world marathon record. "My greatest moment in my career! Without question," he exclaims.

On a perfect day in Berlin, a group of Doctor Rosa's athletes put together a well-executed plan, resulting in Tergat setting a world best of 2:04:55. The only hiccup came when Tergat and the remaining pacemaker, Sammy Korir, passed through the Brandenburg Gate. It looked as though Tergat would again be defeated. "I nearly had a heart attack, I can say," race director Horst Milde recalled of the moment Tergat took an indirect route and inadvertently allowed Korir to close a developing gap. Luckily, however, Tergat triumphed, and took a gargantuan 43 seconds off the previous record.

He ran the race with negative splits. Asked why he said that he had the confidence to do this, based on his training. To approach the race from the angle of not slowing, but speeding up toward the end, he thought, would give him a "better mental boost."

Tergat's Splits: 5K, 15:01; 10K, 29:58 (14:57); 15K, 44:46 (14:48); 20K, 59:45 (14:59); 21.1K, 1:03:04; 25K, 1:14:43 (14:58); 30K, 1:29:25 (14:42); 35K, 1:44:00; 40K, 1:58:38 (14:38); final 2.2K, 6:17 (14:15 pace!)

On Tergat's return to Kenya, thousands came to meet the country's new national hero, the nation's first male ever to hold the world record at the marathon distance. He was given the tradition warrior's garb of animal skins and dress, and drank many a *sortet* (a Kenyan calabash) of *mursiik* (soured milk) in celebration. The greatest honor bestowed by the Tugen tribe, to be named a Tugen Elder, was also given to the champion.

Shortly after claiming the world record in Berlin, Tergat attended an unrelated marathon event, fulfilling duties to his sponsors at the race expo. At a nightclub, where the post-race party was being held, the Kenyan slid into the room unnoticed and moved to the back of the hall, then departed quickly after he had cheered and applauded for the winners. When asked why he did not light up the event by announcing his attendance, he stated modestly, "I don't want to reveal my presence. Today is their night to shine," he indicated, pointing toward his fellow athletes up on the stage. That's Tergat.

Tergat was expected to challenge for the Olympic gold in Athens in 2004. At the previous two Olympics, he had won silvers on the track at 10,000ms. But the marathon in Athens was not to be Tergat's crowning moment. Still he finished a proud tenth, fighting a side stitch, a struggle that probably endeared him to a slew of recreational runners, showing that world record-holders are mortal! "For sure it was not easy. I had to finish, and that made me proud that I did, because you cannot be a champion every day." Tergat smiles as he recalls the day when fluids turned his stomach to a writhing knot, "I would never have dropped out." He insists, "Every success and failure is what inspires me. A real champion is judged not by his best performance but on his ability to rise from his worst performance to rise again. There are no short-cuts in this sport; you either work hard, or you quit. I am not a quitter."

New York, New York

Every champion wants a New York Marathon win on the resumé; Lisa Ondieki said her win in the Big Apple surpassed her Olympic medal. Tergat came to New York looking for Olympic redemption. It was a telling statement he made days before the race. "At the end of the day, if you are not ready after 35 kilometers, then you are not in the race. I think I am a veteran now and have a lot of experience. Most important is to run your own race. My competitors, they know that, too."

The world record-holder's training for this event has been a colossal accumulation of mileage (again up to180 miles per week), with long runs up to 40K and, of course, quality speed work. "Most days, it is two times per day. The marathon is not a 10K race; a high mileage allows me to take the punishment of the event," observes Tergat.

A dramatist could not have scripted a more elegant finish. The final two miles were a picture of beauty yet pain; a show of strength, but with struggle; a battle befitting the ages. "I was running blind," said South African Hendrick Ramaala, who was the defending champion. He and Tergat ran stride, for stride embracing fatigue and anguish. The ride was no easier for Tergat, who remembered, "I was worried I might fall or stumble, I went so deep, so deep." Those who have greatness bestowed upon them are expected to perform great acts.

In a magnificent final charge on Central Park's West Drive, Tergat out-leaned Ramaala by three-tenths of a second. "Ramaala says that it was good for me [winning], But I won't say that it was bad or good. It was the [most] painful win that I've ever witnessed in my life." recalled Tergat after the event.

Tergat's tactics to run major city marathons are:

Don't come into the race over-raced; you must be sharp for the event.

Read the race as it develops; don't have a set plan that cannot be changed en route.

Always remain in contact [with the lead group].

Don't line up unless you are ready to give your best.

Check out the course for tight turns or things that may affect your rhythm.

The Future

Tergat's vocation is unambiguous. "I want to bring awareness. When I travel, I see waste; I see debates on overeating on the TV and seeing how much food one can eat, when people are starving elsewhere. Did you know that for 17 cents, you can provide food for a day for an African child?" He reasons, "Instead of going for that dessert, to donate a few coins can feed someone. Think of that."

Although Tergat's records have been erased from the books, he will indelibly remain, for all time, a legend who looms larger than life.

Comments

"Go into competition with confidence from your training." Paul makes the point about specific training; look at the needs of your event and train accordingly. The balance between family and training is also important. "I live close to the Armed Forces camp, but not with the other runners. This suits me, as if I need training partners, they are there, but it allows me to be with my family. I like to be able to relax with my family in front of the TV, playing with the kids." Determination, sacrifice, and discipline are three key words that crop up often when Tergat talks about his training background. "Without a lot of self-sacrifice I would never have made it. It takes discipline to train day in, day out. If you are not determined to do your best, then it is better not to try at all." Tergat feels that a lot of Western athletes are too quick to erect mental barriers. "In Kenya there is the belief that if you train hard you will succeed. This we have proven. Also focus, focus on the event you are training for. If it is the marathon, then make the training plan for the marathon. If it is cross country then let it be cross county."

Training Sample for Cross Country

High quality is the watchword. The body should be fresh to be able to handle the speed sessions, Tergat believes. This is also the reason that he trains alone. "If I run with others, then all sessions become full-speed burners; thus I prefer to run with others just for speed sessions."

Tergat does no long runs over 1:30, believing that distance kills speed. "I hadn't trained too hard, but I knew I was in good shape," he once said before the World Cross Country. Realizing weeks earlier at the nationals that he was in prime form, Tergat was careful just to maintain form and not tire himself with exhausting training. Basically he trains like the majority of Kenyan runners, mirroring the Armed Forces cross country training during the winter months.

The Week Around the Kenyan Nationals, February 1996

Wednesday	6 AM	60 min. steady
	10 AM	40 min. steady
Thursday	6 AM	40 min. steady
	10 AM	30 min. fartlek
Friday	6 AM	Short jog. Rest day
Saturday	National Cross Country Championships, 1st.	
Sunday	Rest day.	
Monday	10 AM	60 min. steady, hilly terrain
Tuesday	10 AM	60 min. steady, hilly terrain
Wednesday	6 AM	60 min. steady
	10 AM	40 min. fartlek, hard efforts
Thursday	6 AM	60 min. steady
	10 AM	30 min. tempo
Friday	6 AM	Short jog. Rest day.
Saturday	IAAF Nairobi Cross Challenge, 1st.	

Tergat's Marathon Plan

Monday	AM	70 min. steady to fast
	PM	At least 55 min. We have a set route.
Tuesday	AM	90 min steady, progressive
	PM	Same as Monday PM
Wednesday	AM	Fartlek, typically 12-15K
	PM	Same as Monday
Thursday	AM	Long run, 38-45K
	PM	Rest
Friday	AM	70 min.
	PM	Same as Monday
Saturday		Midday Fast 80 min.s, or could be 10 x 1000m (2:45 with 90 sec. rest, down from the 2:30 he would run as a 10,000m runner)
Sunday		70 min. recovery run

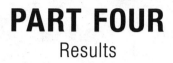

PART FOUR

Results

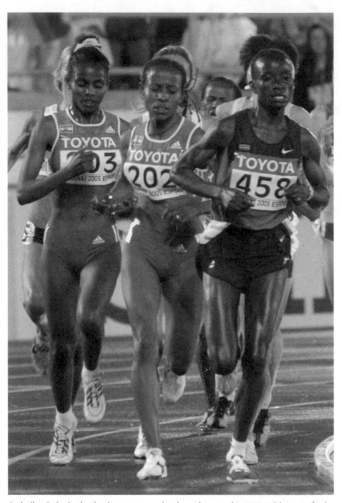

Isabella Ochichi leads the woman who beat her in the 2004 Olympic finals, Meseret Defar, in the IAAF World Championship 5000m heats. (*Flanagan/PrettySporty*)

What Can I Learn From The Kenyans?

After reading my first book, *Train Hard, Win Easy,* many readers wrote and asked if I could write a little about how the "ordinary runner" could adapt his of her training based upon the principles of the Kenyan runners. First and foremost, my books provide inspiration, as the former American record-holder in the marathon, David Morris, and Marla Runyan, Olympian and an American record-holder, were kind enough to mention. Looking at the stories, reading the training profiles, and seeing the results that these athletes have accomplished cannot help but motivate the reader.

On the technical side, there is a current that runs strongly through most Kenyan running, these boys and girls were encouraged to participate in sports while at school. It is never too late to start, but try to surround yourself with supportive, sympathetic people such as one would find in a school environment. Join a club or hook up with other local runners. Kenyans are group-oriented runners, and most neighborhoods in the USA and Europe have a few runners: Meet up!

There is a positive buzz of encouragement throughout the running camps of Kenya. Runners are applauded for going the extra mile or pushing their limits a little higher. Negativity and jealousy, which bring about discouragement, are simply not to be heard. The actual training schedules in this book must be tailored to time availability and individual capabilities. However, taking the bones from a schedule such as Moses Tanui's (see page 236) and reducing the workload can yield a good program for the average runner.

Fifteen Ways to Adopt a Kenyan Training Method

1. Injury prevention. They say the best way to avoid a spear is to stand out of range; this applies to running. Kenyans are excellent at resting up if a possible injury pain is noticed. Do not let that pain get too near you.

2. Study their methods and do not see what may appear as simplicity as a reason for dismissal. Kenyan running is very organic, which in itself is the very essence of the sport. Simple methods are executed with imposing intensity.

3. Group training. After coaching thousand of runners in New York City, I can make the observation that the power of the group never ceases to be underplayed in improving performance.

4. Diet. Try to eat three meals a day. Kenyans rarely eat between meals and seldom have desserts.

5. Don't look for perfection. As a tennis coach would prefer for the perfect game of 6-0, 6-0, the running coach also sets high goals, so do not be disappointed if you do not reach them; 6-4's will win the match. Kenyan athletes do not get down in the dumps after a bad performance or session. Being out there and trying, means you are a winner and that is the Kenyan Way.

6. Don't add up your weekly mileage. Most Kenyans only know their mileage as a need to satisfy Western journalists. The ethic of the focus is to concentrate on the given day.

7. Choose one coach, or training plan, and stick to it. If you chase one chicken, you stand a better chance of catching it than running after two. Kenyans are very good at getting one 12-week program and following it through to a T.

8. Block training: one general striking difference between Kenyan and Western training is the former's use of block work with non-active rest periods. Kenyans are excellent at realizing the most scientific, effective, superb form of resting the body is to do absolutely zilch. After a series of races, the Kenyan then stops running completely. It can be from two to three weeks, to one month or more, but the difference is that during this time the athlete does virtually no training; not even cross-training to keep in shape. Compare this to the American Collegiate cycle, in which where the runner rolls from cross country, straight to the indoor season, to the outdoor track season, to the summer camp, and back into cross country. The term "active rest", where we go to the gym to keep in shape on the rest days and do not rest the body, does not apply to Kenya.

9. Don't push the body when tired. There is always another day.

10. Run off-road. Virtually every single Kenyan criticizes the Western runners for spending too much time on hard surfaces, which, they reason, kills the speed and the natural spring in the legs.

11. Be optimistic. If you never kick the ball, you will not score a goal. Kenyans are extremely positive individuals. Always be willing to take a chance. If you have a bad workout, be happy that it must be proof that your body is tired from the good training that you have done.

12. The secret of Kenyan mechanics appears to be in the foot. Kenyans have very strong ankles, with spring-like qualities that allow the body to bound along with an almost jump-like momentum. Tim Noakes, back in 1996, found an example that exemplifies this theory. "Tergat and the others came by [in the world cross], the ground was hard and the noise of them running by was a tight *tap, tap, tap*. Then a while later the first Europeans came by, *thud, thud, thud!*" Walk around barefoot in the formative years to develop springy levers. The problem is, once the foot has developed and grown, strength training and plyometrics will make the foot stronger, but not springier!

13. Kenyans, if given the choice, tend to lean toward a lightweight, flexible shoe. If you break your arm, after a month in a cast the arm is weak; hence if the foot is put inside a rigid shoe that does not allow each and every muscle in the foot to work, these muscles become weak. There is a trend in the West to wear more and more complicated shoes, with added cushioning; but more is not necessarily better. If you jump out a window and know there is a trampoline below, then your body does not care about the landing, but if you know there is no trampoline. . . learn to use your feet to their fullest.

14. Run to improve running. Yes, as dumb as it sounds. Going to the gym, and cross-training, may be great cardio boosters, but there is a reason Kenyans, for the most part, look good at running; they practice hard! Strengthening muscles through pure running

aligns the body best for the sport. Too much cross-training strengthens non-running muscles that pull Westerners out of natural alignment. Sometimes it pays not to have a gym membership. Think of your muscles; perfect running alignment comes from running, and if you use a leg press to strengthen your leg muscles you will be pulling the legs out of their natural alignment as you build muscle mass irregular to the body's running needs, thus pulling your natural stride out of placement.

15. Nothing comes easy is another slogan of Kenyan running, but what is achieved by pushing your own limits is life's richest reward. To collapse out on the roads with blood in your shoes knowing you gave it your best shot is reward beyond words...

The Basics Explained

All the training, in this book, unless otherwise stated, is run at altitude. The times are far more impressive if you see the tracks the Kenyans run on. Most, being dirt, are subject to the weather. Kenyans very rarely add mileage as is popular in the West; they simply run for time. Diagonals are run across the inner pitch of a running track on the grass; one runs from the "start" to the 200m mark across the infield, then jogs across to the 300m mark and then sprints diagonally again across the infield mark to the 100m mark before jogging back to the 'start.' Hence, the whole session is run on grass. Most Kenyans run at least 90 percent of their training on dirt paths or dirt roads, off the hard asphalt/tarmac.

Long run—Run for time against a set distance. Try and run the long run on a dirt trail, speeding up over the last few miles of the run to as close to competition pace as possible.

Intervals—Be flexible about the amount you are going to run until you feel how strong the body is. Do not be afraid either to extend or shorten the session, and don't feel it imperative to count the number of repeats you perform.

Rest day—Do not necessarily write these days into your program. Instead, take a rest day or two whenever your body tells you a break is needed.

Hill work—Someone following a Kenyan plan in the West may run into problems finding a 22K uphill course, though an adaptation could be to run on a treadmill with a gradient setting. A strong mind will open such doors of thought.

Tempo runs—Start slowly and work into a pace that you feel equates to racing effort. Many Kenyans do not count tempo runs as true speed work, thus an interval session could easily be programmed for the following day. However, ease carefully into this training strategy. Tempo running is commonly the staple ingredient of the Kenyan training plan.

Walking—Strolling, to soften the muscles, can replace an easy run. The East African athlete thinks nothing of going on a three-hour leisurely stroll. The athletes on the American road circuit will quite frequently be seen walking in the evening prior to a race to relax the muscles and prepare the body for sleep.

Racing—Race infrequently to compete at your best. At the 2006 London Marathon, the top two competitors, Martin Lel and Felix Limo, had barely raced one competition between the two of them in the previous few months of build-up. Over-racing rarely leads to a peak performance. Although some athletes in the shorter distances are able to race frequently, the outstanding accomplishments tend to come from the Kenyan athletes who home in on the one key race. In 2006 Paul Tergat raced just twice, running a 59-minute half-marathon and taking third at the ING New York City Marathon; both memorable results.

Easy runs—Isaac Songok and Augustine Choge typically run together in Iten, Kenya. On their easy runs, the pace rarely goes faster than eight-minute miles as they shuffle along the Kenyan roads. This pedestrian pace for these world-class racers allows them to really attack the speed sessions with fresh legs. A principal difference between Western running and Kenyan running is that the Kenyans really do run easy on easy runs. Lornah Kiplagat often runs an easy 10K morning run in 50-52 minutes, yet no woman in history has more sub 31-minute 10K results than Lornah.

Keeping it simple—Kenyans have no desire to reinvent the boring basics. Gimmicks, such as strides per minute, breathing through the nose, and leaning forward are all unheard of in Kenya.

Paul Tergat's Three "Ds" of Running

Dedication. This does not mean giving up the day job, becoming a social hermit, and running 100 miles per week! It means sticking to what task you are doing with a committed level of intensity. The old adage "Whatever you do in life, make sure you do it well" is true for running. If you wish to run well, it is imperative to be dedicated to the sport.

Discipline. Again, do not think of strict rules; instead just focus on giving running the respect it deserves. If you have a 20-miler the next day then try to get to bed early. These should be choices, not sacrifices. If you are training hard, you will find that discipline will go hand in hand with your results.

Determination. This is often thought of as an innate attribute, but it is an asset that can be worked into your running at any time. Try to see the task through; make things happen. Do not wait for moments, create them. Determination can be seen as stubbornness, and as any runner knows, in speed work, or racing, there is always that moment when you want to quit, slow down, pack it in. Do not, and be determined about it!

Most runners have laid great foundations of running over many years. One runner trained for over half a dozen years without prize or praise before finally being selected for the national team. Upon reaching the airport, ready to go and with packed bags, he was told that an official had taken his ticket and he was to be left behind due to "lack of international experience." Turning away from the airport, the dejected athlete resolved to train even harder and thus never be overlooked again. In the following summer, he medaled in the Olympics! The best Kenyan runners have always had their careers immersed in steely determination.

The diet is self-explanatory. In the West, carbohydrates average 45-55 percent of the daily food intake, if one magazine's food check is to be believed. In Kenya they, account for a much larger percentage of the diet. Whether this is a good diet is not up for dispute.

What is conclusive is that there are a lot of Kenyans running exceptionally well on such a diet. Runners such as Paul Tergat, Moses Tanui, and Patrick Konchellah are as careful of their diet as you or I. In our hearts we often know which foods are conductive to a healthy lifestyle.

A typical Kenyan week of training adapted from the specific advice of top Kenyan stars for a runner with a full-time job:

Monday	A long run of 1 hr. 30 min., 2 hrs.
Tuesday	Easy run of 40-60 min., depending on the body
Wednesday	Tempo run. Start slowly; after 20 min. hold your top speed for 30 min. or longer.
Thursday	Hill work. Run hill repeats up and down a steep slope
Friday	Easy run of 40-60 min.
Saturday	Competition, if possible. Otherwise 5 x 1 mile with recoveries long enough to attack the next interval.
Sunday	All the questioned athletes, when asked about this special schedule, were unanimous in agreeing that Sunday should be a rest and family day.

Basically, there *are* no secrets. Very few people enjoy the thought of a grinding set of 400m repeats on the track, and the Kenyans are no exceptions. The general line is that there are no short-cuts to running success. The Kenyans demonstrate rare single-minded devotion to their sport. It depends how badly you want it as to whether or not you can perform to you body's potential. So remember Tergat's "Can you give a little bit more?" the next time when running a session, and try and push harder.

Distraction is a plague. Somebody drops by the house unexpectedly, a film is on the television, night life beckons. The Kenyan runner often distances him/herself from the "bright lights" so as to be able to concentrate solely on running. However, in a working environment this may be hard to do. A compromise can be made; the athlete simply looks at ways to increase the focus toward training during the week.

Shoe4Africa—the Running Charity
Powered by Leppin Sport International

One hundred percent of the author royalties from this book will go directly to Eldoret, Kenya, in our endeavor to build Africa's largest children's hospital.

Ever since I was seven, when I participated in a school project to raise money to buy a tractor for a farm in Boga-Zaire. In 1995, while I was living on the Rift Valley of Kenya I saw the ill-condition of the running shoes of my friends. Here, I knew I could contribute and make a small difference, if only by using my own personal surplus of shoes. I was fortunate, in my first race five years earlier, I had received a sponsorship so that I have never had to buy running shoes to this day (thanks Mizuno). The first "distribution" of shoes was in Eldoret, where I stood with a large box, airmailed over from my apartment in Bromma, Stockholm, and gave out 30 pairs to needy athletes (including a couple of whom went on to great fame).

I ended up leaving Kenya shoeless (and was promptly arrested under the suspicion of vagrancy in the Paris airport). But a simple program developed, as I continued sending boxes of shoes from my home back in Sweden. At first aided by friends who had similar shoe contracts as mine, then by more and more people, until I was receiving shoe donations from-strangers from all over the world. I funded the mailings and distributions myself, and the Shoe Program ran nicely, albeit on a small scale.

I added more countries to receive the free shoes as the shoe count grew. I then began sponsoring races by sending shoes to be given to as many participants as possible at grassroots events in Africa as incentives to entice people to start running. Back in 1999, one 22-year-old told me the pair of shoes was the first present she had ever received, and each day after the morning run she would take a toothbrush and spend an hour meticulously cleaning the shoes. Another person, who would go on to win the Los Angeles Marathon, told me how once a year his family bought bread to celebrate Christmas day—the chance to get a pair of secondhand running shoes (costing 100 times that loaf of bread) would simply never have happened without the Shoe Program.

On December 29, 1999, on the isle of Zanzibar I was attacked by two men wielding a machete and a baseball bat and robbed, ironically, of one shoe. The result left me needing brain surgery. Fully repaired, with metal plates in my skull, the charity changed its name from the Shoe Program to Shoe4Africa. I pushed on with greater effort: if people were close to killing people for used shoes, well. . . I needed to send a lot more!

In 2001, a box was sent to my friend Max Iranqhe, a coach in Amsha, Kenya. He gave a pair to a 14-year-old boy and told him to "start running." A few years later that boy, Fabiano Joseph, won the World Half Marathon Championship.

Shoe4Africa was born of a very straightforward and powerful concept: by giving someone the most basic sports gear, their life can change for the better—and this can happen at nominal costs. In the last few years, interest in Shoe4Africa has grown exponentially, and with that interest, so have the donations of running shoes. The overwhelming amount of sports gear given to the organization was an indication that Shoe4Africa could—and should—expand its scope. The next logical step was to hold signature races where instead of only promoting basic running, Shoe4Africa could begin holding events to address community health issues, in particular, awareness of HIV/AIDS, and to help empower African women.

The idea of using Shoe4Africa events as a means to deliver information on HIV/AIDS came when the organization received a disturbing email from one of the teams I was sponsoring. The coach wrote apologetically, stating that the athletes had been given routine physicals, and it turned out that half of these seemingly healthy athletes were HIV+. The coach assumed that all sponsorship would cease, as the stigma around HIV/AIDS was so severe in that community.

Instead of dropping the team's sponsorship, I realized there was an opportunity—in fact, an obligation—to do something about this problem.

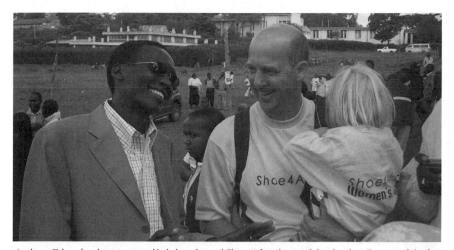

Anthony Edwards, whose input and help has elevated Shoe4Africa, here with his daughter Poppy and the former world record holder Paul Tergat at a Shoe4Africa event. (*Author*)

We immediately held the largest women-only race in Kenya, and then as this signature event spread, we held one in Tanzania. At only our second event we attracted 2,900 women and more than 3,000 spectators. Our platform for health awareness was comprehensive. We began each event with speeches from Olympic and world champion athletes, we had theater with a health theme, and a similar performance from a dance group, and ended with AIDS testing. We also printed AIDS awareness papers in the native Kalenjin tongue where our biggest events were held. We were the first organization to do so.

In America, the HIV/AIDS epidemic has been partially controlled though successful public health education campaigns. Through the media, a strong message was sent out that HIV/AIDS is nothing to be ashamed of, and it is important to talk openly about it. The concept of "safe sex" took hold, and people learned how to prevent infection. This same knowledge needs to be brought to African towns and villages, towns like Kisii, Kenya, where the prevalence of HIV infection reached 35 percent in 2000 according to the World Bank. That is one in every three people.

Sadly, the HIV/AIDS figures disproportionately fall to women. A recent report from the World Bank indicates that 65 percent of those living with HIV/AIDS in Kenya are women. This is due, in part, to the obstacles African women face getting access to basic education and health care.

Shoe4Africa is in a unique position to address the silence and denial that shrouds AIDS/HIV in many African nations. In 2006, Shoe4Africa held six highly attended run/walk events that specifically included an HIV/AIDS awareness component. In Iten, Kenya, a health educator was at the finish line to speak to participants as a group and one-on-one, about the disease and how to prevent it. (Given that a high percentage of women in that area have limited reading skills, oral communication was preferable to flyers or

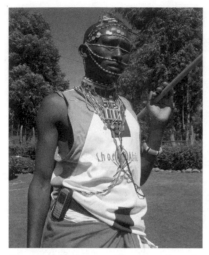

One hundred dancers, with a group from the Maasi, provide a festival setting at the Shoe4Africa races. Leonard was the Maasai in charge. (*Author*)

brochures.) In Tanzania, free t-shirts were given out that read: "Shoe4Africa: Promoting AIDS Awareness Through Sports." The fact that 1,500 Tanzanians were wearing—and discussing—an item of clothing that mentioned AIDS is a victory in itself. Likewise, in Morocco, the fact that more than 350 women (all of whom were non-athletic types) finished a Shoe4Africa race and were willing to attend an event linked to health and HIV/AIDS was a success beyond what anyone thought possible.

At our Nyamira event in Western Kenya the winner of our health walk was a 50-year-old woman who had not done a single sporting activity since leaving school; but not by choice! She said she had been waiting for years to take part in a fun run. Her grandson came out to watch and was so inspired by his grandmother that he laced up a pair of running shoes, and last year he reached the national level of running!

We introduced a program to schools in Kenya and Tanzania where we would sponsor girls only on the condition that the schools agreed to hold each term an AIDS awareness day. We sponsor a running camp in the Marakwet district of Kenya under the same guidelines, asking the coaches to add a health component to the athletics agenda. The first girl in the program, Farida Makula, went on to win the 1500 and 5000m national titles and was named the Tanzanian female athlete of the year.

In December 2006, now with the backing of our sponsor Leppin Sport International, we were granted a not-for-profit status. Anthony Edwards, a dear friend of mine over the past few years, became the chairman of the board of directors; he immediately elevated the organization from a lickety-spickity hobby to a real organization. His kitchen became our office, and although we are a staff of two, we set off to conquer the world fueled on his wife (Jeanine) Zoegas's coffee. Here's to you Tony!

In the fall of 2007, we held a shoe collection on the streets of New York after the city's marathon, collecting 11,000 pairs in a little over six hours! Our plan was to hold a running race to empower women in Kibera, Africa's largest slum. Unfortunately a couple of months before the festival was to be held violence broke out in Kenya and the country was in flames. We adapted, holding the first peace race using the athletes of the clashing tribes to send a powerful message. Six hundred schoolchildren wielding olive branches marched behind over 40 international star athletes led by Douglas Wakiihuri, a Kikuyu, and Luke Kibet, a Kalenjin—the two tribes that had been fighting only weeks earlier were now singing songs of peace.

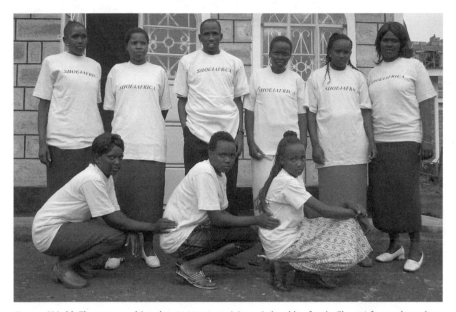

Former World Champion and London 2007 winner Martin Lel and his family, Shoe4Africa ambassadors. (*Author*)

Weeks later we held another peace race at Martin Lel's house; then two days later, again using the concept of the athletes to promote peace, Ben Jipcho of the Kalenjin tribe (who is now disabled after being shot in the leg during the clashes) and John Ngugi of the Kikuyu walked along with 250 Kalenjin school children into Kenya's largest "no-go" refugee camp to greet 250 Kikuyu children. They shook hands, each Kalenjin child gave a spare t-shirt to a new friend, and then in front of 20,000 displaced citizens, the children ran together through and around the camp.

This is in large part why we are building the Shoe4Africa Children's Hospital. For 13-years Shoe4Africa has *never* fund raised. Now, needing $15-million, things have changed. Charities often hold big running races where the race entry fees generated are used to support the program—for us, all of our events are not only free to enter, but participants get free refreshments, free t-shirts, prizes such as computers, cell phones, and cash, and running shoes! Thus to maintain these programs, support running camps, sponsor school fees, and establish a new children's hospital, we need to raise money. We need your help if we are to get this job done. Shoe4Africa does not have an overhead like other charities—100 percent of all donations go straight to our programs; not a <u>single penny</u> is used for administration or travel expenses. I will close this book with these words of encouragement:

> "I am always ready to do anything for Shoe4Africa because you are always doing the right things. Just call me and let me know the place. We run together!"—Ezekiel Kemboi, 2004 Olympic Steeplechase Champion.

"You are running a very nice project, the Shoe4Africa work works."—Matthew Birir, Olympic Steeplechase Champion 1992.

"Shoe4Africa is a great initiative, really helping a lot of people in Kenya."—Paul Tergat, world record holder, marathon. (Paul also has his own effective charity, the Paul Tergat Foundation, www.paultergatfoundation.org)

"Congratulations on your great work with Shoe4Africa. I have seen your races and they are amazing."—Tegla Loroupe, two time world record holder, marathon; three times world champion.

"Shoe4Africa is a wonderful thing for Kenya and the people of Kenya really hope that Shoe4Africa will continue to do these wonderful things you are doing here in Africa."—Isaiah Kiplagat, CEO/Chairman of Athletics Kenya

"Very good work, please keep it up. Kenya needs these things."—President Daniel Toroitich Arap Moi (1978-2002)

To learn more about Shoe4Africa, please visit our Web site at www.shoe4africa.org

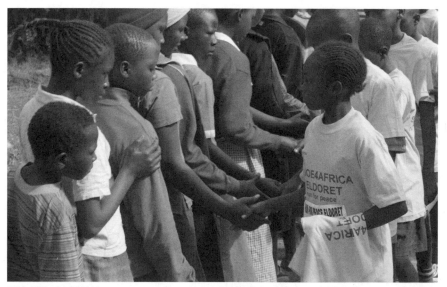

The children of Eldoret town meet and bring t-shirts for the kids of a refugee camp before running together for peace after the Kenyan post-election violence.

About The Author

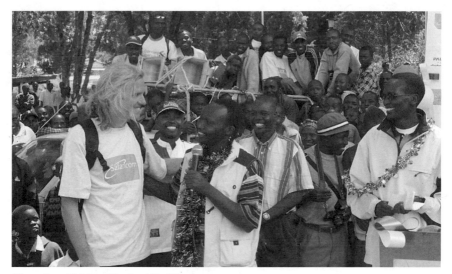

The author with Moses Tanui and Paul Tergat.

Toby Tanser is director of Shoe4Africa which he founded in 1995, and a director of both the New York Road Runners, the world's largest running organization, and Achilles International, the world's largest organization for athletes with disabilities. He sits on the coaches advisory board of *Runner's World*. A former professional runner, Tanser has not only lived and trained with the top runners in Kenya for more than a decade, but also traveled to meets in Europe, Asia, and the Americas with the Africans. His first book, *Train Hard, Win Easy* (TAF News), was published in 1997. It was favorably reviewed in over 17-countries, reprinted in foreign languages, and has become, in the words of Jonathan Beverly of *Running Times*, "a cult classic." Tanser also wrote *The Essential Guide to Running the New York City Marathon* (Pedigree Penguin) and, while working in for the athletics federation in Stockholm, Sweden, a training manual for "boosting the country's athletic impact through studying the world's most successful runners." Tanser's articles about running have appeared in journals worldwide as well as in *Runner's World*, *New York Runner*, and *Metrosports* magazines. He coaches New York City's largest running team, the NY Flyers, and is the track and cross country coach at the Fashion Institute in Manhattan. In addition, he coaches various charity organizations, including Team Lifeline, and is the race director of the Hope & Possibility, an annual race in New York City that supports athletes with disabilities. Tanser wrote and co-produced the global Puma Trainaway series and the New York Road Runners audio guide for the ING New York City Marathon. He has also done TV and Web commentary for marathons in America and Europe.

Acknowledgements

Many, many thanks to each and every athlete mentioned in this book. Your lessons in warmth, humility, and humanity travel with me each day. Thanks for teaching me so much more than the obvious.

For every photographer whose art in this book, thank you so much—that you donated is a blessing for these pages: Don Wilkinson, Dave Drennan, The New York Road Runners, Ivy League Archives, Cinque Mulini Archives, Alison Wade, Parker Morse, Bob Burgess, Leo Kulinski Jr., Jeroen Deen, Giuliano De Portu, Cheryl Flanagan (aka Flanagan/Pretty Sporty), Martijn Venhuizen, Pieter Langerhorst, Robert Lejeune, Omega Fotocronache/ Giancarlo Colombo, Mike Kobal, and Randy Lefko. To my friend Stuart Calderwood who read through the draft and grammatically fixed up my mistakes. Thanks to my publisher, Bruce H. Franklin, for believing in *More Fire*.

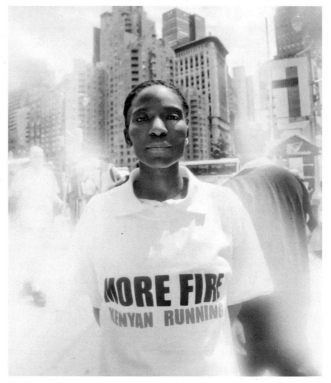

Catherine Ndereba runs with More Fire. (*Mike Kobal*)